Study Guide

Pharmacology
A Nursing Process Approach

6th Edition

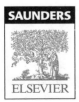

Joyce LeFever Kee, MS, RN
Associate Professor Emerita
School of Nursing
College of Health Sciences
University of Delaware
Newark, Delaware

Evelyn R. Hayes, PhD, MPH, FNP-BC
Professor
School of Nursing
College of Health Sciences
University of Delaware
Newark, Delaware

Linda E. McCuistion, PhD, RN, ANP, CNS
Professor
Division of Nursing
Our Lady of Holy Cross College
New Orleans, Louisiana

SAUNDERS

ELSEVIER

ELSEVIER
SAUNDERS

11830 Westline Industrial Drive
St. Louis, Missouri 63146

STUDY GUIDE FOR PHARMACOLOGY:
A NURSING PROCESS APPROACH

ISBN: 978-1-4160-5290-6

Copyright © 2009, 2006, 2003, 2000, 1997, 1993 by Saunders, an imprint of Elsevier Inc.

NOTICE

Knowledge and best practice in this field are constantly changing. As new research and experience broaden our knowledge, changes in practice, treatment and drug therapy may become necessary or appropriate. Readers are advised to check the most current information provided (i) on procedures featured or (ii) by the manufacturer of each product to be administered, to verify the recommended dose or formula, the method and duration of administration, and contraindications. It is the responsibility of the practitioner, relying on their own experience and knowledge of the patient, to make diagnoses, to determine dosages and the best treatment for each individual patient, and to take all appropriate safety precautions. To the fullest extent of the law, neither the Publisher nor the Authors assumes any liability for any injury and/or damage to persons or property arising out of or related to any use of the material contained in this book.

The Publisher

Previous editions copyrighted 1993, 1997, 2000, 2003, and 2006.

ISBN: 978-1-4160-5290-6

Senior Acquisitions Editor: Kristin Geen
Developmental Editor: Jamie Horn
Editorial Assistant: Jennifer Stoces
Publishing Services Manager: Jeff Patterson
Senior Project Manager: Clay S. Broeker
Design Direction: Teresa McBryan

Working together to grow
libraries in developing countries

www.elsevier.com | www.bookaid.org | www.sabre.org

ELSEVIER   BOOK AID International   Sabre Foundation

Printed in the United States

Last digit is the print number: 9 8 7 6 5 4 3 2 1

Preface

This comprehensive *Study Guide* is designed to provide the learner with clinically based situation practice problems and questions. This book accompanies the text *Pharmacology: A Nursing Process Approach,* sixth edition, and may also be used independently of the text.

Opportunities abound for the enhancement of critical thinking and decision-making abilities. Hundreds of study questions and answers are presented on nursing responsibilities in therapeutic pharmacology. For example, Chapter 3 details the principles of drug administration. Chapter 4 is composed of six sections, each devoted to a specific area of medications and calculations. Multiple practice opportunities are provided in the areas of measurement, methods of drug calculations, calculation of oral and injectable dosages (including pediatrics), and calculation of intravenous fluids. Each chapter follows a new format that includes study questions (including multiple choice, matching, word searches, crossword puzzles, and completion exercises), NCLEX review questions (including alternate item format questions), and critical thinking exercises.

There are more than 160 drug calculation problems and questions, many relating to actual client care situations and enhanced with actual drug labels. The learner is also expected to recognize safe dosage parameters for the situation. The combination of the instructional material in the text and the multiplicity of a variety of practice problems in this *Study Guide* preclude the need for an additional drug dosage calculation book.

The nursing process is used throughout the client situation-based questions and critical thinking exercises. Chapters have questions that relate to assessment data, including laboratory data and side effects, planning and implementing care, client/family teaching, cultural and nutritional considerations, and effectiveness of the drug therapy regimen.

Because of the ever-expanding number of drugs available, pharmacology can be an overwhelming subject. To help students grasp essential content without becoming overwhelmed, chapters have been divided into multiple smaller sections. The result is a revised layout that will be much more user-friendly. In addition, one new chapter has been added, covering questions related to drugs of abuse.

Answers to all questions are presented in the Answer Key. In addition to the answers for the drug dosage calculation problems, the thought process and actual solving of the problems are outlined in many instances.

Additional resources are found in the appendixes, including a basic math review and a prototype drug chart format for your use.

The *Study Guide* is part of a comprehensive pharmacology package including the text, *Companion CD,* and *Instructor's Electronic Resource.* The *IER* is a CD containing the instructor's manual, ExamView test bank, PowerPoint lecture slides, and an image collection. Additional resources are also available on the companion Evolve website at http://evolve.elsevier.com/KeeHayes/pharmacology/.

This comprehensive package and each of its components were designed to promote critical thinking and learning. We are excited about this edition of the *Study Guide* because it offers the learner a variety of modalities for mastering the content.

Acknowledgments

We extend most sincere appreciation to the many professionals who facilitated the development of this *Study Guide for Pharmacology: A Nursing Process Approach,* sixth edition. We especially thank the following for their assistance, past and present, with questions for their respective chapters: Margaret Barton-Burke, PhD, RN; Joseph Boullata, PharmD, BCNSP; Michelle M. Byrne, MS, PhD, CNOR; Robin Webb Corbett, PhD, RN, C; Sandy Elliott, CNM, MSN; Linda Goodwin, RNC, MEd; Judith W. Herrman, PhD, RN; Kathleen J. Jones, RN-C, MS, ANP; Robert J. Kizior, BS, RPh; Paula R. Klemm, PhD, RN, OCN; Anne E. Lara, RN, MS, AOCN, APRN,BC; Linda Laskowski-Jones, RN, MS, APRN, BC, CEN; Ronald J. Lefever, RPh; Patricia S. Lincoln, BSN, RN; Patricia O'Brien, MA, MSN; Laura K. Williford Owens, PharmD; Lisa Ann Plowfield, PhD, RN; Larry D. Purnell, PhD, RN, FAAN; Nancy C. Sharts-Hopko, RN, PhD, FAAN; Jane Purnell Taylor, RN, MS; Lynette M. Wachholz, MN, APRN, IBCLC; and Gail Wilkes, MS, RNC, AOCN.

We are most grateful to pharmaceutical companies for permission to use their drug labels in the drug dosage calculation problems. Pharmaceutical companies that extended their courtesy to this book include Abbott Laboratories, American Home Products, American Regent Products Co., AstraZeneca Pharmaceuticals, Bayer Corporation, Bristol-Myers Squibb Co., DuPont/Merck Pharmaceuticals, Eli Lilly and Co., Elkins-Sinn Inc., Glaxo-SmithKline Inc., Marion Merrell Dow Inc., McNeilab Inc., Merck and Co. Inc., Mylan Pharmaceuticals, Pfizer Labs, Warner-Lambert Co., and Wyeth-Ayerst Laboratories.

We are indebted to the students and clients we have had the privilege of knowing during our many years of professional nursing practice. From you we have learned many important aspects about the role of therapeutic pharmacology in nursing practice.

To the staff at Elsevier, especially Kristin Geen, Senior Acquisitions Editor; Jamie Horn, Developmental Editor; Clay Broeker, Senior Project Manager; and Jeff Patterson, Publishing Services Manager, we thank you for your reviews and suggestions.

We offer our appreciation and love to my husband, Edward D. Kee (JLK), to my parents Margaret K. and Justin F. Hayes (ERH), and to Robert Ekas, Jr. (LEM), for their ongoing love and support.

Joyce LeFever Kee
Evelyn R. Hayes
Linda E. McCuistion

Contents

1 Drug Action: Pharmaceutic, Pharmacokinetic, and Pharmacodynamic Phases

Study Questions

Crossword puzzle: Use the definition to determine the pharmacologic term.

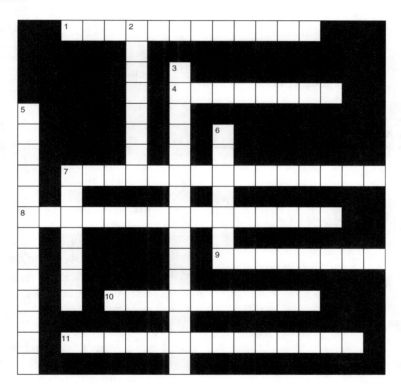

Across

1. Dissolution of the drug
4. One-half of the drug concentration to be eliminated
7. Effect of drug action because of hereditary influence
8. Four processes of drug movement to achieve drug action
9. Toxic effect as a result of drug dose or therapy
10. Drug that blocks a response without a chemical structure
11. Drug bound to protein

Down

2. Located on a cell membrane to enhance drug action
3. Effect of drug action on cells
5. Drug tolerance to repeated administration of a drug
6. Drug that produces a response
7. Psychologic benefit from a compound

Match the following terms with their descriptions.

_____ 12. protein-bound drug

_____ 13. unbound drug

_____ 14. hepatic first pass

_____ 15. dissolution

_____ 16. passive absorption

_____ 17. nonselective receptors

a. breakdown of a drug into smaller particles

b. proceeds directly from intestine to the liver

c. drugs that affect various receptors

d. free active drug causing a pharma-cologic response

e. causes inactive drug action/response

f. drug absorbed by diffusion

g. drug requiring a carrier for absorption

NCLEX Review Questions

Select the best response.

18. Which drug form is most rapidly absorbed from the gastrointestinal (GI) tract?
    a. tablet
    b. enteric-coated tablet
    c. suspension
    d. poultice

19. Enteric-coated tablets are absorbed from the:
    a. stomach.
    b. intestine.
    c. mouth.
    d. esophagus.

20. Usually food has what effect on drug dissolution and absorption?
    a. enhances
    b. interferes with
    c. does not affect
    d. catalytic

21. The sequence of the four processes of pharmacokinetics is:
    a. absorption, metabolism, distribution, excretion.
    b. distribution, absorption, metabolism, excretion.
    c. distribution, metabolism, absorption, excretion.
    d. absorption, distribution, metabolism, excretion.

22. Drugs that pass rapidly through the GI membrane include:
    a. lipid-soluble and ionized.
    b. lipid-soluble and non-ionized.
    c. water-soluble and ionized.
    d. water-soluble and non-ionized.

23. The factors that most commonly affect drug action are:
    a. poor circulation, pain, stress, hunger, fasting.
    b. stress, hunger, weather, pH of drug.
    c. poor circulation, hunger, stress, BMI.
    d. BMI, pH of drug, stress, poor circulation.

24. E.T. is taking a drug that is highly protein-bound. Several days later, E.T. takes a second drug that is 90% protein-bound. What happens to the first drug?
    a. The first drug remains highly protein-bound.
    b. The first drug becomes increasingly inactive.
    c. More of the first drug is released from the protein and becomes more pharmacologically active.
    d. The first drug is excreted in the urine.

25. The major site of drug metabolism is the:
    a. kidney.
    b. liver.
    c. lung.
    d. skin.

26. The route for drug absorption that has the greatest bioavailability is:

  a. oral.

  b. intramuscular.

  c. subcutaneous.

  d. intravenous.

27. The serum half-life of a drug is the time required:

  a. for half of a drug dose to be absorbed.

  b. after absorption for half of the drug to be eliminated.

  c. for a drug to be totally effective.

  d. for half the drug dose to be completely distributed.

28. Drugs with a half-life of 24 to 30 hours would probably be administered on a dose schedule of:

  a. three times a day.

  b. twice a day.

  c. once a day.

  d. every other day.

29. For elimination through the kidneys to be possible, a drug must:

  a. be lipid-soluble.

  b. be water-soluble.

  c. be protein-bound.

  d. have a long half-life.

30. Mrs. T. has a renal disorder. Her creatinine clearance is 40 ml/min. Her drug dose should be:

  a. increased.

  b. decreased.

  c. the same for 1 week.

  d. discontinued.

31. The biologic activity of a drug is determined by the:

  a. fit of the drug at the receptor site.

  b. misfit of the drug at the receptor site.

  c. inability of the drug to bind to a specific receptor.

  d. ability of the drug to be rapidly excreted.

32. Drugs that prevent or inhibit a response are known as:

  a. antagonists.

  b. agonists.

  c. depressants.

  d. antiseptics.

33. A receptor located in different parts of the body may initiate a variety of responses depending on its anatomic site. The receptor is:

  a. nonselective.

  b. instigating a drug-enzyme interaction.

  c. initiating a primary response.

  d. nonspecific.

34. The valid indicator that measures the margin of safety of the drug is its:

  a. therapeutic range.

  b. therapeutic index.

  c. duration of action.

  d. biologic half-life.

35. Drugs with narrow therapeutic ranges, such as digoxin (0.5-2 mcg/ml), require plasma/serum drug level monitoring to avoid drug toxicity:

  a. yearly.

  b. daily.

  c. at periodic intervals.

  d. weekly.

36. After drug administration, the highest plasma/serum concentration of the drug at a specific time is called:

  a. peak level.

  b. trough level.

  c. half-life.

  d. minimum effective concentration (MEC).

37. Before the administration of a medication, the nurse should check a drug reference book or the drug pamphlet to obtain all the following pertinent data EXCEPT the:

  a. protein-binding effect.

  b. half-life.

  c. therapeutic range.

  d. maximum efficacy.

38. Physiologic effects not related to the desired effect(s) that can be predictable or associated with the use of a drug are called:
    a. severe adverse reactions.
    b. side effects.
    c. synergistic effects.
    d. toxic effects.

39. When an immediate drug response is desired, a large initial dose is given to rapidly achieve an MEC in the plasma. This is called the:
    a. peak level.
    b. trough level.
    c. loading dose.
    d. therapeutic range.

40. A time-response curve evaluates three parameters of drug action, which does NOT include:
    a. therapeutic range.
    b. onset of action.
    c. peak action.
    d. duration of action.

41. Nursing interventions concerning drug therapy include the following EXCEPT:
    a. assessing for side effects of drugs, especially those that are nonselective.
    b. checking drug reference books for dosage ranges, side effects, protein-binding percentage, and half-life.
    c. teaching the client to wait a week after the occurrence of signs and symptoms to see if they disappear.
    d. checking the client's serum therapeutic range of drugs that are more toxic or have a narrow therapeutic range.

42. A low protein level in the blood decreases the number of protein-binding sites and causes an increase in amount of free drug in the plasma, potentially resulting in drug overdose. Examples of causes of low protein levels include the following: *Select all that apply.*
    a. low potassium level
    b. malnutrition
    c. high potassium level
    d. infants
    e. elderly

43. Which of the following statements are true? *Select all that apply.*
    a. Drugs are absorbed faster in acidic fluid.
    b. The very young have decreased gastric acidity.
    c. The elderly have increased gastric acidity.
    d. Liquid drugs are more rapidly available for GI absorption than solids.
    e. Tablets are 100% drug.

Critical Thinking Exercises

Use a separate sheet of paper for your answers.

J.R., an elderly client, has been taking digoxin 0.25 mg daily and warfarin (Coumadin) 5 mg daily for several months. J.R. noticed that large purple spots (purpura) developed on her hands, arms, and ankles. She tells the nurse that she has never had these types of "spots" before.

1. What is purpura?

2. Can purpura occur because of protein-binding percentage and half-life of the drug, drug dosages, and/or drug interaction? Explain.

3. What are the nursing responsibilities related to J.R.'s clinical problem?

4. What is an appropriate response by the nurse to J.R.'s concerns?

5. J.R.'s serum digoxin level is 2.5 mcg/ml. Her urine output has decreased. Is J.R.'s serum digoxin level within the normal therapeutic range? Explain the possible cause of her serum digoxin level.

6. What effects might occur as a result of J.R.'s urine output and drug therapy?

7. What are the recommended nursing interventions related to her serum digoxin level and urine output?

2   Nursing Process and Client Teaching

Study Questions

Define the following:

1. Assessment

2. Planning

3. Implementation/intervention

4. Evaluation

Match the step of the nursing process in Column II with the phrases in Column I.

	Column I		Column II
_____ 5.	nursing diagnosis	a.	assessment
_____ 6.	current health history	b.	planning
_____ 7.	goal setting	c.	implementation/intervention
_____ 8.	client's environment	d.	evaluation
_____ 9.	action to accomplish goals		
_____ 10.	drug allergies or reactions		
_____ 11.	referral		
_____ 12.	client/significant other education		
_____ 13.	use of teaching drug cards		
_____ 14.	laboratory test results		
_____ 15.	effectiveness of health teaching and drug therapy		

Complete the following:

16. List two possible nursing diagnoses commonly associated with drug therapy:

   a.

   b.

17. List four essential qualities of an effective goal:

   a.

   b.

   c.

   d.

18. Write two goals incorporating the essential qualities:

   a.

   b.

19. List the four suggested categories for client teaching related to pharmacotherapeutics:

    a.

    b.

    c.

    d.

20. Teaching plans that stimulate multiple senses and require active participation by the client and significant others enhance learning. List four teaching tips to be considered in each teaching plan:

    a.

    b.

    c.

    d.

21. Identify at least two questions to ask the client or significant others that will elicit unique information to help the nurse to enhance adherence to the drug therapy regimen:

    a.

    b.

NCLEX Review Questions

Select the best response.

22. *Risk for injury* is included in which phase of the nursing process?
    a. assessment
    b. potential nursing diagnoses
    c. planning
    d. implementation

23. *Obtain client's weight to be used for future comparison* is included in which phase of the nursing process?
    a. assessment
    b. potential nursing diagnoses
    c. planning
    d. evaluation

24. *The client will receive adequate nutritional support through enteral feedings* is included in which phase of the nursing process?
    a. assessment
    b. potential nursing diagnoses
    c. planning
    d. implementation

25. *The client will be free from hyperactivity* is included in which phase of the nursing process?
    a. assessment
    b. potential nursing diagnoses
    c. planning
    d. evaluation

26. *Instruct client to avoid caffeine-containing foods* is included in which phase of the nursing process?
    a. potential nursing diagnoses
    b. planning
    c. implementation
    d. evaluation

27. *Evaluate effectiveness of drug therapy* is included in which phase of the nursing process?
    a. assessment
    b. potential nursing diagnoses
    c. implementation
    d. evaluation

28. *Sleep pattern disturbance* is included in which phase of the nursing process?
    a. assessment
    b. potential nursing diagnoses
    c. planning
    d. implementation

29. *Advise client to report adverse reactions such as nausea and severe vomiting to health care provider; drug choice or dosage may need modification* is included in which phase of the nursing process?
    a. assessment
    b. potential nursing diagnoses
    c. planning
    d. implementation

30. *Anxiety* is included in which phase of the nursing process?
    a. potential nursing diagnoses
    b. planning
    c. implementation
    d. evaluation

31. *Instruct client not to discontinue medication abruptly* is included in which phase of the nursing process?
    a. assessment
    b. potential nursing diagnoses
    c. planning
    d. implementation

32. The nurse is developing a teaching plan for the client. Which of the following are suggested to be included? *Select all that apply.*
    a. Actively involve client.
    b. Provide written instructions at appropriate level for client.
    c. Consider using a variety of media.
    d. Discourage questions from client and family.
    e. Provide for return demonstration.

33. Factors commonly resulting in nonadherence with a drug therapy plan include: *Select all that apply.*
    a. Forgetfulness
    b. Knowledge deficit
    c. Motivation
    d. Side effects
    e. Language barrier

3 Principles of Drug Administration

Study Questions

Define the following:

1. Absorption

2. Cumulative effect

3. Distribution

4. Informed consent

5. Metabolism

6. Toxicity

Complete the following:

7. Identify at least two specific nursing interventions when administering drugs to pediatric clients: _____ and _____.

8. List the "five plus five rights" of drug administration and nursing implications for each:

Right	Nursing Implications
a.	
b.	
c.	
d.	
e.	
f.	
g.	
h.	
i.	
j.	

9. Identify six factors modifying drug response and specific nursing implications for each:

	Factor	**Nursing Implications**
a.		
b.		
c.		
d.		
e.		
f.		

10. In the following table, the routes for parenteral administration of drugs are identified. For each route of administration, provide the following: (a) common needle size, (b) angle of insertion, and (c) common site(s).

Route	Needle Size	Angle of Insertion	Site(s)
ID			
SubQ			
IM			
IV			

Complete the following word search. Clues are given in questions 11-15. Circle your responses.

```
S  I  L  A  R  E  T  A  L  S  U  T  S  A  V
O  M  D  V  Z  T  W  G  G  K  N  E  Y  I  E
B  U  D  L  E  A  M  F  L  O  H  S  C  P  N
J  I  R  D  O  N  O  T  U  D  X  Q  M  U  T
D  O  R  S  O  G  L  U  T  E  A  L  G  H  R
E  F  B  D  I  O  T  L  E  D  W  A  N  B  O
S  B  E  I  M  C  R  L  A  F  Z  I  Y  K  G
D  C  O  P  A  J  T  I  L  Q  O  T  R  N  L
R  E  F  U  S  A  L  R  E  A  S  O  N  A  U
D  E  N  E  P  O  E  M  I  T  E  T  A  D  T
S  L  A  I  T  I  N  I  F  Y  M  W  H  J  E
B  N  T  U  O  X  R  N  T  R  L  D  A  P  A
T  D  E  M  N  T  R  W  I  G  Q  M  H  U  L
```

11. The injection site that is well-defined by bony anatomic landmarks is _____.

12. The preferred site for intramuscular injections for infants and children is _____.

13. The site that is easily accessible but not suitable for repeated injections or injections more than 2 ml is _____.

14. The preferred site for the Z-track technique is _____.

15. The site (not visible to the client) that has the danger of injury if incorrect technique is used is _____.

Match the letter from Column II with the correct response in Column I.

	Column I		**Column II**
____ 16.	drugs poured by others	a.	do not administer
____ 17.	client states that drug is different than usual	b.	do administer
____ 18.	offer ice to numb tastebuds for distasteful drugs		
____ 19.	drugs transferred from one container to another		
____ 20.	record fluids taken with medications on the intake and output sheet		
____ 21.	medications left with visitors		

NCLEX Review Questions

Select the best response.

22. The order to "give multivitamins ii caps po daily" is an example of what category of drug order?
    a. STAT
    b. standing
    c. single
    d. PRN

23. J.T. has an order to receive Demerol 100 mg, IM, STAT. This is an example of what category of drug order?
    a. PRN
    b. standing
    c. STAT
    d. single

24. When you calculate the dosage for J.B.'s cardiac medication, the drug dose is "large." The best initial action for you to take is:
    a. check client's name band and give medication.
    b. check your calculations.
    c. call health care provider.
    d. withhold medication and document as not given.

25. The preferred way to correct a charting error is to:
    a. draw a single line through incorrect information and initial.
    b. scratch out incorrect information and initial.
    c. white out incorrect information.
    d. write that the information is incorrect.

26. You read in the chart that R.T. is allergic to one of his prescribed medications. Your first nursing action is to:
    a. withhold the medication.
    b. withhold the medication and call health care provider.
    c. ask client about his drug allergy.
    d. give medication and document.

27. One of A.A.'s medications is in a liquid form. You pour the medication with the container at eye level and read the meniscus at what point?

    a. low part of curve
    b. high part of curve
    c. marker on container
    d. side of curve

28. Your client is not wearing an ID band. What should be your first nursing action?

    a. Call the health care provider and document.
    b. Give the medication and document.
    c. Report your finding and have ID band put on client.
    d. Ask client where his ID band is.

29. Universal precautions require that you do all of the following EXCEPT:

    a. do not cap needles.
    b. cap needles.
    c. wash hands.
    d. wear gloves.

30. Before storing unused stable solutions from open vials in the refrigerator, the nurse should write the following information on the label:

    a. date and time vial opened; initials.
    b. date and time vial opened and client's name.
    c. date and number of remaining doses.
    d. date and initials.

31. When a client refuses to take a medication, the nurse must:

    a. call the health care provider.
    b. document reason not taken.
    c. contact the supervisor.
    d. reinforce the importance of taking medication.

32. For clients who are vomiting or comatose, medication administration is contraindicated via which route?

    a. intravenous
    b. intradermal
    c. oral
    d. suppository

33. When is the best time to administer oral medications if food interferes with absorption of the medication?

    a. 15 minutes after meals
    b. 15 minutes before meals
    c. 1 hour after eating
    d. on an empty stomach

34. When applying medication topically, the nurse, to avoid skin contact with the medication, should use all of the following EXCEPT:

    a. applicator.
    b. gloves.
    c. straw.
    d. hands.

35. If a glucocorticoid is ordered with a bronchodilator, you need to wait how many minutes between administering medications?

    a. 1
    b. 2
    c. 3
    d. 5

36. When administering ear drops, the client should be sitting with the head tilted toward which side?

    a. affected
    b. unaffected

37. In an adult, gently pull the auricle in what direction before instilling ear drops?

    a. up
    b. down

38. Ear drops are best administered:
    a. at room temperature.
    b. directly after removal from the refrigerator.
    c. slightly heated.

39. Which of the following are not allowed by The Joint Commission? *Select all that apply.*
    a. IM
    b. U
    c. IU
    d. Trailing zero
    e. qd

40. The "right to education" includes which of the following? *Select all that apply.*
    a. client receives correct information about the drug and how it relates to situation
    b. possible side effects
    c. laboratory monitoring
    d. data collected before administration of drug
    e. evaluation of client response

4   Medications and Calculations

Introduction

The medications and calculations' chapter in this Study Guide is subdivided into six sections: (4A) Systems of Measurement; (4B) Methods for Calculation; (4C) Calculations of Oral Dosages; (4D) Calculations of Injectable Dosages; (4E) Calculations of Intravenous Fluids; and (4F) Pediatric Drug Calculations. Before reading and working the drug calculation problems, the student/nurse may find it helpful to review Appendix A: Basic Math Review, located near the end of this book.

Numerous drug labels appear in the drug calculation problems. The purpose is to familiarize the student/nurse with reading drug labels and calculating drug dosages from the information provided on the drug labels.

Drug calculation practice problems in each of the six sections provide an opportunity for the student/nurse to gain skill and competence in collecting and organizing the required data.

Practice problems have examples of the administration of medications via a variety of routes including both oral and parenteral (subcutaneous, intramuscular, and intravenous).

It is recommended that the student/nurse first read the practice problem and estimate an answer. The student/nurse should select one of the four methods (basic formula, ratio and proportion, fractional equation, or dimensional analysis) for drug calculations that are presented in the pharmacology textbook. After completing the required calculations, the student/nurse can compare the estimate with the calculated answer. In the event of a discrepancy, the student/nurse should review both the thought process used in answering the problem and the actual mathematical calculation. It may be necessary to review the related section in Chapter 4 of the text. Practice problems provide reinforcement for the student/nurse to gain expertise in the process of actually calculating drug dosages.

SECTION 4A—SYSTEMS OF MEASUREMENT

Metric, Apothecary, and Household Systems

Complete the following:

1.   The system of international units of measurement is _____. The units of these measurements are: weights _____; volume _____; and length _____.

2.   In the metric system, to convert larger units to smaller units, move the decimal point to the (right/left) for each unit changed. (Circle correct answer.)

3.   In the metric system, to convert smaller units to larger units, move the decimal point to the (right/left) for each unit changed. (Circle correct answer.)

4.   With the apothecary system, the unit of weight is _____, and units of volume are _____, _____, and _____.

5.   When are household measurements used? _____

6.   Household measurements include _____, _____, and _____.

Give the abbreviations for the following units:

7.   _____ gram

8.   _____ milligram

9.   _____ liter

10.   _____ milliliter

11.   _____ kilogram

12.   _____ microgram

13.   _____ nanogram

14.   _____ meter

15.   _____ grain

16.   _____ fluid ounce

17.   _____ fluid dram

18.   _____ quart

19.   _____ pint

20.   _____ minim

21.   _____ cup

22.   _____ tablespoon

23.   _____ teaspoon

24.   _____ drops

25.   The most frequently used conversions within the metric system are:
   a.   1 g = _____ mg
   b.   1 L = _____ ml
   c.   1 mg = _____ mcg

Complete the unit equivalent for the following measurements:

26.　　3 grams = _____ milligrams

27.　　1.5 liters = _____ milliliters

28.　　0.1 gram = _____ milligrams

29.　　2500 milliliters = _____ liters

30.　　250 milliliters = _____ liter

31.　　500 milligrams = _____ gram

32.　　2 quarts = _____ pints

33.　　2 pints = _____ fluid ounces

34.　　1½ quarts = _____ fluid ounces

35.　　32 fluid ounces = _____ pints

36.　　2 fluid ounces = _____ fluid dram

37.　　Complete the chart on household measurements:

　　　　1 medium-sized glass = _____ ounces

　　　　1 coffee cup　　　　= _____ ounces

　　　　1 ounce　　　　　　= _____ tablespoons

　　　　1 tablespoon　　　　= _____ teaspoons

　　　　1 drop　　　　　　= _____ minim

Conversion Among the Metric, Apothecary, and Household Systems

38.　　When converting a unit of measurement from one system to another, convert to the unit on the drug container.

　　　　Example:

　　　　Order: V-Cillin K 0.5 g, PO, q8 h.

　　　　Available:

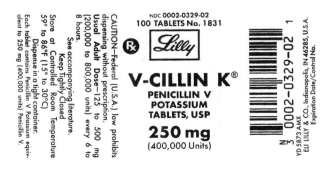

　　　　Convert _____ to _____ .

Convert the following units of measurement to metric, apothecary, and household equivalents. Refer to Table 4A-4 in text as needed.

39.   1 g = _____ mg, or _____ gr

40.   _____ g = 500 mg, or _____ gr

41.   0.1 g = _____ mg, or _____ gr

42.   1 gr = _____ mg

43.   0.4 mg = _____ gr

44.   _____ L = 1000 ml, or _____ qt

45.   240 ml = _____ fl oz, or _____ glass

46.   30 ml = _____ oz, or _____ T, or _____ t

47.   5 ml = _____ t

48.   1 ml = _____ m, or _____ gtt

49.   3 T = _____ oz, or _____ t

50.   5 oz = _____ ml, or _____ T

SECTION 4B—METHODS FOR CALCULATION

Complete the following:

1.   Before calculating drug dosages, all units of measurement must be converted to one system. Convert to the system used on the _____ .

Give the following metric and apothecary equivalents. Refer to Tables 4A-4 and 4B-1 as needed.

2.   1000 mg = _____ g

3.   1 g = _____ gr

4.   30 mg = _____ gr

5.   0.25 g = _____ mg

6.   300 (325) mg = _____ gr

7.   0.3 mg = _____ gr

8.   2½ ounces = _____ ml, or _____ T

9.   15 ml = _____ ounce, or _____ T, or _____ t

10.   4 T = _____ t

11.   30 gtt = _____ ml

12.   10 ml = _____ t

Interpretation of Drug Label

Give information concerning the following drug label:

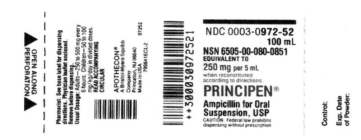

13.   Brand name _____

14.   Generic name _____

15.   Dosage _____

16.   Drug form _____

Methods for Drug Calculation

Use the basic formula, ratio and proportion, or dimensional analysis method to calculate the following drug problems:

17.   Order: codeine gr 1, q4-6 h, PRN.
       Available:

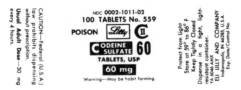

The drug is in grains and the unit on the bottle is in milligrams. Conversion to the same unit is necessary to work the problem. Conversion is to (grains/milligrams). (Circle correct answer.) Refer to Table 4A-4 in text as needed. gr 1 = 60 mg.

Basic Formula

$$\frac{D}{H} \times V = \frac{\overset{1}{\cancel{60}} \text{ mg}}{\underset{1}{\cancel{60}}} \times 1\,\text{tab} = 1\,\text{tablet}$$

Ratio and Proportion

$$H \quad : V \quad :: D \quad : X$$
$$60\,\text{mg} : 1\,\text{tab} :: 60\,\text{mg} : X\,\text{tab}$$
$$60X = 60$$
$$X = \frac{\cancel{60}}{\cancel{60}} = 1\,\text{tablet}$$

Dimensional Analysis

$$V = \frac{V(\text{vehicle}) \times C(H) \times D(\text{desired})}{H(\text{on hand}) \times C(D) \times 1} =$$

(drug label) (conversion factor, (desired order)

$$\text{tab} = \frac{1\,\text{tab} \times 1000\,\text{mg} \times 1\,\text{gr}}{60\,\text{mg} \times 15\,\text{gr} \times 1} = \frac{1000}{900} = 1.1 \text{ or } 1\,\text{tablet}$$

Refer to Table 4A-4 in text as needed. gr 1 = 60 mg.
NOTE—1.1 tablet should be rounded off to 1 tablet.

18. Order: Norvir (ritonavir) 0.2 g, PO, b.i.d.
    Available:

Exp. Lot 02-7878-2/R2 Store in refrigerator between 36° - 46°F (2° - 8°C). Protect from light.

NDC 0074-9492-54
84 Capsules

NORVIR™
RITONAVIR CAPSULES
100 mg

Caution: Federal (U.S.A.) law prohibits dispensing without prescription.

TM-Trademark

Do not accept if seal over bottle opening is broken or missing.

Dispense in a USP tight, light-resistant container.

Each capsule contains: 100 mg ritonavir.

See enclosure for prescribing information.

©Abbott
Abbott Laboratories
North Chicago,
IL 60064, U.S.A.

a. Is conversion needed? Explain.

b. $\text{BF}: \dfrac{D}{H} \times V = \quad \text{RP}: H : V : D : \quad \text{or} \quad \text{DA}: V = \dfrac{V \times C(H) \times D}{H \times C(D) \times 1} =$

19. Order: Benadryl (diphenhydramine) 25 mg, PO, q6 h, PRN.
Available: Benadryl 12.5 mg/5 ml

a. Is conversion needed? Explain.

b. How many ml would you give? Calculate the drug problem using the method you selected.

20. Order: Biaxin (clarithromycin) 0.25 g, PO, b.i.d.
Available:

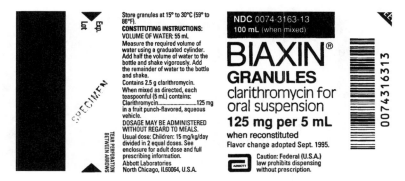

a. Is conversion needed? Explain.

b. How many ml would you give?

21. Order: hydroxyzine (Vistaril) 100 mg, IM, q6 h.
Available:

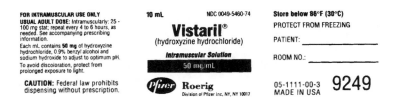

a. Is conversion needed? Explain.

b. How many ml would you give?

22.   Order: cefazolin (Kefzol) 500 mg, IM, q8h.

Available: (NOTE—Redi-vial container has diluent in a separate compartment of the vial. Push plug to release diluent for reconstitution.)

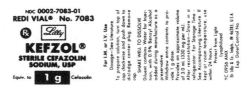

a.   Is conversion needed? Explain.

b.   How many ml would you give?

Additional Dimensional Analysis

23.   Order: Precose (acarbose) 50 mg, PO, t.i.d.

Available:

a.   How many tablets would you give?

b.   Which drug label(s) would you select? Explain.

24. Order: Losartan potassium (Cozaar) 0.1 g, daily.
    Available:

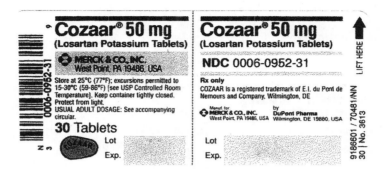

How many tablets should the client receive per day?

Abbreviations

Define the following abbreviations.

25. gr _____

26. g _____

27. gtt _____

28. l, L _____

29. mcg _____

30. mEq _____

31. ml _____

32. mg _____

33. kg _____

34. fl oz _____

35. $\overline{ss}$ _____

36. T _____

37. t _____

38. supp _____

39. T.O. _____

40. IM _____

41. IV _____

42. KVO _____

43. SL _____

44. Sub Q _____

45. PO, po _____

46. AC, ac _____

47. PC, pc _____

48. $\overline{c}$ _____

49. $\overline{s}$ _____

50. NPO _____

51. PRN _____

52. q8h _____

53. b.i.d. _____

54. t.i.d. _____

55. What is the difference between q.i.d. and q6h? _____

56. What is the difference between mg and mcg?
    _____

SECTION 4C—CALCULATIONS OF ORAL DOSAGES

The drug calculation problems include oral dosages for adults.

1.   Order: benztropine (Cogentin) 1 mg, PO, daily.
      Available:

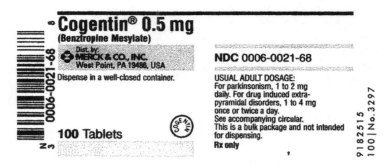

How many tablets would you give?

2.   Order: codeine sulfate 60 mg, PO, q6h, PRN.
      Available: Tablets are available at your institution in two forms (see drug labels).
      Which container would you use? Why?

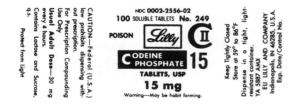 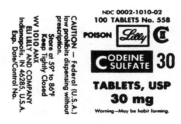

How many tablets would you give?

3. Order: propranolol (Inderal) 15 mg, PO, q6h.

    Available: propranolol 10 mg and 20 mg tablets.

    Which tablet strength would you use? How many tablets would you give?

4. Order: penicillin V potassium 250 mg, PO, q6h.

    Available: (NOTE—The generic name of the drug may be given instead of the brand name. Check the label for both names.)

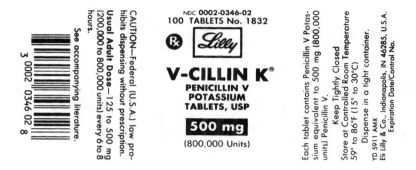

    How many tablets would you give?

5. Order: cimetidine (Tagamet) 600 mg, PO, hour of sleep.

    Available:

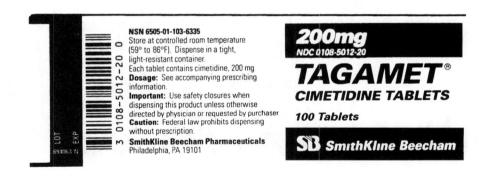

    How many tablets would you give?

6.   Order: verapamil 60 mg, PO, q.i.d.

    Available:

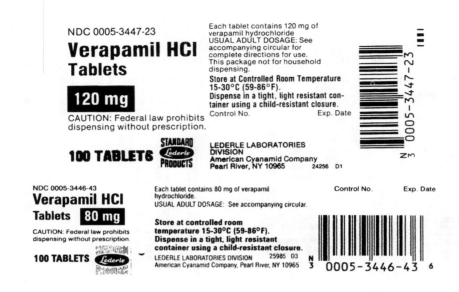

Which strength of verapamil would you select?

Tablets are scored. How many tablets would you give?

7.   Order: Artane SR 10 mg, PO, daily.

    Available:

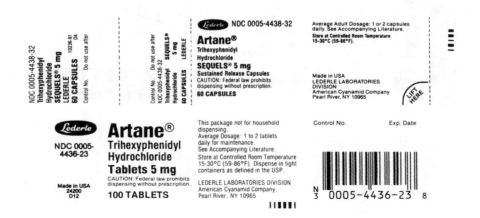

Which container of Artane 5 mg would you select? Why? How many tablet(s)/sequel(s) would you give?

8.   Order: trazodone (Desyrel) 150 mg, PO, daily.

Available: Desyrel in 50 mg tablets and 100 mg tablets.

How many tablets would you give if the 50 mg (strength) tablet is used? If the 100 mg tablet is used?

9.   Order: Coumadin (warfarin) 7.5 mg, PO, daily.

Available: (NOTE—Tablet is scored.)

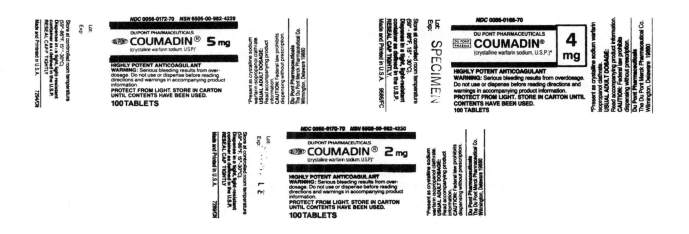

Which container of Coumadin would you select? How many tablets would you give?

10.   Order: lithium carbonate, 300 mg, PO, t.i.d.

Client's serum lithium level is 1.8 mEq/L (normal value is 0.5-1.5 mEq/L).

Available: lithium carbonate in 150 and 300 mg capsules, and 300 mg tablets. Because the serum lithium level is 1.8 mEq/L, would you:

a.   give 150 mg (half the dose)?

b.   give 300 mg tablet and not the capsule?

c.   advise the client not to take the dose for a week?

d.   withhold the drug and contact the health care provider?

11. Order: nitroglycerin gr ½₀₀, PO, SL, STAT.
    Available:

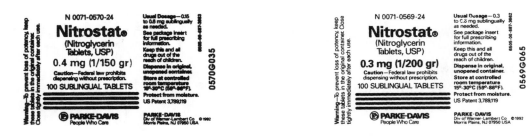

Which nitroglycerin container would you select, the 0.4 mg or the 0.3 mg? Why?

12. Order: Coreg (carvedilol) 25 mg, PO, b.i.d.
    Available:

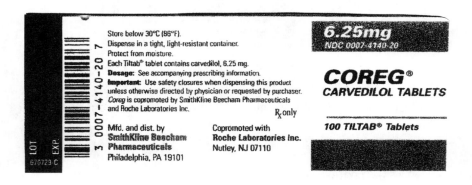

a. How many tablets would you give per dose?

b. How many tablets should the client receive in 24 hours?

13.   Order: azithromycin (Zithromax) 400 mg, daily first day, then 200 mg, daily next 4 days.
      Available:

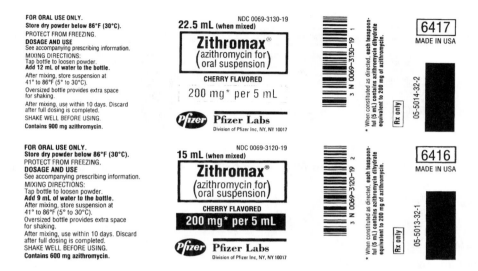

Which bottle would you select? Why?

How many ml would you give the first day and how many ml per day for the next 4 days?

14.   Order: Artane (trihexyphenidyl) Elixir 1 mg, PO, b.i.d.
      Available: Artane 2 mg/5 ml.

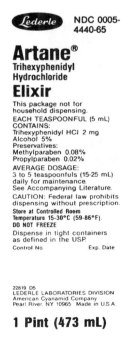

How many ml would you give?

15.   Order: doxycycline (Vibra-Tabs), 0.2 g, PO first day, then 0.1 g, PO daily for 6 days.
      Available:

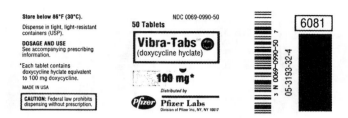

How many tablets should the client receive the first day, then how many tablets per day for 6 days?

16.   Order: digoxin 0.25 mg, PO, daily.

Available: Lanoxin (digoxin) 0.125 mg tablets. The drug comes in 0.25 mg tablets, but that strength tablet is not available.

How many tablets would you give? If the client questions the tablets, what should your response be?

17.   Order: Augmentin, 400 mg, PO, q6 h.
      Available:

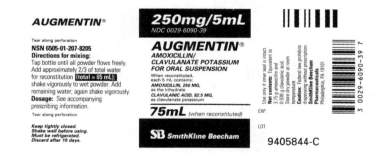

How many ml would you give?

18.   Order: cefadroxil (Duricef) 1 g, PO, daily.
        Available:

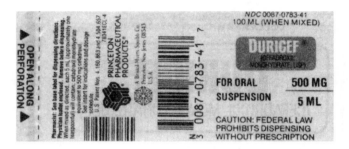

How many ml would you give?

19.   Order: prazosin (Minipress) 10 mg, PO, daily.
        Available: prazosin 1 mg, 2 mg, and 5 mg tablets.
        Which tablet would you select and how much would you give?

20.   Order: carbidopa-levodopa (Sinemet), 12.5-125 mg, PO, b.i.d.
        Available: Sinemet 25-100 mg, 25-250 mg, and 10-100 mg tablets.
        Which tablet would you select and how much would you give?

21.   Order: Ceclor 150 mg, PO, q8 h.
        Available:

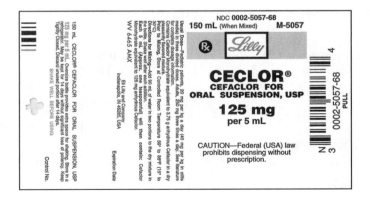

How many ml should the client receive per dose?

22.   Order: ampicillin (Principen) 0.5 g, PO, q6 h.

Available:

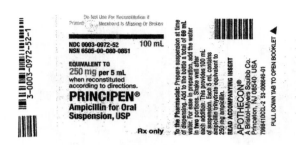

How many ml should the client receive per dose?

SECTION 4D—CALCULATIONS OF INJECTABLE DOSAGES

Complete the following:

1.   Methods for administering medications by parenteral routes include _____, _____, and _____

2.   Insulin and heparin may be administered by the routes of _____ and _____ .

3.   Vials are glass containers with (self-sealing rubber tops/tapered glass necks). Vials are usually (discarded/reusable if properly stored). (Circle correct answers.)

4.   Before drug reconstitution, the nurse should check the drug circular and/or drug label for instructions. After a drug has been reconstituted and additional dose(s) are available, the nurse should write on the drug label _____, _____, and _____ .

5.   Tuberculin syringes are usually used for _____ and _____. A tuberculin syringe (is/is not) used for insulin administration. (Circle correct answer.)

6.   Insulin syringes are calibrated in (units/ml). (Circle correct answer.)

7.   After use of a prefilled cartridge and Tubex injector, which of the following should be discarded?

    a.   cartridge

    b.   Tubex injector

    c.   cartridge and Tubex injector

    d.   neither cartridge nor Tubex injector

8.   The nurse is preparing an IM injection for an adult. The needle gauge and length should be:

    a.   20, 21 gauge; ½, 58 inch in length.

    b.   23, 25 gauge; ½, 58 inch in length.

    c.   19, 20, 21 gauge; 1, 1½, 2 inches in length.

    d.   25, 26 gauge; 1, 1½ inches in length.

9. The two parts of a syringe that must remain sterile are:
    a. outside of syringe and plunger.
    b. tip of the syringe and plunger.
    c. both the tip and outside of the syringe.
    d. tip and outside of syringe and plunger.

10. Subcutaneous injections can be administered in which of the following degree angle(s)?
    a. 10° and 15° angles
    b. 45°, 60°, and 90° angles
    c. 45° angle only
    d. 90° angle only

11. You calculate the drug dosage to be 0.25 ml. What type of syringe should you select?
    a. 3 ml syringe
    b. insulin syringe
    c. tuberculin syringe
    d. 10 ml syringe

12. To mix 4 ml of sterile saline solution in a vial containing a powdered drug, which size syringe should you select?
    a. tuberculin syringe
    b. insulin syringe
    c. 3 ml syringe
    d. 5 ml syringe

Determine how many ml to give:

13. Order: heparin 3000 units, subQ, q6 h.
    Available: Which heparin would you select?

    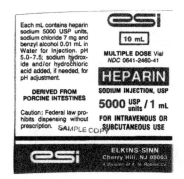   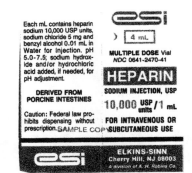

    How many ml would you give?

14. Order: codeine gr s̄s̄, q4-6 h, subQ, PRN.
    Available: Prefilled drug cartridge contains 60 mg/1 ml.
    How many ml would you give?

15.   Order: morphine sulfate gr ⅙ subQ, STAT.
       Available:

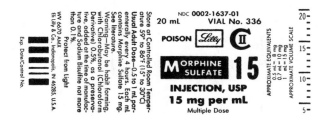

       How many ml would you give?

16.   Order: Humulin L insulin 36 units, subQ, qAM.
       Available:

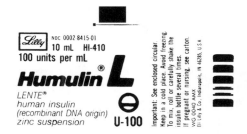

       Indicate on the insulin syringe the amount of insulin to be withdrawn.

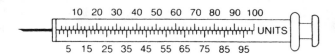

17.   Order: regular insulin 8 units and NPH 44 units, subQ, qAM.
       Available: (NOTE—These insulins can be mixed together in the same insulin syringe.)

       Indicate on the insulin syringe the amount of each insulin to be withdrawn. Which insulin should
       be drawn up first?

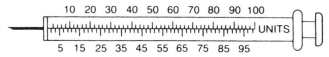

18.   Order: digoxin 0.25 mg, IM, STAT. (NOTE—Usually digoxin is administered intravenously; however, in this problem, IM is indicated.)

Available:

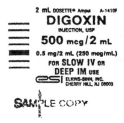

How many ml would you give?

19.   Order: vitamin B$_{12}$ (cyanocobalamin) 400 mcg, IM, daily for 5 days.

Available:

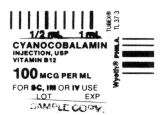   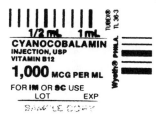

Which prefilled cartridge would you select?

How many ml would you give?

20.   Order: clindamycin 300 mg, IM, q6h.

Available:

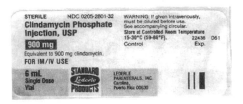

How many ml would you give?

21.   Order: meperidine (Demerol) 60 mg, IM, and atropine 0.5 mg, IM, preoperatively.

       Available: (NOTE—These drugs are compatible and can be mixed in the same syringe.)

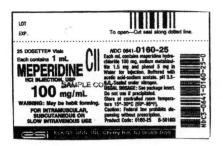 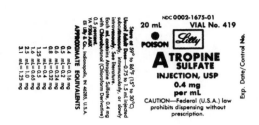

How many ml of meperidine would you discard?

How many ml of meperidine and how many ml of atropine would you give?

22.   Order: naloxone (Narcan) 0.8 mg, IM, for narcotic-induced respiratory depression. Repeat in 3 minutes if needed.

       Available:

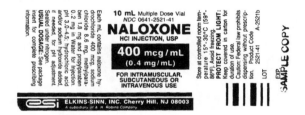

How many ml would you give?

23.   Order: hydroxyzine (Vistaril) 35 mg, IM, preoperatively.

       Available:

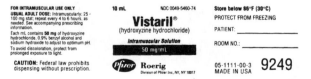

How many ml would you give?

24.   Order: oxacillin sodium 500 mg, IM, q6h.

Available: Drug in powdered form. (NOTE—Convert to the unit system on the bottle.)

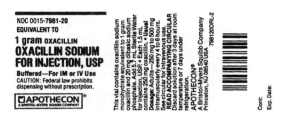

How many ml would you give?

25.   Order: oxacillin sodium 300 mg, IM, q6h.

Available:

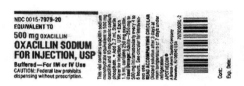

You are to add _____ ml of sterile water to yield _____ ml of drug solution.
How many ml would you give?

26.   Order: nafcillin (Nafcil) 250 mg, IM, q4h.

Available:

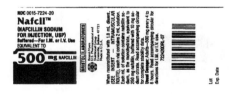

You are to add _____ ml of diluent to yield _____ ml of drug solution.
How many ml would you give?

27.   Order: trimethobenzamide (Tigan) 100 mg, IM, STAT.

Available: trimethobenzamide (Tigan) ampule, 200 mg/2 ml.

How many ml would you give?

28.   Order: chlorpromazine (Thorazine) 20 mg, deep IM, t.i.d.
      Available:

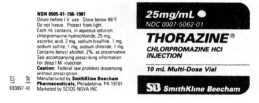

      How many ml would you give?

29.   Order ticarcillin (Ticar) 400 mg, IM, q6 h.
      Available:

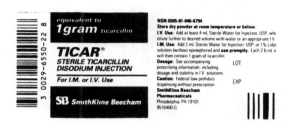

      You are to add _____ ml of diluent to yield _____ ml of drug solution.
      How many ml would you give?

30.   Order: cefonicid (Monocid) 750 mg, IM, daily.
      Available:

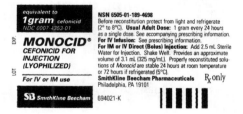

   a.   How many gram(s) is 750 mg?

   b.   How many ml of diluent should be injected into the vial? (See drug label.)

   c.   How many ml of cefonicid should the client receive per day?

31.   Order: cefotetan disodium (Cefotan) 750 mg, IM, q12 h.

Available: (Note—Mix 2 ml of diluent; drug solution will equal 2.4 ml.)

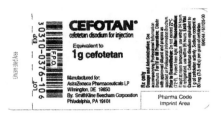

a.   How many ml would you give per dose?

b.   Can the remainder of the solution be used later? Explain.

32.   Order: Unasyn (ampicillin sodium/sulbactam sodium) 1 g, IM, q6 h.

Available: (Note—Mix 2.2 ml of diluent; drug solution will equal 2.6 ml.)

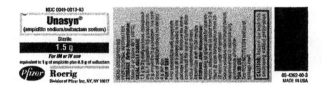

How many ml would you give per dose?

SECTION 4E—CALCULATIONS OF INTRAVENOUS FLUIDS

Complete the following:

1.   The health care provider orders the type and amount of intravenous (IV) solutions per 24 hours, and the nurse calculates the IV flow rate according to _____, _____, and _____.

2.   Macrodrip infusion sets deliver _____ gtt/ml; microdrip infusion sets deliver _____ gtt/ml.

3.   If the infusion rate is less than 100 ml/hr, the preferred IV set is (macrodrip/microdrip). (Circle correct answer.)

4.   KVO means _____. The preferred size of IV bag for KVO is (1000 ml/500 ml/250 ml). (Circle correct answer.)

5.   When should drugs such as potassium chloride (KCl) and multiple vitamin solutions be injected into the IV bag or bottle? _____

Give the abbreviations for the following solutions:

6.   5% dextrose in water _____

7.   Normal saline solution or 0.9% sodium chloride (NaCl) _____

8.   5% dextrose in ½ normal saline solution (0.45% NaCl) _____

9.   5% dextrose in lactated Ringer's _____

Complete the following:

10.   Intermittent IV administration is prescribed when a drug is administered in a (small/large) volume of IV fluid over a (long/short) period of time. (Circle correct answers.)

11.   The Buretrol is a (calibrated cylinder with tubing/small IV bag of solution with short tubing). (Circle correct answer.) It is used in administering _____.

12.   The pump infusion regulator that delivers ml/hr is a (volumetric/nonvolumetric) IV regulator. (Circle correct answer.)

13.   Patient-controlled analgesia (PCA) is a method used to administer drug intravenously. The purpose/objective is to provide a _____.

Continuous Intravenous Administration

Select step method I, II, or III from the text to calculate the continuous IV flow rate. Memorize the step method.

14.   Order: 1 liter or 1000 ml of D_5W to infuse over 6 hours.
      Available: Macrodrip set: 10 gtt/ml.
      a.   The IV flow rate should be regulated as _____ gtt/min.

15.   Order: 1000 ml of D_5 ½ NS with multiple vitamins and KCl 10 mEq to infuse over 8 hours.
      Available: Macrodrip set: 15 gtt/ml.
                KCl (potassium chloride) 20 mEq/10 ml ampule.
                Multiple vitamin (MVI) vial.
      a.   When should KCl and MVI be injected into the IV bag?

      b.   Calculate the IV flow rate in gtt/min. _____

16.   Order: 1 liter of 0.9% NaCl (normal saline solution) to infuse over 12 hours.

Available: Macrodrip set: 10 gtt/ml

Microdrip set: 60 gtt/ml

a.   Which IV set would you use? _____

b.   Calculate the IV flow rate in gtt/min according to the IV set selected. _____

17.   Order: 2.5 liters of IV fluids to infuse over 24 hours. This includes 1 liter of D_5W, 1 liter of D_5 ½ NS, and 500 ml of 5% D/LR.

Available: The three above solutions.

a.   One liter is equal to _____ ml.

b.   Total number of ml of IV solutions to infuse in 24 hours is _____ ml.

c.   Approximate amount of IV solution to administer per hour
        is _____ ml.

d.   Which type of IV set would you select?

e.   Calculate the IV flow rate according to the IV set you selected. _____ gtt/min

18.   A liter of IV fluid was started at 7:00 AM and was to run for 8 hours. The IV set delivers 10 gtt/ml. At 12:00 PM only 500 ml were infused.

a.   How much IV fluid is left? _____

b.   Recalculate the flow rate for the remaining IV fluids. Keep in mind that if the client has a cardiovascular problem, rapid IV flow rate may not be desired.

Intermittent Intravenous Administration

(NOTE—Only add the volume of drug solution ≥ 5 ml to IV fluid to determine final drip rate.)

19.   Order: cimetidine (Tagamet) 200 mg, IV, q6h.

Available:

Set and solution: Buretrol (calibrated cylinder set) with drop factor 60 gtt/ml; 500 ml of NSS.

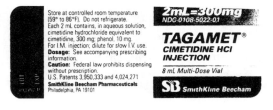

Instruction: Dilute cimetidine 200 mg in 50 ml of NSS and infuse in 20 minutes.

Drug calculation:

IV flow calculation (determine gtt/minute):

20.   Order: cefamandole (Mandol) 500 mg, IV, q6 h.

Available:

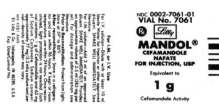

How many ml of diluent would you add?

Drug solution equals: _____.

Set and solution: Calibrated cylinder with drop factor, 60 gtt/ml; 500 ml of D_5W.

Instruction: Dilute cefamandole 500 mg reconstituted solution in 50 ml of D_5W and infuse in 30 minutes.

Drug calculation (convert to the unit on the drug label):

IV flow calculation (determine gtt/minute):

21.   Order: nafcillin (Nafcil) 1000 mg, IV, q6 h.

Available:

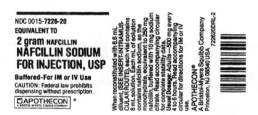

How many ml of diluent would you add?

Drug solution equals: _____

Set and solution: Secondary set with drop factor 15 gtt/ml; 100 ml of D_5W.

Instruction: Dilute nafcillin 1000 mg in 100 ml of D_5W and infuse in 40 minutes.

Drug calculation (convert to the unit on the drug label):

IV flow calculation (determine gtt/minute):

22.   Order: kanamycin (Kantrex) 250 mg, IV, q6 h.

Available:

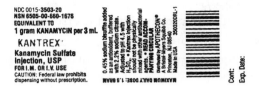

Set and solution: Secondary set with drop factor 15 gtt/ml; 100 ml of D_5W.

Instruction: Dilute kanamycin 250 mg in 100 ml of D_5W and infuse in 45 minutes.

Drug calculation (convert to the unit on the drug label):

IV flow calculation (determine gtt/minute):

23.   Order: ticarcillin (Ticar) 750 mg, IV, q4 h.

Available:

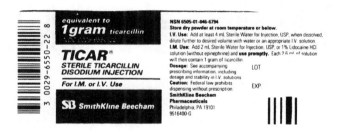

How many ml of diluent would you add?

Drug solution equals: _____

Set and solution: Buretrol set with drop factor 60 gtt/ml; 500 ml of D_5W.

Instruction: Dilute ticarcillin 750 mg solution in 75 ml of D_5W and infuse in 30 minutes.

Drug calculation (convert to the unit on the drug label):

IV flow calculation (determine gtt/minute):

Volumetric IV Regulator

24. Order: Septra (trimethoprim 80 mg and sulfamethoxazole 400 mg), IV, q12 h.

 Available: Septra (trimethoprim 160 mg and sulfamethoxazole 800 mg/10 ml).

 How many ml would equal the drug order? _____

 Set and solution: Volumetric pump regulator and 125 ml of D_5W.

 Instruction: Dilute Septra 80/400 mg in 125 ml of D_5W and infuse in 90 minutes.

 Drug calculation:

 Volumetric pump regulator (How many ml/hr?):

25. Order: doxycycline (Vibramycin) 75 mg, IV, q12 h.

 Available: Add 8 ml of diluent = 10 ml.

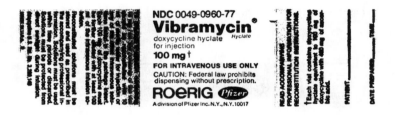

 How many ml would equal the Vibramycin 75 mg? _____

 Set and solution: Volumetric pump regulator; 100 ml of D_5W.

 Instruction: Dilute Vibramycin 75 mg solution in 100 ml of D_5W and infuse in 1 hour (60 minutes).

 Drug calculation:

 Volumetric pump regulator (How many ml/hr?):

26.   Order: amikacin sulfate 400 mg, IV, q12 h.

Adult weight: 64 kg

Adult drug dosage: 7.5 mg/kg/q12 h

Available:

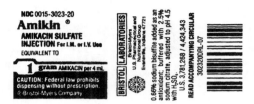

How many ml would equal amikacin 400 mg? _____

Set and solution: Volumetric pump regulator; 125 ml of D_5W.

Instruction: Dilute amikacin 400 mg in 125 ml of D_5W and infuse in 1 hour.

Drug calculation:

Volumetric pump regulator (How many ml/hr?):

27.   Order: minocycline 75 mg, IV, q12 h.

Available: Add 5 ml of diluent

How many ml would equal minocycline 75 mg? _____

Set and solution: Volumetric pump regulator; 500 ml of D_5W.

Instruction: Dilute minocycline 75 mg in 500 ml of D_5W and infuse in 2 hours.

Drug calculation:

Volumetric pump regulator (How many ml/hr?):

28.   Order: cefepime hydrochloride (Maxipime) 500 mg, IV, q12 h.

Available:

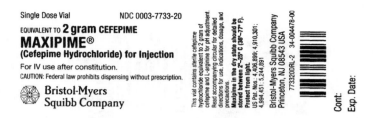

Set and solution: Calibrated cylinder set with drop factor.

Instruction: 60 gtt/ml; 100 ml of D_5W.

a.   How many ml of drug solution should the client receive?

The drug label does not indicate the amount of diluent to use. This may be found in the pamphlet insert. Usually if you inject 2.6 ml of diluent, the amount of drug solution should be 3.0 ml. If you inject 3.4 or 3.5 ml of diluent, the amount of drug solution should be 4 ml.

b.   Dilute cefepime 500 mg in 50 ml of D_5W and infuse in 30 minutes.

29.   Order: Unasyn (ampicillin sodium/sulbactam sodium) 1.5 g, IV, q6 h.

Available: (NOTE—Mix 3 g in 10 ml of diluent.)

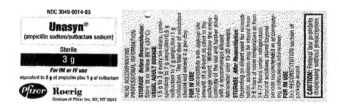

Set and solution: Buretrol or like set with drop factor of 60 gtt/ml; 500 ml of D_5W.

Instruction: Dilute Unasyn 1.5 g solution in 100 ml of D_5W and infuse in 30 minutes.

Drug calculation:

IV flow calculation (determine gtt/minute):

30. Order: Mefoxin (cefoxitin) 500 mg, IV, q6 h.
     Available: (NOTE—Mix 1 g in 10 ml of diluent.)

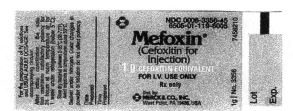

Set and solution: Volumetric pump regulator; 100 ml of D$_5$W.

Instruction: Dilute Mefoxin 500 mg in 100 ml of D$_5$W and infuse in 45 minutes.

Drug calculation:

Volumetric pump regulator (How many ml/hr?):

SECTION 4F—PEDIATRIC DRUG CALCULATIONS

Orals

1. Order: penicillin V potassium (V-Cillin K) 200,000 units, PO, q6 h.
    Child weighs 46 pounds or 21 kg.
    Child's drug dosage: 25,000-90,000 units/kg/day in 3-6 divided doses.
    Available: (NOTE—The dosage per 5 ml is in mg and units.)

Is the prescribed dose safe?

How many ml should the child receive for each dose?

2.   Order: cefuroxime axetil (Ceftin), 200 mg, PO, q12 h.

Child's age: 8 years; weight: 75 pounds.

Child's drug dosage (3 months-12 years): 10-15 mg/kg/day.

Available:

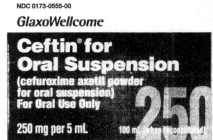

Is the prescribed dose safe?

How many ml should the child receive per dose?

3.   Order: amoxicillin 75 mg, PO, q6 h.

Child weighs 5 kg.

Child's drug dosage: 50 mg/kg/day in divided doses.

Available:

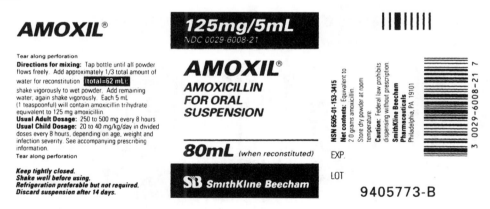

Is the prescribed dose safe?

According to the drug order, how many ml should the child receive per day (24 hours)?

4.   Order: acetaminophen 250 mg, PO, PRN.

     Available: 160 mg/5 ml.

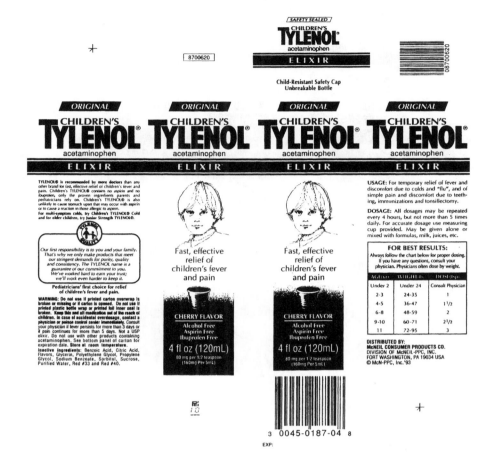

How many ml would you give? Round off numbers when necessary.

5.   Order: cloxacillin 100 mg, PO, q6h.

     Child weighs 8 kg.

     Child's drug dosage: 50-100 mg/kg/day in 4 divided doses.

     Available: cloxacillin (Tegopen), 125 mg/5 ml.

     Is the prescribed dose safe?

     How many ml should the child receive per dose?

6.   Order: erythromycin suspension 160 mg, PO, q6 h.

Child weighs 25 kg.

Child's drug dosage: 30-50 mg/kg/day in divided doses, q6 h.

Available:

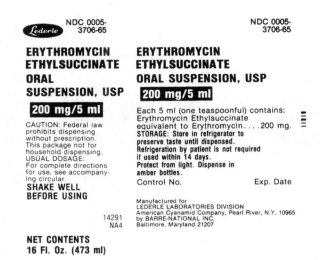

Is the prescribed dosage within dose parameters?

Explain.

7.   Order: cefaclor (Ceclor) 75 mg, PO, q8 h.

Child weighs 22 pounds.

Child's drug dosage: 20-40 mg/kg/day in 3 divided doses.

Available:

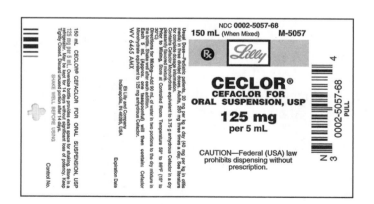

How many ml per dose should be given?

8.   Order: Augmentin 150 mg, PO, q8 h.

Child weighs 26 pounds.

Child's drug dosage: 40 mg/kg/day in 3 divided doses.

Available:

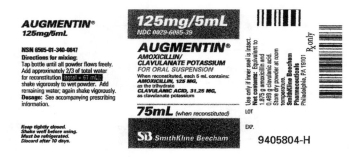

How many kg does the child weigh?

Is the prescribed dosage within dose parameters?

How many ml of Augmentin should the child receive per dose?

9.   Order: cyclophosphamide (Cytoxan).

Child's height is 48 inches; weight is 60 pounds.

Child's body surface area (BSA) is _____ m^2. Determine BSA by plotting the child's height and weight on the nomogram (p. 50).

Child's drug dosage: 60–250 mg/m^2.

What is the safe dosage range?

10.   Order: phenytoin (Dilantin).

Child's weight is 50 pounds; height is unknown.

Child's BSA is _____ m^2. Use the center graph of the nomogram (p. 50) because the height is unknown.

Child's drug dosage: 250 mg/m^2 in 3 divided doses.

Available: Dilantin 30 mg/5 ml.

How many ml should be given per dose? Round off numbers.

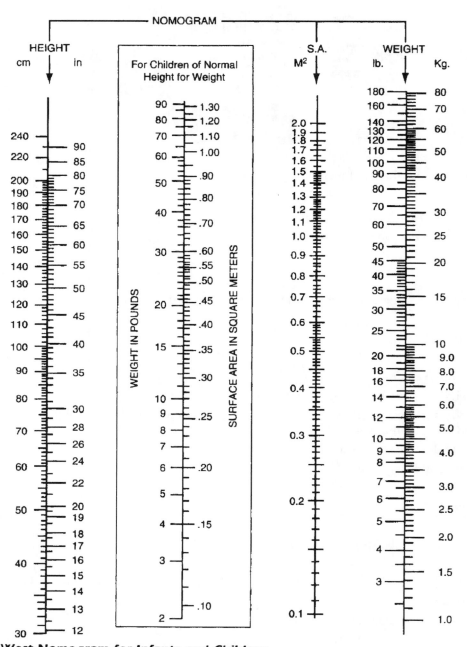

West Nomogram for Infants and Children

Directions: (1) Find height. (2) Find weight. (3) Draw a straight line connecting the height and weight. Where the line intersects on the SA column is the body surface area (m²). (Modified from data by Boyd E, West CD. In Behrman RE, Kliegman RM, Jensen HB: *Nelson textbook of pediatrics*, ed 18, Philadelphia, 2007, Saunders.)

Injectables

11. Order: ampicillin (Polycillin-N) 100 mg, IM, q6 h.

 Child's weight: 26 pounds. (Convert pounds to kilograms [kg].)

 Child's drug dosage: 25-50 mg/kg/day.

 Available:

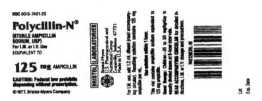

 Is the drug dose safe?

 How many ml per dose should the child receive?

12. Order: pentobarbital (Nembutal) 25 mg, IM, preoperatively.

 Child's weight: 40 pounds. (Convert pounds to kilograms.)

 Child's drug dosage: 3-5 mg/kg

 Available: Nembutal 50 mg/ml

 Is the drug dose safe?

 How many ml per dose should the child receive?

13. Order: kanamycin (Kantrex) 50 mg, IM, q12 h.

 Child's weight: 10 kg.

 Child's drug dosage: 15 mg/kg/day in 2 divided doses.

 Available:

 Is the drug dose safe?

 How many ml per dose should the child receive?

14.   Order: amikacin sulfate (Amikin) 50 mg, IM, q12 h.
Child's weight: 9 kg.
Child's drug dosage: 5 mg/kg/q8 h OR 7.5 mg/kg/q12 h.
Available:

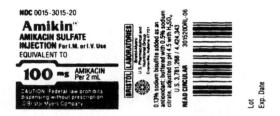

Is the drug dose safe?

How many ml per dose should the child receive?

15.   Order: cefazolin sodium (Kefzol) 125 mg, IM, q6 h.
Child's weight: 48 pounds.
Child's drug dosage: 25-50 mg/kg/day in 3-4 divided doses.
Available:

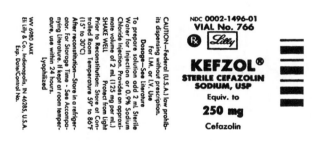

You are to add _____ ml of diluent to yield _____ ml of drug solution.

Is the drug dose safe?

How many ml per dose should the child receive?

16.   Order: tobramycin (Nebcin) 25 mg, IM, q8h.

Child's weight: 22 kg.

Child's drug dosage: 3-5 mg/kg/day in 3 divided doses.

Available:

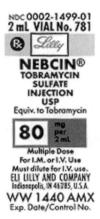

Is the drug dose safe?

How many ml per dose should the child receive?

5   The Drug Approval Process

Study Questions

Define the following:

1. Controlled substance

2. Malfeasance

3. Misfeasance

4. Nonfeasance

Match the letter from Column II with the applicable description in Column I.

	Column I		Column II
_____ 5.	trade name	a.	chemical name
_____ 6.	owned by manufacturer	b.	generic name
_____ 7.	drug's chemical structure	c.	brand name
_____ 8.	official; nonproprietary		
_____ 9.	registered trademark		

Complete the following:

10. What is the approval seal of reputable online pharmacies?

11. List at least two drugs that children take that may be toxic in large doses:

    a.

    b.

12. List four provisions of the Comprehensive Drug Abuse Prevention and Control Act of 1970:

    a.

    b.

    c.

    d.

13. Both the American Nurses Association (ANA) and the Canadian Nurses Association (CNA) have a Code of Ethics, which are standards for ethical practice in nursing. Identify at least six of these standards:

    a.

    b.

    c.

    d.

    e.

    f.

NCLEX Review Questions

Select the best response.

14. What resource provides the basis for standards in drug strength and composition throughout the world?
    a. U.S. Pharmacopeia/National Formulary
    b. Physicians' Desk Reference
    c. Drug Facts and Comparisons
    d. International Pharmacopeia

15. The current authoritative source for drug standards is:
    a. Nurse Practice Acts.
    b. U.S. Pharmacopeia/National Formulary.
    c. Physicians' Desk Reference.
    d. Controlled Substances Act.

16. The primary purpose of federal legislation related to drug standards is:
    a. to provide consistency.
    b. to establish cost controls.
    c. to ensure safety.
    d. to act as an information resource.

17. The FDA's mandate to monitor and control the manufacture and marketing of drugs comes from:
    a. the Food, Drug, and Cosmetic Act of 1938.
    b. the Controlled Substances Act.
    c. the Kefauver-Harris Amendment.
    d. the Durham-Humphrey Amendment.

18. Which legislation identified those drugs that required a prescription and a new prescription for refill?
    a. Food, Drug, and Cosmetic Act of 1938
    b. Controlled Substances Act
    c. Kefauver-Harris Amendment
    d. Durham-Humphrey Amendment

19. The Kefauver-Harris Amendment was established to improve safety by requiring which of the following in the literature?
    a. recommended dose
    b. pregnancy category
    c. side effects and contraindications
    d. adverse effects and contraindications

20. What state law controls drug administration by nurses?
    a. Nurse Practice Act
    b. FDA
    c. Food, Drug, and Cosmetic Act
    d. State Board of Nursing

21. Controlled substances are grouped in Schedules/categories; what is the number of Schedules?
    a. 3
    b. 5
    c. 7
    d. 9

22. Which of the following Schedule drugs have accepted medical use?
    a. I through IV
    b. I through V
    c. II through V
    d. III through V

23. What is correct about Schedule drugs' potential for abuse?
    a. V > IV
    b. III > I
    c. I > III
    d. V > III

24. Your client abuses drugs. LSD and heroin belong to which Schedule?
    a. I
    b. II
    c. III
    d. IV

25. The nurse needs to know that codeine in cough syrup belongs to which Schedule?
    a. II
    b. III
    c. IV
    d. V

26. In institutions/agencies, controlled substances must be stored:
    a. in a medicine cabinet.
    b. in a locked location.
    c. near the nurses' station.
    d. double wrapped and labeled.

27. Drugs in Canada's Schedule G have moderate potential for abuse and require a prescription both for initial allocation and for refills. These drugs are similar to what Schedule in the United States?
    a. II
    b. III
    c. IV
    d. V

28. In Canada, OTC preparations are administered by what group of the respective provinces?
    a. Pharmacy Acts
    b. Canadian Food and Drug Act
    c. 1961 Narcotic Control Act
    d. Health Protection Act

29. According to the FDA, drugs in which pregnancy category are considered not to present a risk to the fetus?
    a. A
    b. B
    c. C
    d. D

30. Two advantages associated with use of generic drugs are:
    a. lower cost.
    b. same active ingredients.
    c. different active ingredients.
    d. same price.

31. Two disadvantages associated with generic drugs are:
    a. less extensive testing.
    b. similar testing.
    c. variation in response.
    d. no disadvantages.

32. Which drug resource is published annually and updated monthly?
    a. U.S. Pharmacopeia
    b. Physicians' Desk Reference
    c. American Hospital Formulary
    d. Internet Drug Index

33. Which legislation decreased the time for approval of drugs used for treating AIDS and cancer?
    a. Drug Regulation Act of 1992
    b. Controlled Substances Act
    c. Durham-Humphrey Amendment
    d. Kefauver-Harris Amendment

34. The nurse must be alert to counterfeit prescription drugs. The following are clues to counterfeit products: *Select all that apply.*
    a. variation in labeling
    b. different taste
    c. different appearance
    d. different dose

35. Implications of HIPAA include the following: *Select all that apply.*
    a. release of information only to client
    b. private area for pharmacy consultation
    c. client receives report of each visit
    d. client signs for copy of privacy statement

6   Transcultural and Genetic Considerations

Study Questions

Define the following:

1. Paralanguage

2. Biocultural ecology

3. Ethnocultural

4. Ethnopharmacology

5. Spatial distancing

6. Temporality

NCLEX Review Questions

Select the best response.

7. Most drug testing in the United States has which ethnic group for research participants?
    a. Chinese
    b. African American
    c. Polynesian
    d. European American

8. African Americans:
    a. are less responsive to beta blockers than are European Americans and Hispanics.
    b. are more responsive to beta blockers than are European Americans and Hispanics.
    c. experience fewer toxic side effects with psychotropic medications than do European Americans.
    d. experience fewer toxic side effects with antidepressant medications than do European Americans.

9. Many cultural groups have lactose intolerance. Symptoms of lactose intolerance include:
    a. constipation.
    b. palpitations.
    c. elevated enzymes.
    d. bloating.

10. Jose Gonzalez, age 45, has developed lactose intolerance. Dietary counselling to meet calcium requirements includes encouraging him to eat:
    a. leafy green vegetables.
    b. chicken.
    c. flour tortillas.
    d. gelatin.

11. Communication, one of the domains of culture, includes:
    a. maintenance of eye contact.
    b. use of traditional health care providers.
    c. use of complementary/alternative medicine.
    d. primary occupation.

12. Lisa, age 22, is from the Caribbean. She is 6 months pregnant. At her mother's request, she eats red clay to provide minerals for the fetus, a practice she intends to continue. You would:
    a. insist that she stop the practice immediately.
    b. determine the amount of clay she eats daily.
    c. ask her to substitute corn starch for the clay.
    d. double her daily iron supplement.

13. Pablo de Omedo is newly diagnosed with diabetes and is taking an oral hypoglycemic. His curandero has recommended that he drink sabila tea three times a day to improve his nutrition. As his home health nurse, you would:
    a. encourage him to drink it four times a day.
    b. discourage the practice; sabila tea potentiates oral hypoglycemics.
    c. discourage the practice; sabila tea decreases the effects of oral hypoglycemics.
    d. encourage him to drink the tea but also be sure he continues taking his oral hypoglycemic medication.

14. Factors that affect clients' physiologic responses to medications include:
    Select all that apply.
    a. genetics.
    b. diet.
    c. age.
    d. values.

15. Factors that affect clients' adherence with medication prescriptions include:
    Select all that apply.
    a. heredity.
    b. poverty.
    c. trust in health care provider.
    d. access to health care.

Critical Thinking Exercises

Use a separate sheet of paper for your answers.

A Chinese couple, Foua and Nao Liu, bring their 6-year-old daughter, Lia Liu, to the emergency department. The child had a pulmonary infection and was last seen in the emergency department 2 days ago. At that time, Lia was prescribed erythromycin 150 mg. She does not seem to be improving. The parents bring the bottle of liquid erythromycin with them in a plastic bag. Included in the bag is a porcelain Chinese soup spoon, which is about the size of a tablespoon. The instructions on the bottle read: Take 1 teaspoon every 6 hours for 10 days. The bottle is almost half empty.

1. If the parents do not make eye contact with the nurse, how would you interpret this behavior?

2. The parents were giving Lia a tablespoon of erythromycin each time instead of a teaspoon. How much more erythromycin was the child receiving than prescribed?

3. Is this a potentially dangerous dose?

4. How might this over-dosage have been prevented?

5. If the parents only speak in the present tense, how will this affect your nursing care and discharge teaching?

6. If you had needed an interpreter, who would be the "ideal interpreter"?

7. If you needed an interpreter and one was not available, how might you have communicated with the parents?

7 Drug Interaction and Over-the-Counter Drugs

Study Questions

Define the following:

1. Addiction

2. Drug abuse

3. Drug incompatibility

4. Drug interaction

5. Withdrawal

Match the following terms with the letter of the definition.

	Term		Definition
_____ 6.	drug inter-action	a.	undesirable drug effect
_____ 7.	drug incom-patibility	b.	changes that occur in the absorption, distribution, metabolism, or excretion of one or more drugs
_____ 8.	adverse drug reac-tion		
_____ 9.	pharma-cokinetic interaction	c.	altered effect of a drug as a result of interaction with other drugs
_____10.	pharmaco-dynamic interaction	d.	reaction that occurs in vitro
		e.	interaction that results in addi-tive, synergistic, or antagonistic drug effects

Match the following agents with the letter of the action.

	Agent		Action
_____ 11.	laxatives	a.	decrease drug absorption
_____ 12.	aspirin	b.	increase drug absorption
_____ 13.	antacids		
_____ 14.	food	c.	block drug absorption
_____ 15.	narcotics	d.	change urine pH to alkaline
		e.	change urine pH to acidic
		f.	increase or decrease absorp-tion
		g.	increase drug excretion

Complete the following:

16. E.J., 4 years old, is complaining of a sore throat, a cough productive of green sputum, and bilateral knee pain. Her mother is about to administer several OTC preparations. Four concerns about OTC drugs in this situation include:

    a.

    b.

    c.

    d.

NCLEX Review Questions

Select the best response.

17. Which of the following drug groups is primarily absorbed by the small intestine?
    a. barbiturates
    b. salicylates
    c. anticonvulsants
    d. theophylline

18. Your client is receiving two analgesics for pain relief. Two drugs with similar action are administered to achieve which of the following effects?
    a. additive
    b. synergistic
    c. agonistic
    d. antagonistic

19. Your client had surgery yesterday. He is taking two drugs at the same time: a narcotic and an antihistamine. This is an example of which of the following drug effects?
    a. additive
    b. synergistic
    c. agonistic
    d. antagonistic

20. When two drugs that have opposite effects are administered (e.g., stimulant and beta blocker), the drug effects are cancelled. This is an example of which of the following effects?
    a. additive
    b. synergistic
    c. agonistic
    d. antagonistic

21. A major drug-food interaction occurs between monoamine oxidase (MAO) inhibitors and foods rich in which of the following?
    a. caffeine
    b. fiber
    c. tyramine
    d. acetylcholine

22. Your client is taking digoxin and a diuretic. You need to be aware of digitalis toxicity and which of the following serum levels?
    a. potassium
    b. sodium
    c. calcium
    d. chloride

23. Which of the following is NOT a sign of digitalis toxicity?
    a. nausea
    b. vomiting
    c. bradycardia
    d. tachycardia

24. As a nurse, you know that increased drug metabolism results in _____ drug elimination and _____ concentration of the drug.
    a. decreased; increased
    b. decreased; decreased
    c. increased; decreased
    d. increased; increased

25. Most drugs are excreted through which of the following?
    a. lungs
    b. urine
    c. saliva
    d. feces

26. What amendment approved drugs safe for consumption that may be sold as OTC drugs?
    a. Durham-Humphrey
    b. Kefauver-Harris
    c. Drug Modernization
    d. Food and Cosmetic

27. What amendment requires proof of efficacy and safety of the drug?
    a. Durham-Humphrey
    b. Kefauver-Harris
    c. Drug Modernization
    d. Food and Cosmetic

28. Based on review by the FDA, the OTC drugs are assigned to one of how many categories?
    a. two
    b. three
    c. four
    d. five

29. Drugs not included in nonprescription products because they are unsafe or ineffective are assigned to which OTC category?
    a. I
    b. II
    c. III
    d. IV

30. Most drug-induced photosensitivity reactions can be avoided by the following actions: *Select all that apply.*
    a. using sunscreen
    b. eating foods high in vitamin C
    c. wearing protective clothing
    d. avoiding excessive sunlight

31. Clients with impaired renal function should avoid the following: *Select all that apply.*
    a. aspirin
    b. acetaminophen
    c. Milk of Magnesia
    d. ibuprofen

32. The nurse is caring for a client receiving prescription drugs including an anticoagulant. The nurse is aware that anticoagulants have an increased effect with the following drugs: *Select all that apply.*
    a. lovastatin
    b. aminoglycosides
    c. propranolol
    d. ibuprofen
    e. fibrates

8   Drugs of Abuse

Study Questions

Define the following:

1. Drug abuse

2. Drug misuse

3. Addiction

4. Dependence

5. Tolerance

6. Intoxication

7. Detoxification

8. Withdrawal

Complete the following.

9. It is important that nurses be aware of the early signs of alcohol withdrawal syndrome, including:

    a.

    b.

    c.

    d.

NCLEX Review Questions

Select the best response.

10. Several students are brought to the emergency department after the police interrupted their cocaine party. Which of the following most accurately describes the effects of cocaine?
    a. insomnia and fine tremors
    b. dilated pupils and diaphoresis
    c. hypotension and tachycardia
    d. depression and pinpoint pupils

11. Your cocaine-using client is also taking digoxin daily. What is the interaction of these two drugs?
    a. no interaction
    b. reciprocal increase in effects
    c. bradycardia
    d. dysrhythmias

12. It is essential that nurses anticipate withdrawal syndrome in clients because alcohol withdrawal delirium can usually be prevented with the administration of which of the following drugs?
    a. naloxone (Narcan)
    b. methadone (Dolophine)
    c. disulfiram (Antabuse)
    d. lorazepam (Ativan)

13. Wernicke's encephalopathy is one of many effects of chronic alcohol use. The drug of choice to treat this is:
    a. IV thiamine.
    b. IV glucose.
    c. IV KCl.
    d. IV plasma expanders.

14. The only FDA-approved cannabis preparation is which of the following drugs?

    a. dronabinol

    b. lorazepam

    c. methadone

    d. naloxone

15. John, your client, has chosen to use Commit lozenges to aid him with smoking cessation. Health teaching for John includes which of the following?

    a. Avoid food and drink for 15 minutes before taking the lozenge.

    b. This product is not advised for those with asthma.

    c. Chewing and swallowing the lozenge increase GI side effects.

    d. Avoid food and drink for 15 minutes after taking the lozenge.

16. What percentage of nurses abuse drugs and demonstrate related impaired practice?

    a. 3%-6%

    b. 7%-10%

    c. 11%-15%

    d. >15%

17. Severe pain in drug-dependent clients should be treated with opioids at much higher doses than those used with drug-naive clients.

    a. true

    b. false

18. The nurse is caring for a client experiencing withdrawal from alcohol. Which of the following clinical manifestations are related to a major withdrawal syndrome? *Select all that apply.*

    a. gross tremors

    b. seizures

    c. hyperreflexia

    d. nausea

    e. hallucinations

19. A health care provider just ordered Chantix for the client. Which of the following are appropriate interventions to include in the care plan for this client? *Select all that apply.*

    a. Set quit date with client.

    b. Instruct client about nicotine replacement systems.

    c. Provide client information on support group.

    d. Contact client every 2 days.

    e. Evaluate effectiveness of cessation plan.

9 Herbal Therapy with Nursing Implications

Study Questions

Match the description with the letter of the reference.

Description

_____ 1. "Reasonable certainty" reported on specific herbal remedy

_____ 2. The authoritative source for therapeutic substances

_____ 3. Supports study of alternative therapies

_____ 4. Supportive of 1976 resolution for health care for world's population by 2000

_____ 5. Plant-based remedies

_____ 6. Two primary types of herbal monographs

_____ 7. Clarified marketing regulations for herbal remedies

Reference

a. United States Pharmacopeia

b. World Health Organization

c. Phytomedicine

d. German Commission E

e. Office of Alternative Medicine

f. Dietary Supplement Health and Education Act of 1994

g. Therapeutic and qualitative

Complete the following word search. Clues are given in questions 8-13. Circle your responses.

O	M	D	V	Z	T	W	A	E	T
F	R	E	S	H	H	E	R	B	C
J	I	R	D	O	S	L	I	O	A
D	S	B	I	D	Y	C	U	T	R
E	J	B	D	I	R	T	L	E	T
T	I	N	C	T	U	R	E	A	X
D	A	O	P	A	P	T	R	E	E
R	P	F	U	S	A	L	R	E	A
D	E	N	Y	P	S	E	U	I	W
S	X	A	K	T	I	L	I	F	Y

8. Adding a sweetener to an herb and cooking it results in a _____.

9. Soaking dried or fresh herbs in boiling water makes a _____.

10. _____ are derived from soaking fresh or dried herbs in a solvent.

11. _____ have more reliable dosing by isolating certain components.

12. Soaking dried herbs in oil and heating for a long time result in an _____.

13. Enzyme activity may cause _____ to decay in a few days.

Match the herb with the letter of its description.

Herb		Description
____ 14.	ginkgo biloba	a. provides muscle relaxation
____ 15.	peppermint oil	b. widely used as laxative and with Crohn's disease
____ 16.	yarrow	c. immune enhancer
____ 17.	saw palmetto	d. may be helpful in Raynaud's and Alzheimer's diseases
____ 18.	kava kava	e. relief from stiffness and pain of osteoarthritis and rheumatoid arthritis
____ 19.	goldenseal	
____ 20.	psyllium	f. tonic, astringent, and to relieve congestion of common cold
____ 21.	echinacea	
____ 22.	ginger	g. may be effective treatment for tension headache
____ 23.	St. John's wort	h. stops wound bleeding
		i. "herbal Prozac"
		j. "plant catheter"

NCLEX Review Questions

Select the best response.

24. An herb commonly used for external treatment of insect bites and minor burns is:
    a. feverfew.
    b. yarrow.
    c. aloe vera.
    d. licorice.

25. A popular tea for relief of digestive and gastrointestinal distress is:
    a. chamomile.
    b. licorice.
    c. St. John's wort.
    d. kava kava.

26. Which herb is popularly known as "herbal valium"?
    a. saw palmetto
    b. valerian
    c. echinacea
    d. St. John's wort

27. Frequently mixed with fillers, a popular all-purpose women's tonic herb is:
    a. kava kava.
    b. dong quai.
    c. ginseng.
    d. elderberry.

28. An herb frequently used for relief of migraine headache is:
    a. garlic.
    b. feverfew.
    c. peppermint oil.
    d. yarrow.

29. Worldwide, the most commonly prescribed herbal remedy is:
    a. gingko biloba.
    b. echinacea.
    c. ginger.
    d. licorice.

30. The extract of which herb may prevent damage to liver cells?
    a. peppermint
    b. psyllium
    c. milk thistle
    d. ginkgo biloba

31. An herb that is a natural estrogen promoter and that may lower the seizure threshold if taken with anticonvulsants is:
    a. ginger.
    b. psyllium.
    c. feverfew.
    d. evening primrose.

32. The herb of endurance is:
    a. echinacea.
    b. ginger.
    c. garlic.
    d. ginseng.

33. An herb used for CNS sedation without loss of mental acuity or memory and no risk of tolerance as well as used to treat anxiety and insomnia is:
    a. licorice.
    b. kava kava.
    c. peppermint.
    d. milk thistle.

34. Current good manufacturing practices (CGMPs) include all of the following EXCEPT:
    a. quality of all contents.
    b. strength of all contents.
    c. long shelf-life.
    d. free of contaminants and impurities.

35. You assess your client for ginseng abuse syndrome, which includes all of the following EXCEPT:
    a. urinary retention.
    b. edema.
    c. insomnia.
    d. hypertonia.

36. Health teaching for your client taking an anticoagulant would include evidence of which of the following herbal products?
    a. echinacea
    b. garlic
    c. evening primrose
    d. sage

37. Which of the following statements reflect prudent use of herbs: *Select all that apply.*
    a. Okay to use when breast-feeding.
    b. Do not take a large quantity of any one herbal product.
    c. Give herb time to work for a persistent symptom before seeking care from a health care provider.
    d. Do not give herbs to infants or young children.
    e. Brands of herbal products are interchangeable.

38. The nurse is caring for a client who takes a variety of herbal products and will start to take a prescription antidiabetic medication. Which of the following herbs will change the effect of the antidiabetic drug? *Select all that apply.*
    a. cocoa
    b. dandelion
    c. evening primrose
    d. feverfew
    e. garlic

Critical Thinking Exercises

Use a separate piece of paper for your answers.

J.C., a 24-year-old male teacher, visits his health care provider for a pre-employment physical examination. During the nursing history, J.C. tells you that he has several questions about the use of herbs. His questions/statements are:

1. "How do I know what to take? There are so many varieties, almost as many as cough meds." What advice would be appropriate for you to give J.C.?

2. "My friend tells me that if I take echinacea, St. John's wort, and valerian every day, I will live longer." What cautions (with rationale) would you give J.C. about this combination?

3. "Oh yes, and what about the use of ma huang for weight loss and as an energy booster?" What would be an appropriate response?

10 Pediatric Pharmacology

Study Questions

Define the following:

1.   Developmental age

2.   Chronologic age

Complete the following:

3.   Identify two reasons that pediatric drugs are less researched than those used in the adult population.

    a.

    b.

4.   Infants have _____ protein sites than adults, so _____ dosages of medications are needed.
    a.   more, higher
    b.   more, lower
    c.   fewer, higher
    d.   fewer, lower

5.   Describe two methods of calculating pediatric medication dosages:

    a.

    b.

6.   Describe one cognitive element that needs to be considered when administering medications to children in each of the following age groups:
    a.   Infant
    b.   Toddler
    c.   Preschool
    d.   School age
    e.   Adolescent

7.   Describe the procedure for applying EMLA to a 6-year-old child:

8.   Discuss why a plastic bandage is so important to the preschool child following an injection.

9.   List five elements of medication administration that are key in teaching families to give medications to their children.

    a.

    b.

    c.

    d.

    e.

NCLEX Review Questions

Select the best response.

10. You are administering an acidic medication to a 2-week-old infant. What is the impact of the client's age on the absorption of this medication?
    a. increase
    b. decrease
    c. no effect
    d. protective

11. A 2-year-old child is to receive a water-soluble medication. Based on your knowledge of medication distribution, how may the dosage need to be modified for this client in order to reach therapeutic levels?
    a. increased
    b. decreased
    c. no change
    d. alternate route

12. The blood-brain barrier in infants allows medication into the nervous system more easily than in adults. This increases the likelihood in children of which of the following?
    a. side effects
    b. protection
    c. toxicity
    d. quicker recovery

13. What is the rate of absorption of topical drugs by children compared with adults?
    a. faster
    b. slower
    c. no difference
    d. depends on age

14. The components of pharmacokinetics include: *Select all that apply.*
    a. absorption.
    b. distribution.
    c. onset.
    d. metabolism.
    e. excretion.

15. Strategies to involve parents/significant other family members in the administration of medications to pediatric clients include: *Select all that apply.*
    a. restraining the child.
    b. administering the medication.
    c. evaluating the effectiveness of the medication.
    d. providing comfort to the child after medication administration.
    e. preparing the medication for the nurse to administer.

Critical Thinking Exercises

Use a separate piece of paper for your answers.

You are a nurse on a busy pediatric unit. You need to provide medications for five clients. These five clients include a 10-month-old receiving oral elixir antibiotics for an ear infection, a 10-year-old receiving subcutaneous insulin for diabetes mellitus, a 4-year-old receiving a topical anesthetic in preparation for insertion of an IV, a 2-year-old receiving eye drops for an infection, and a 16-year-old receiving intramuscular pain medication on a one-time basis. Answer the following questions about these clients:

1. What are the ways to most successfully administer the oral medications to the 10-month-old client?

2. What special considerations exist for the child receiving a topical anesthetic?

3. Describe the procedure for administering the intramuscular and subcutaneous injections to those two children.

4. In what ways do the pharmacokinetics and pharmacodynamics differ with each route?

5. In what ways do the pharmacokinetics and pharmacodynamics differ with each age group?

11 Geriatric Pharmacology

Study Questions

Define the following:

1. Biotransformation

2. Compliance

3. Noncompliance

4. Polypharmacy

Indicate the direction of change for each of the physiologic changes in the adult therapeutic regimen.

5. pH of gastric secretions

6. Cardiac output and blood flow

7. Hepatic enzyme function

8. Glomerular filtration rate

9. When the efficiency of hepatic and renal systems is decreased, the half-life of the drug shows a(n) _____.

    a. increase
    b. decrease

10. List four reasons commonly given by the elderly for nonadherence with drug therapy and a specific nursing intervention for each.

Reason	Nursing Intervention
a.	
b.	
c.	
d.	

NCLEX Review Questions

Select the best response.

11. An indicator of the glomerular filtration rate and the normal value (ml/min) for an adult are:
    a. creatinine clearance: 80-130.
    b. SGOT: 4-12.
    c. troponin: 80-120.
    d. urea: 1.2-4.5.

12. In older adults, drug dosages are adjusted based on all of the following EXCEPT:
    a. laboratory test results.
    b. amount of adipose tissue.
    c. height.
    d. health problems.

13. Choice antihypertensive agents for the elderly have a low incidence of which of the following?
    a. electrolyte imbalance
    b. central nervous system side effects
    c. loss of appetite
    d. vision changes

14. Digoxin (Lanoxin), a cardiac glycoside, has a long half-life. In older adults, especially those more than 80 years old, digoxin accumulation might cause which of the following?
    a. weakness
    b. increased appetite
    c. urinary retention
    d. digitalis toxicity

15. The dose of antidepressants for the elderly is usually what percentage of the dose for middle-age adults?
    a. 10-30
    b. 30-50
    c. 50-70
    d. 70-90

16. When administering drugs to the elderly, the nurse must have all of the following information EXCEPT:
    a. whether the drug is highly protein-bound.
    b. the half-life of the drug.
    c. the availability of the drug.
    d. the serum levels of drugs with narrow therapeutic ranges.

17. Factors contributing to adverse reactions in the elderly include all of the following EXCEPT:
    a. loss of protein-binding sites.
    b. decline in hepatic first-pass metabolism.
    c. prolonged half-life of the drug.
    d. increase in hepatic first-pass metabolism.

18. Which drug would have fewer adverse and toxic effects?
    a. fat-soluble, half-life of 50 hours
    b. fat-soluble, 90% protein-bound
    c. half-life of 4 hours, 50% protein-bound
    d. half-life of 30 hours, 90% protein-bound

19. Which of the following organs are especially significant in drug therapy of the elderly and should be monitored?
    a. kidney and pancreas
    b. kidney and liver
    c. liver and pancreas
    d. kidney and lungs

20. E.B. reports dizziness every morning when he gets out of bed. E.B. is probably experiencing:
    a. bradycardia.
    b. orthostatic hypotension.
    c. intermittent claudication.
    d. hyperventilation.

21. The nurse should recommend that E.B.:
    a. take his pulse rate before getting out of bed.
    b. take deep breaths.
    c. move a chair close to the bed.
    d. change position slowly.

Situation: Following hospitalization, A.E. receives a home visit from the nurse. A.E. asks questions concerning her medications.

22. A.E. asked if she should continue to take the medications she took before hospitalization. What is the most appropriate response?
    a. "Yes, you should continue to take the drugs that you took before going to the hospital."
    b. "You should take one-half the dosage of each drug that you took prior to hospitalization."
    c. "You should take only the drugs that have been prescribed on discharge and not drugs that you took prior to hospitalization unless otherwise indicated."
    d. "You should continue to take those drugs that have been helpful to you."

23. A.E. says that before hospitalization, she was taking digoxin 0.125 mg per day. The new prescription is digoxin 0.25 mg per day. What should she do? Your response would be for A.E. to take:

    a. digoxin 0.125 mg per day.

    b. digoxin 0.25 mg per day.

    c. digoxin 0.125 mg in the morning and 0.25 mg in the evening.

    d. both digoxins at least 1 hour apart.

24. A.E. says she has problems opening the bottle tops of the drugs. An appropriate response is to:

    a. ask the pharmacist to place the drugs in bottles with non–child-proof caps.

    b. tell A.E. to put her medications in glass cups and place them in the cabinet.

    c. put the drugs in individual envelopes.

    d. ask a family member to help her daily with the medications.

25. A.E. says that she is to take the newly prescribed drugs at different times. She has vision problems. What would your suggestion be so that she would comply with her medication regimen?

    a. Line up the bottles of medications on a table and instruct her to take them in that order.

    b. Obtain a daily (preferably) or weekly pill container from the drug store and fill the container the day or week before with the drugs.

    c. Ask a neighbor to give her daily medications.

    d. Tell her to write down drugs that she has taken that day.

26. The 80-year-old client begins taking a tricyclic antidepressant. What clinical manifestations represent side effects of this class of drug? *Select all that apply.*

    a. tachycardia

    b. bradycardia

    c. constipation

    d. hypotension

    e. urinary retention

27. The nurse is reviewing the 85-year-old client's list of medications and is aware that the following antibacterials are not frequently prescribed for clients older than 75 years of age. *Select all that apply.*

    a. anticoagulants

    b. diuretics

    c. aminoglycosides

    d. fluoroquinolones

    e. vancomycin

Critical Thinking Exercises

Use a separate piece of paper for your answers.

M.Z., a basically healthy octogenarian, visits her health care provider for her annual checkup. During the health history, she complains of "trouble falling asleep and staying asleep and having to get up to go to the bathroom several times each night." She thinks her current medications are HydroDIURIL and Halcion. "I try to remember to take my meds, and sometimes I take an extra one, just in case I missed a dose."

1. What laboratory tests would be helpful to determine if M.Z. was having kidney problems, especially because of her frequent nocturia?

2. How might M.Z.'s sleep deprivation be corrected?

3. What information, if any, needs to be reported to the health care provider?

4. What are M.Z.'s health teaching needs?

12 Medication Administration in Community Settings

Study Questions

Complete the following word search. Clues are given in questions 1-7. Circle your responses.

```
S  N  O  I  T  A  R  E  D  I  S  N  O  C  P  N  L  D  E  T  S  A
B  W  U  O  G  Z  H  K  L  Y  C  D  V  R  T  L  E  N  L  E  C  Q
S  T  C  E  F  F  E  E  D  I  S  L  T  A  C  L  S  F  L  G  T  O
V  A  R  U  I  M  T  S  D  L  A  E  G  J  E  L  B  F  L  I  P  M
H  E  T  B  V  P  X  I  K  N  R  G  R  B  T  S  A  F  E  T  Y  R
F  M  I  K  B  S  A  U  O  Y  T  A  A  C  X  D  E  M  J  L  K  D
I  G  C  J  G  F  U  I  M  H  J  L  L  R  M  O  Y  P  L  I  B  A
R  E  O  B  E  X  S  C  S  U  T  B  H  I  D  I  E  T  O  N  E  B
J  H  I  B  N  S  C  E  Y  A  M  K  N  P  I  A  V  J  H  Q  O  D
Y  T  P  M  E  E  T  O  B  J  E  I  D  F  O  L  K  M  O  L  A  S
A  S  D  F  R  E  T  N  U  M  S  W  I  M  V  D  I  U  Q  E  R  Y
N  Y  O  E  A  T  M  J  K  T  Y  R  O  T  A  L  U  G  E  R  U  H
B  R  P  W  L  I  Y  R  R  A  F  G  N  H  T  E  L  L  I  A  C  U
P  E  Y  B  V  R  I  A  K  L  J  C  H  I  L  D  S  A  F  E  M  N
A  G  O  C  U  L  T  U  R  A  L  B  H  T  E  S  S  C  P  O  L  Q
L  K  K  R  E  I  E  P  E  R  S  O  N  A  L  B  E  L  I  E  F  S
R  E  J  N  O  R  I  G  I  N  A  L  I  T  B  O  P  E  M  Y  E  V
T  Q  I  N  P  R  T  R  A  D  I  T  I  O  N  A  L  V  U  A  S  F
```

1. Medication administration in any community setting must be consistent with _____, _____, and _____ requirements.

2. Communication and tracking are required to _____ untoward responses and medication errors.

3. The five areas of suggested client teaching are _____, _____, _____, _____, and _____.

4. In all aspects of medication administration, client _____ is of primary concern.

5. Two necessary qualities related to the storage of medications are _____, _____ containers; with _____ caps, as necessary.

6. As part of the cultural assessment, the nurse initially assesses the client's _____.

7. Nurses may demonstrate respect for cultural diversity by including _____ and _____ practices in the health care plan.

Complete the following:

8. Labeling of the medication must be by the _____ or the _____.

9. In the event of a medication error, the nurse's role is to report it to the _____ and participate in a plan to prevent future occurrences.

10. When a narcotic order is discontinued in the home setting, the health care provider is notified of any _____ narcotics.

11. The home health aides have involvement only with the medications that the client _____ ; this involvement may only be of assistance.

12. Health care providers permitted to give medications in the home include _____ nurses.

NCLEX Review Questions

Select the best response.

13. Clients allergic to medications are advised to do which of the following?
    a. Wear medic-alert identification.
    b. Take extra vitamin C.
    c. Avoid use of penicillin.
    d. Have annual CBC.

14. Administration of medication is ultimately regulated by which of the following?
    a. guidelines of the agency
    b. state's Nurse Practice Act
    c. ANA guidelines
    d. state nurses' association

15. A nurse at the work site may be responsible for identifying self-care centers for specific conditions. Which of the following conditions are best suited for this level of service?
    a. abdominal pain and low-grade fever
    b. common cold and chest pain
    c. common cold and minor cuts
    d. headache and numbness in arm

16. A complete prescription for a medication includes the following: *Select all that apply.*
    a. date
    b. drug
    c. dose
    d. frequency
    e. route
    f. health care provider signature
    g. number of refills
    h. generic, if available

17. Commonly used OTC preparations that frequently may not be compatible with prescription medications include the following: *Select all that apply.*
    a. cough and cold preparations
    b. diet aids
    c. antacids
    d. fat-soluble vitamins

18. Areas of diet teaching typically include advice about the following: *Select all that apply.*
    a. drug-food interactions
    b. foods rich in vitamin C
    c. alcohol use
    d. foods to avoid

Critical Thinking Exercises

Use a separate piece of paper for your answers.

Chris is an 8-year-old carefree second grader who was recently prescribed an inhaler PRN for exercise-induced asthma. As the school nurse, what information would you discuss with Chris and his family about the requirements of the medication order and labeling of the medication that will be kept at school?

13 The Role of the Nurse in Drug Research

Study Questions

Define the following:

1. Informed consent

2. Control group

3. Experimental group

4. Placebo

Match the letter from Column II to the applicable description in Column I.

Column I		Column II
_____ 5. descriptive design	a.	comparison of effectiveness of two antibiotics using two groups: clients receiving antibiotic A and clients receiving antibiotic B
_____ 6. quasi-experimental design		
_____ 7. intervening variables		
_____ 8. probability sampling	b.	subjects randomly selected from the population
_____ 9. crossover design	c.	subject is its own control
_____ 10. matched pair design	d.	a chart review of hospitalized clients who received ritodrine at Evergreen Hospital in 1992
_____ 11. double and triple design		
_____ 12. independent variable	e.	preferred for drug research

_____ 13. control group

_____ 14. experimental group

_____ 15. dependent variable

f. subjects matched on intervening variables and randomly assigned to experimental or control group

g. may include disease and state of severity, age, and weight

h. participant receives treatment

i. the drug itself

j. provides a baseline to measure the effects

k. subjects' clinical reactions

Complete the following:

16. Describe two roles of the nurse in clinical drug trials: _____ and _____.

17. Identify at least three new drugs and explain the purpose of each.
    a.

    b.

    c.

18. Identify at least three medications that have been FDA-approved for expanded indications.
    a.

    b.

    c.

NCLEX Review Questions

Select the best response.

19. An integral component of respect for person is:
    a. risk.
    b. beneficence.
    c. autonomy.
    d. justice.

20. Duty not to harm others is referred to as which of the following?
    a. risk
    b. beneficence
    c. autonomy
    d. justice

21. Objective allocation of social benefits and burdens is included in the principle of which of the following?
    a. risk
    b. beneficence
    c. autonomy
    d. justice

22. Few potential drugs are actually used in clinical situations based on the findings of the research and development process. The number is approximately which of the following?
    a. 1 in 1000
    b. 1 in 5000
    c. 1 in 10,000
    d. 1 in 20,000

23. Identification of the safe therapeutic dose and drug-related abnormal changes in animal organs are the objectives of which of the following?
    a. human clinical experimentation
    b. toxicity screening
    c. risk-to-benefit ratio
    d. peak levels

24. A multidisciplinary team ensures that data will answer the clinical questions in which phase of human experimentation?
    a. I
    b. II
    c. III
    d. IV

25. Long-term use of a drug is addressed in which phase of human experimentation?
    a. I
    b. II
    c. III
    d. IV

26. A standard for the many aspects of clinical trials is which of the following?
    a. Declaration of Helsinki
    b. institutional review boards
    c. good clinical practice (GCP)
    d. self-determination

27. The experimental study design requires the following: *Select all that apply.*
    a. researcher controls treatment
    b. alternate treatment methods
    c. control groups
    d. random assignment

28. The nurse is working on a clinical drug trial. Which interventions are appropriate for the nurse to provide the client? *Select all that apply.*
    a. Obtain informed consent.
    b. Screen subjects.
    c. Adhere to protocols.
    d. Monitor selected parameters.
    e. Document data.
    f. Record subject's own evaluation.
    g. Evaluate significance of findings.

14 Vitamin and Mineral Replacement

Study Questions

Define the following:

1. Fat-soluble vitamins

2. Megavitamin

3. Minerals

4. Water-soluble vitamins

Match the letter of fat- or water-soluble vitamins in Column II with the appropriate word or phrase in Column I.

Column I

_____ 5. vitamin A

_____ 6. vitamin B complex

_____ 7. vitamin C

_____ 8. vitamin D

_____ 9. vitamin E

_____ 10. vitamin K

_____ 11. toxic in excessive amounts

_____ 12. metabolized slowly

_____ 13. minimal protein binding

_____ 14. readily excreted in urine

_____ 15. slowly excreted in urine

Column II

a. fat-soluble vitamins

b. water-soluble vitamins

Match the letter of the common food sources with the appropriate vitamin.

Vitamin

_____ 16. vitamin A

_____ 17. vitamin B$_{12}$

_____ 18. vitamin C

_____ 19. vitamin D

_____ 20. vitamin E

Food Sources

a. fermented cheese, egg yolk, milk

b. wheat germ, egg yolk, liver

c. fish, liver, egg yolk

d. green and yellow vegetables

e. tomatoes, pepper, citrus fruits

f. whole grains and cereals

g. milk and cream

Complete the following:

21. List two nursing interventions related to the administration of vitamins: _____ and _____.

22. List three health teaching suggestions for a client taking or contemplating taking an OTC iron preparation.

a.

b.

c.

NCLEX Review Questions

Select the best response.

23. Inappropriate indications for vitamin therapy include which of the following?
    a. feeling tired
    b. debilitating illness
    c. improvement of overall health
    d. a and c only

24. The USDA's Food Guide Pyramid recommends that fat be limited to what percentage of caloric intake?
    a. 10%
    b. 20%
    c. 30%
    d. 40%

25. Regulation of calcium and phosphorus metabolism and calcium absorption from the intestine is a major role of which of the following vitamins?
    a. A
    b. B_{12}
    c. C
    d. D

26. Synthesis of prothrombin and other clotting factors is a role of which of the following vitamins?
    a. E
    b. K
    c. A
    d. D

27. Protection of red blood cells from hemolysis is a role of which of the following vitamins?
    a. E
    b. K
    c. A
    d. D

28. This acid is required for body growth. There is a disruption in cellular division without which of the following acids?
    a. pyloric
    b. lactic
    c. folic
    d. gastric

29. Which of the following minerals is essential for regeneration of hemoglobin?
    a. copper
    b. selenium
    c. chromium
    d. iron

30. Sixty percent of iron is found in which component of red blood cells?
    a. hemoglobin
    b. hematocrit
    c. plasma
    d. blastocysts

31. Egg yolks, dried beans, and fruits are foods rich in what vitamin/mineral?
    a. vitamin C
    b. zinc
    c. iron
    d. vitamin D

32. Antacids and vitamin C have which of the following effects on iron absorption?
    a. decrease
    b. increase
    c. no change
    d. synergetic

33. The client is advised to drink a liquid iron preparation through a straw because it may do which of the following?
    a. cause bleeding gums
    b. discolor tooth enamel
    c. corrode tooth enamel
    d. cause esophageal varices

Situation: J.P., 15 years old, has a skin disorder that is diagnosed as acne. J.P. is taking large doses of vitamin A. The next four questions refer to this situation.

34. Vitamin A is essential for maintaining the following body tissues EXCEPT:
    a. skin.
    b. hair.
    c. ovaries.
    d. eyes.

35. Vitamin A is stored in the liver, kidneys, and fat. It is excreted:
    a. rapidly from the body.
    b. slowly from the body.
    c. only in the bile and feces.
    d. several hours after ingestion.

36. Massive doses of vitamin A may be toxic; therefore client teaching for J.P. should include all of the following EXCEPT:
    a. encouraging J.P. to contact the health care provider concerning drug dosing.
    b. informing J.P. that high doses of vitamin A could cause toxicity (hypervitaminosis A).
    c. teaching J.P. not to exceed the recommended dietary allowance without health care provider approval.
    d. instructing J.P. that massive doses of vitamin A are needed for months to alleviate acne.

37. Which vitamin would be considered less toxic than vitamin A?
    a. vitamin K
    b. vitamin D
    c. vitamin E
    d. vitamin C

38. Which of the following statements is/are true about zinc?
    a. found in lamb, eggs, and leafy vegetables
    b. to be taken 2 hours after antibiotic
    c. adult RDA is 12-19 mg
    d. all of the above

39. Chromium is thought to be helpful in control of:
    a. non–insulin-dependent diabetes.
    b. common cold.
    c. Raynaud's phenomenon.
    d. Alzheimer's disease.

40. Which of the following statements is/are true about copper?
    a. deficiency corrected by iron supplements
    b. deficiency associated with Wilson's disease
    c. found in shellfish, legumes, and cocoa
    d. all of the above

41. Vitamin K is used to treat which of the following? *Select all that apply.*
    a. peripheral neuritis
    b. antidote for oral anticoagulant overdose
    c. hypoprothrombinemia or vitamin K deficiency
    d. anemia

42. Vitamins are organic chemicals that are most necessary for which of the following? *Select all that apply.*
    a. tissue healing
    b. tissue growth
    c. metabolic functions
    d. eyesight

43. Vitamin intake should be increased in the presence of which of the following conditions? *Select all that apply.*
    a. alcoholism
    b. balanced diet
    c. fad diets
    d. breast-feeding

Critical Thinking Exercises

Use a separate sheet of paper for your answers.

P.J., a 48-year-old attorney, is an avid weight lifter and takes multiple vitamin and mineral supplements. He indicates that he tries to eat one full meal a day and "catches bites" as time permits.

1. What dietary suggestions do you have for P.J.?

2. What vitamins and minerals would you recommend for P.J.?

15 Fluid and Electrolyte Replacement

Study Questions

Define the following:

1. Hypercalcemia

2. Hyperkalemia

3. Hypernatremia

4. Hypocalcemia

5. Hypokalemia

6. Hyponatremia

7. Osmolality

8. Tonicity

Match the terms in Column II with the descriptions in Column I.

Column I	Column II
_____ 9. similar to plasma concentration	a. osmolality
	b. osmolarity
_____ 10. based on milliosmoles per kilogram of water	c. iso-osmolar
	d. hypo-osmolar
	e. hyperosmolar
_____ 11. fluids contain fewer particles and more water	
_____ 12. fluids have a higher solute/particle concentration	

Give the normal serum level ranges for the following electrolytes:

Electrolyte	Serum Range
13. potassium	
14. sodium	
15. calcium	
16. magnesium	

Match the electrolyte in Column II with the related drug in Column I.

Column I	Column II
_____ 17. normal saline	a. potassium
_____ 18. potassium chloride	b. sodium
_____ 19. Maalox	c. calcium
_____ 20. Epsom salt	d. magnesium
_____ 21. calcium chloride	
_____ 22. Slow-K	

Give the rationale for the nursing interventions related to potassium drug administration.

Nursing Intervention	Rationale
23. Give oral potassium with a sufficient amount of water or juice (6-8 ounces) or at mealtime.	23.
24. Dilute IV potassium chloride in the IV bag several times to promote thorough mixing of potassium in the IV solution.	24.
25. Check the IV site for infiltration, especially when potassium chloride is in the IV fluids.	25.
26. Monitor the amount of urine output, hourly and at 24 hours.	26.
27. Monitor the serum potassium level.	27.
28. Monitor the ECG.	28.
29. Instruct the client who is taking potassium-wasting diuretics or a cortisone preparation to eat foods rich in potassium or take a potassium supplement as needed.	29.
30. Instruct the client to report signs and symptoms of hypokalemia or hyperkalemia, which are _____.	30.
31. Assess for signs and symptoms of digitalis toxicity when the client is taking digoxin and a potassium-wasting diuretic and/or cortisone.	31.

NCLEX Review Questions

Select the best response.

32. Normal serum osmolality is:
    a. 175-195 mOsm/kg.
    b. 275-295 mOsm/kg.
    c. 375-395 mOsm/kg.
    d. 475-495 mOsm/kg.

33. The serum osmolality can be calculated by:
    a. doubling the serum sodium level.
    b. halving the serum sodium level.
    c. doubling the serum calcium level.
    d. halving the serum calcium level.

34. When the serum osmolality is 285 mOsm/kg, the body fluid is:
    a. hypo-osmolar.
    b. iso-osmolar.
    c. hyperosmolar.
    d. neo-osmolar.

35. An IV solution with an osmolality of 540 mOsm is considered to be what type of solution?
    a. hypotonic
    b. isotonic
    c. hypertonic
    d. neotonic

36. IV solutions used for fluid replacement include all of the following EXCEPT:
    a. crystalloids.
    b. blood products.
    c. lipids.
    d. urea.

37. Electrolytes necessary for the transmission of nerve impulses include all of the following EXCEPT:
    a. potassium.
    b. sodium.
    c. zinc.
    d. magnesium.

38. The majority of potassium is excreted:
    a. by the liver.
    b. by the kidneys.
    c. by the lungs.
    d. in the feces.

39. When administering potassium orally, the nurse knows that it must be taken with at least how many ounces of water or juice?
    a. 2
    b. 4
    c. 6
    d. 8

40. You include in your health teaching that vitamin D is needed for calcium absorption from the:
    a. GI tract.
    b. liver.
    c. colon.
    d. kidneys.

41. Calcium is distributed intercellularly and intracellularly in what proportions?
    a. 25%; 75%
    b. 75%; 25%
    c. 50%; 50%
    d. 90%; 10%

42. Thiazide diuretics such as hydrochlorothiazide (HydroDIURIL) have what effect on the serum calcium level?
    a. decrease
    b. increase
    c. no change
    d. marked decrease

Situation: B.Z. is receiving 2 liters of IV fluids: 1000 ml (1 liter) of D_5W and 1000 ml of D_5 /0.45% NaCl (D_5 /½ NS). Questions 43 to 48 relate to this situation.

43. These IV solutions are classified as:
    a. colloids.
    b. crystalloids.
    c. lipids.
    d. blood products.

44. One liter (1000 ml) of 5% dextrose in ½ normal saline solution (D_5/0.45% NaCl) is what type of IV fluid?
    a. isotonic
    b. hypotonic
    c. hypertonic
    d. isohypotonic

45. If D_5W is used continuously over several days, the IV solution becomes:
    a. hypotonic.
    b. hypertonic.
    c. isotonic.
    d. isohypertonic.

46. What is B.Z.'s serum osmolality according to the following current laboratory values: serum sodium 140 mEq/L; BUN 15 mg/dl; blood glucose 110 mg/dl?
    a. 280 mOsm
    b. 285 mOsm
    c. 291 mOsm
    d. 296 mOsm

47. B.Z.'s serum osmolality is:
    a. iso-osmolar.
    b. hypo-osmolar.
    c. hyperosmolar.
    d. isohyperosmolar.

48. Lactated Ringer's IV solution has similar composition to:
    a. white blood cells.
    b. plasma.
    c. body tissue.
    d. skin.

Situation: E.R., 43 years old, is taking Slow-K. She is taking hydrochlorothiazide 50 mg daily to control her hypertension. Questions 49 to 53 relate to this situation.

49. E.R.'s serum potassium level was 3.2 mEq/L. Her serum potassium level was:
    a. increased.
    b. decreased.
    c. normal.
    d. extremely low.

50. The Slow-K should be given:
    a. when the client's stomach is empty.
    b. at bedtime.
    c. with 8 ounces of water.
    d. 2 hours before meals.

51. E.R. complains of nausea, vomiting, and abdominal distention. These are probably related to:
    a. hyponatremia.
    b. hypernatremia.
    c. hyperkalemia.
    d. hypokalemia.

52. You advise E.R. to eat foods rich in potassium. All of the following foods are rich in potassium EXCEPT:
    a. dry fruits.
    b. bananas and prunes.
    c. broccoli and peanut butter.
    d. eggs and whole-grain breads.

53. E.R. asks why she has to take potassium. The best response would include all of the following EXCEPT:
    a. "Your diuretic causes not only water and sodium to be excreted but also potassium."
    b. "Your serum potassium level is low, and Slow-K helps to prevent a potassium deficit."
    c. "Your health care provider should discontinue the potassium supplement after a week."
    d. "The potassium supplement should maintain a normal potassium level in your body while you are taking the diuretic (potassium-wasting diuretic)."

Situation: P.H., 65 years old, is hospitalized with hyperkalemia. P.H.'s urine output has been markedly decreased. Questions 54 to 56 relate to this situation.

54. Which of the following serum potassium levels would indicate hyperkalemia?
    a. 5.9 mEq/L
    b. 4.6 mEq/L
    c. 3.8 mEq/L
    d. 2.9 mEq/L

55. All of the following may cause hyperkalemia EXCEPT:
    a. renal insufficiency.
    b. administration of IV solutions with large doses of potassium chloride in each solution.
    c. potassium-wasting diuretics.
    d. poor urine output for days.

56. P.H.'s serum potassium level is 6.1 mEq/L. The nurse should observe for signs and symptoms of hyperkalemia, which include all of the following EXCEPT:
    a. abdominal cramps.
    b. muscle weakness.
    c. tachycardia and later bradycardia.
    d. oliguria.

Situation: I.Q., 68 years old, has a calcium deficit. Her serum calcium level is 3.6 mEq/L. Questions 57 to 59 refer to this situation.

57. I.Q.'s serum calcium level is:
    a. slightly low.
    b. severely low.
    c. low average.
    d. normal.

58. The health care provider orders calcium chloride in 5% dextrose and 0.45% sodium chloride (D$_5$/½ NS). What effect may saline solution have on calcium chloride?
    a. It may increase the effects of calcium.
    b. It has little or no effect on the calcium additive.
    c. Calcium additives should always be added to IV solutions containing sodium chloride.
    d. Sodium encourages calcium loss; calcium should not be mixed with a saline solution.

59. The best response by the nurse to this IV order is to:
    a. explain to the client that she should not accept this IV fluid.
    b. suggest to the health care provider to change the IV order to 5% dextrose in water (D5W) and explain why.
    c. do nothing, because this solution would not have any effect on the calcium chloride additive.
    d. report the health care provider to the chiefs of both nursing and medicine.

60. The following drugs are used to treat hyperkalemia: *Select all that apply.*
    a. glucagon
    b. IV sodium bicarbonate, calcium gluconate
    c. insulin and glucose
    d. Kayexalate and sorbitol

61. Which of the following statements are true of chloride? *Select all that apply.*
    a. It is a cation in the extracellular fluid.
    b. It contributes to tooth formation.
    c. It is irritating to gastric mucosa.
    d. Normal serum level is 95-108 mEq/L.

62. Which of the following statements are true of phosphorus? *Select all that apply.*
    a. It is a major anion in the intracellular fluid.
    b. It inhibits acid-base balance.
    c. It is necessary for neuromuscular activity.
    d. Normal serum level is 0.7-3.6 mEq/L.

Critical Thinking Exercises

Use a separate piece of paper for your answers.

A.F. is taken to the emergency department after an automobile accident. He is losing large amounts of blood. Vital signs (VS) are BP 100/60 mm Hg; P 112 beats/min; R 32 breaths/min.

1. What are the advantages of the use of crystalloids versus colloids when there is an acute blood loss?

2. What are the advantages of the use of whole blood versus packed red blood cells (RBCs)?

3. Explain the significance of A.F.'s VS.

A.F. is admitted to the hospital after receiving 2 L of crystalloids and 2 units of whole blood. After receiving the IV fluids, his VS are BP 122/65 mm Hg; P 92 beats/min; R 28 breaths/min. His urine output is 400 ml in 8 hours.

4. Describe the pathophysiology of A.F.'s vital signs.

5. Why did A.F.'s VS improve?

During the next 23 hours, A.F. receives 3 L of D_5W with 20 mEq of potassium chloride in two of the liters. His serum potassium level is 3.3 mEq/L.

6. What type of IV solution is missing with this 24-hour IV fluid order? Explain.

7. What is the difference in the fluid osmolalities of the following crystalloids: D_5W, D_5/0.45% NaCl, and lactated Ringer's solution?

8. What may occur if all of the IV solutions are hypertonic?

9. What is the purpose of the potassium chloride (KCl)? What effect does the potassium order have on A.F.'s serum potassium level?

10. What should the nursing assessment for A.F. include related to his IV therapy?

16 Nutritional Support

Study Questions

Define the following:

1. TPN

2. Valsalva maneuver

3. Intermittent enteral feedings

4. Nutritional support

5. Label the routes for enteral feedings:

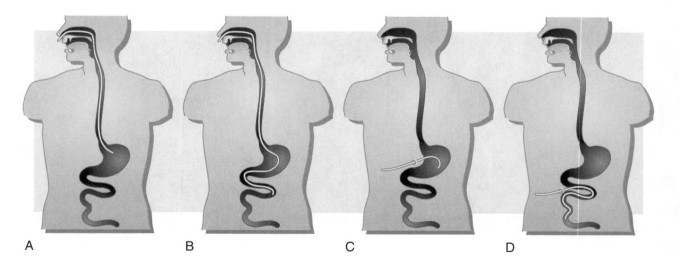

A   B   C   D

a. _____

b. _____

c. _____

d. _____

Complete the following:

6. Identify at least four ways that nutritional support aids the client.

   a.

   b.

   c.

   d.

NCLEX Review Questions

Select the best response.

7. Your client has diabetes mellitus. He is most likely to receive which of the following enteral formulas?
   a. Glucerna
   b. Respalor
   c. Nepro
   d. NutriHep

8. Your client has COPD. He is most likely to receive which of the following enteral formulas?
   a. Glucerna
   b. Respalor
   c. Nepro
   d. NutriHep

9. A type of solution used for nutritional support is:
   a. 5% dextrose in water (D5W).
   b. 0.9% sodium chloride (normal saline).
   c. lactated Ringer's.
   d. Ensure.

10. Ensure and Sustacal are examples of:
    a. blenderized solutions.
    b. polymeric, lactose-free solutions.
    c. polymeric, milk-based solutions.
    d. elemental or monomeric solutions.

11. What type of enteral feeding is administered over 30-60 minutes by drip or pump infusion?
    a. bolus
    b. intermittent
    c. gravity
    d. continuous

12. Blended enteral solutions include all of the following EXCEPT:
    a. Osmolite.
    b. Compleat B (Sandoz).
    c. baby food with water added.
    d. foods blenderized into liquid consistency.

13. TPN is administered:
    a. orally.
    b. via a peripheral vein.
    c. via a central venous line.
    d. via a subcutaneous line.

14. The percentage of dextrose in TPN is approximately:
    a. 5%.
    b. 10%.
    c. 25%.
    d. 50%.

15. Continuous feedings into the small intestine are commonly infused at which of the following rates per hour?
    a. 25-50 ml
    b. 50-125 ml
    c. 100-175 ml
    d. 150-200 ml

16. Diarrhea associated with enteral feedings may be managed by which of the following?
    a. changing the enteral solution
    b. decreasing the rate of infusion
    c. diluting the solution
    d. all of the above

17. A residual of greater than what percentage of previous feeding indicates delayed gastric emptying?
    a. 30
    b. 40
    c. 50
    d. 60

18. Enteral feeding should be used before TPN for the following reasons: *Select all that apply.*
    a. It is less costly.
    b. It poses less risk of infection.
    c. It maintains gastrointestinal (GI) integrity.
    d. There is less risk of aspiration.

19. Which of the following are complications associated with use of TPN? *Select all that apply.*
    a. pneumothorax
    b. aspiration
    c. air embolism
    d. infection

20. Sequence the steps of transitional parenteral to enteral feeding:
    a. Stop parenteral feeding when about 75% of nutritional needs are met via enteral nutrition.
    b. Introduce small amount of enteral feeding at a slow rate of 25-40 ml/hour.
    c. Reduce parenteral feeding by appropriate amount.
    d. Determine GI tolerance.
    e. Increase amount of enteral feeding q 8-12 hours.

Critical Thinking Exercises

Use a separate piece of paper for your answers.

T.A. is unable to swallow fluids. She received IV parenteral fluids for 1 week. A nasogastric tube was inserted for intermittent enteral feedings. The family asked how long T.A. would receive "tube feeding."

1. What are some of the advantages and disadvantages of each of the four methods used to administer enteral feedings?

2. Cite possible reasons that T.A.'s IV therapy was discontinued.

3. How often should T.A. receive enteral feedings? Explain.

4. How would you respond to the family's question about the length of time T.A. will be receiving enteral feedings?

5. How can aspiration be prevented?

T.A. developed diarrhea after receiving Ensure Plus for 36 hours. The order for Ensure Plus was changed to 300 ml of a 70% solution of Ensure Plus every 6 hours.

6. How can diarrhea be managed?

7. What amount of the Ensure Plus and water mixture is needed to produce a 70% enteral solution? (See Chapter 4, Section 4C in text if necessary.)

17 Adrenergics and Adrenergic Blockers

Study Questions

Define the following:

1. Alpha blockers

2. Beta blockers

3. Selectivity

4. Sympathomimetic

5. Sympatholytic

Complete the following word search. Clues are given in questions 6-16. Circle your responses.

```
A  V  N  O  I  S  N  E  T  R  E  F  Y  H  H
D  T  A  B  P  P  G  U  H  J  X  Q  T  T  S
R  X  C  M  E  R  T  N  X  Q  F  M  O  Y  I
E  S  N  H  H  T  S  K  I  N  M  O  M  B  A
N  P  J  B  Y  T  A  M  Q  T  M  P  H  G  L
E  U  C  E  X  P  S  B  U  S  A  Z  P  T  P
R  G  Y  T  K  F  O  A  L  T  R  W  H  F  H
G  N  X  A  L  Q  P  T  H  O  O  G  X  X  A
I  I  O  1  Z  Z  R  O  E  1  C  P  U  J  2
C  T  W  L  X  S  L  B  Q  N  A  K  P  Q  Y
A  T  C  C  2  Y  I  M  H  T  S  H  E  G  E
V  I  S  A  T  I  B  I  O  P  F  I  P  R  Z
Y  S  T  I  Y  N  I  Z  D  T  L  D  O  L  S
P  E  C  Z  O  E  N  I  T  I  G  E  R  N  A
B  S  M  H  M  W  S  S  E  R  P  I  N  I  M
```

6. Adrenergic receptors are located on the cells of _____ muscle.

7. Urinary retention may occur with high doses of _____ drugs.

8. Nasal sprays should be used with the client (sitting up/lying down). *(Circle correct answer.)*

9. Sympathomimetics (do/do not) pass into the breast milk. *(Circle correct answer.)*

10. Adrenergic blockers are the same as _____.

11. The antidote for IV infiltration of alpha- and beta-adrenergic drugs such as norepinephrine and dopamine is _____.

12. The alpha blocker that may cause impotence or a decrease in libido is _____.

13. Mood changes such as depression and suicidal tendencies are possible when taking which type of adrenergic blocker? _____

14. Abruptly stopping a beta blocker can cause rebound _____.

15. Nonselective beta blockers such as Inderal are contraindicated in clients with _____ and _____.

16. What is most likely to occur if a client is taking an adrenergic agonist with an adrenergic blocker? _____

Match the letter of the receptor with the associated adrenergic response.

Adrenergic Response	Adrenergic Receptor
____ 17. increases gastrointestinal relaxation	a. alpha$_1$
____ 18. increases force of heart contraction	b. alpha$_2$
____ 19. dilates pupils	c. beta$_1$
____ 20. decreases salivary secretions	d. beta$_2$
____ 21. inhibits release of norepinephrine	
____ 22. dilates bronchioles	
____ 23. increases heart rate	
____ 24. promotes uterine relaxation	
____ 25. dilates blood vessels	

Complete the following:

26. List four nursing implications associated with adrenergic medications:

    a.

    b.

    c.

    d.

27. List four nursing implications associated with adrenergic blocker medications:

    a.

    b.

    c.

    d.

NCLEX Review Questions

Select the best response.

Situation: N.F. has asthma and is taking isoproterenol (Isuprel) for control of this condition. Questions 28 to 31 refer to this situation.

28. The desired effect of this drug is:
    a. decreased heart rate.
    b. bronchodilation.
    c. increased urinary output.
    d. increased state of alertness.

29. Isoproterenol also stimulates beta$_1$ receptors, resulting in:
    a. increased heart rate.
    b. bronchospasm.
    c. acute heart block.
    d. nasal congestion.

30. You assess N.F. for all of the following common side effects of adrenergic drugs EXCEPT:
    a. tachycardia.
    b. palpitations.
    c. tremors.
    d. decreased blood pressure.

31. You advise N.F. that adrenergic drugs should be administered _____ to avoid nausea and vomiting.
    a. at bedtime
    b. with food
    c. 2 hours after meals
    d. with extra fluids

32. Over-the-counter drugs for cold symptoms have sympathetic properties and are contraindicated in clients with:
    a. hypertension.
    b. diabetes mellitus.
    c. coronary artery disease.
    d. all of the above.

33. (See Table 17-2.) The adrenergic drug used to treat acute hypotension that does NOT decrease renal function is:
    a. epinephrine.
    b. norepinephrine bitartrate.
    c. metaraminol bitartrate.
    d. dopamine hydrochloride.

34. For a client with asthma, beta$_2$-adrenergic drugs are more desirable than those that have beta$_1$ and beta$_2$ properties. The advantage of a beta$_2$ (selective) adrenergic agonist is that the drug:
    a. increases heart rate.
    b. increases blood pressure.
    c. dilates bronchial tubes.
    d. increases urine output.

35. Which of the following is NOT a beta$_2$-adrenergic agonist?
    a. albuterol
    b. dopamine
    c. terbutaline
    d. isoetharine chloride

Situation: K.R., 64 years old, is receiving prazosin (Minipress) for dysrhythmias. Questions 36 through 38 refer to this situation.

36. The nurse should assess K.R. for which common side effect of Minipress:
    a. constipation.
    b. decreased heart rate.
    c. excessive saliva.
    d. hypertension.

37. The usual dose of Minipress is:
    a. 0.5-1 mg t.i.d.
    b. 1-5 mg t.i.d.
    c. 6-10 mg t.i.d.
    d. 10-15 mg t.i.d.

38. Which of the following would NOT be included in K.R.'s teaching plan?
    a. Warning signs of hypoglycemia may be masked.
    b. Rise slowly to avoid orthostatic hypotension.
    c. Increase fluid intake.
    d. Report "stuffy nose" and/or dizziness.

39. Which of the following is NOT included in health teaching specific to diabetes mellitus?
    a. Warning signs of hypoglycemia may be masked.
    b. Add two snacks to the daily diet.
    c. Monitor blood sugar monthly and follow the diet.
    d. The insulin dose may need to be adjusted.

40. (See Table 17-4 in the text if necessary.) A beta blocker used to decrease blood pressure and pulse (heart) rate in asthmatic clients with little effect on bronchial tubes is:
    a. propranolol hydrochloride.
    b. nadolol.
    c. pindolol.
    d. atenolol.

41. The four types of adrenergic receptors are: *Select all that apply.*
    a. $alpha_1$.
    b. $alpha_2$.
    c. $beta_1$.
    d. $beta_2$.
    e. $delta_1$.
    f. $delta_2$.
    g. $gamma_1$.
    h. $gamma_2$.

42. Common side effects/adverse effects of albuterol (Proventil) include: *Select all that apply.*
    a. tremors.
    b. dizziness.
    c. somnolence.
    d. bradycardia.
    e. palpitations.

Critical Thinking Exercises

Use a separate sheet of paper for your answers.

K.S. is taking propranolol (Inderal) 40 mg t.i.d. for angina pectoris and cardiac dysrhythmias. During the nursing assessment, the nurse records that the client stated, "I'm troubled at times with asthma." Vital signs (VS) are BP 126/84 mm Hg; P 62 beats/min; R 24 breaths/min.

1. Propranolol hydrochloride blocks which receptor site(s)?

2. Is K.S.'s drug dose within the safe range? Explain.

3. Could propranolol affect K.S.'s asthma? Explain.

4. What effect could propranolol have on K.S.'s heart rate? Why?

5. K.S. may experience certain side effects when using propranolol over a long period. What are the client teaching aspects that should be explained to K.S.?

6. If K.S. abruptly stopped taking propranolol, would rebound tachycardia or rebound hypertension occur? Explain.

7. If K.S. had diabetes, what effect might this drug have on his blood sugar?

8. What other beta blockers might K.S. take that might cause fewer side effects?

18 Cholinergics and Anticholinergics

Study Questions

Define the following:

1. Acetylcholine

2. Anticholinergic

3. Cholinergic

4. Cholinesterase

5. Muscarinic receptors

6. Adrenergic receptors

7. Parasympathomimetics

8. Parasympatholytics

Complete the following:

9. Cholinergic drugs and anticholinergic drugs have (similar/opposite) effects. (Circle correct answer.)

10. Nicotinic receptors affect the _____ muscles.

11. Indirect-acting cholinergic drugs inhibit the release of _____.

12. The classic anticholinergic drug is _____.

13. List four purposes of cholinergic drugs.

   a.

   b.

   c.

   d.

14. List four nursing interventions associated with bethanechol:

    a.

    b.

    c.

    d.

15. List four nursing implications associated with anticholinergic medications:

    a.

    b.

    c.

    d.

NCLEX Review Questions

Select the best response.

16. The receptor that stimulates smooth muscle and slows the heart rate is:
    a. nicotinic.
    b. muscarinic.
    c. acetylcholine.
    d. sympathomimetic.

17. The cholinergic drug used primarily to increase urination is:
    a. bethanechol chloride (Urecholine).
    b. metoclopramide hydrochloride (Reglan).
    c. edrophonium chloride (Tensilon).
    d. neostigmine (Prostigmin).

18. Anticholinesterases are used to produce pupillary:
    a. dilation.
    b. constriction.
    c. nonresponsiveness.
    d. dilation and constriction (one pupil dilated and one constricted).

19. Anticholinergic drugs are contraindicated for clients having what disease of the eye?
    a. cataracts
    b. glaucoma
    c. retinopathy
    d. macular degeneration

Situation: J.R. has difficulty urinating. He was prescribed bethanechol chloride (Urecholine) 25 mg t.i.d. Questions 20 to 25 relate to this client situation.

20. Bethanechol is a:
    a. cholinergic agonist.
    b. anticholinergic.
    c. cholinesterase inhibitor.
    d. sympatholytic.

21. The mode of action of bethanechol is to:
    a. stimulate nicotinic receptors.
    b. stimulate muscarinic receptors.
    c. inhibit muscarinic receptors.
    d. inhibit nicotinic receptors.

22. J.R.'s drug dose is:
    a. higher than the therapeutic range.
    b. lower than the therapeutic range.
    c. within the suggested therapeutic range.
    d. an extremely low daily therapeutic dose.

23. The action of bethanechol that corrects J.R.'s clinical problem of urinary retention is to:
    a. promote contraction of the bladder.
    b. inhibit bladder contraction.
    c. stimulate kidney secretion.
    d. decrease bladder tone.

24. Which of the following is NOT a clinical action of bethanechol?
    a. increased gastrointestinal peristalsis
    b. increased gastrointestinal secretion
    c. increased heart rate
    d. pupillary constriction

25. Which of the following is NOT a tissue response to large doses of cholinergic drugs?
    a. increased bronchial secretions
    b. increased salivation
    c. urinary retention
    d. decreased heart rate

26. The drug used to treat myasthenia gravis by increasing muscle strength is:
    a. bethanechol (Urecholine).
    b. pilocarpine (Pilocar).
    c. neostigmine bromide (Prostigmin).
    d. edrophonium chloride (Tensilon).

27. Which of the following is NOT an effect of anticholinergic drugs?
    a. diarrhea
    b. urinary retention
    c. mydriasis
    d. dilated bronchi

28. Atropine is frequently prescribed in all of the following situations EXCEPT:
    a. as a preoperative medication.
    b. as an antispasmodic.
    c. to treat bradycardia.
    d. to treat urinary retention.

29. Atropine-like drugs are contraindicated in clients with:
    a. parkinsonism.
    b. peptic ulcer.
    c. glaucoma.
    d. cirrhosis.

Situation: C.G., 70 years old, is admitted for evaluation of peptic ulcers. She is taking propantheline (Pro-Banthine) three times a day. Questions 30 to 33 relate to this situation.

30. The usual dose of Pro-Banthine is:
    a. 0.5-15 mg t.i.d.
    b. 7.5-15 mg t.i.d.
    c. 75-150 mg t.i.d.
    d. 150-250 mg t.i.d.

31. You would encourage C.G. to eat foods that are:
    a. high in fiber.
    b. high in protein.
    c. low in fat.
    d. low in salt.

32. Your health teaching plan for C.G. would include all of the following EXCEPT:
    a. avoid alcohol.
    b. use artificial tears.
    c. decrease fluids.
    d. avoid constipation.

33. Anticholinergic drugs are contraindicated in clients with all of the following conditions EXCEPT:
    a. asthma.
    b. urinary retention.
    c. gastrointestinal obstruction.
    d. heart block.

34. A specific group of anticholinergics may be prescribed in the early treatment of which of the following neuromuscular disorders?
    a. myasthenia gravis
    b. parkinsonism
    c. multiple sclerosis
    d. muscular dystrophy

35. Which of the following is NOT an action of anticholinergics?

    a. suppressing tremors

    b. decreasing muscular rigidity

    c. increasing gastrointestinal peristalsis

    d. decreasing salivation and drooling

36. Which of the following drugs is used to treat an overdose of organophosphate pesticides that causes paralysis?

    a. neostigmine

    b. edrophonium chloride

    c. pralidoxime chloride

    d. tacrine hydrochloride

37. Advice for the client taking anticholinergic drugs would include which of the following?

    a. Increase intake of vitamins A and C.

    b. Increase intake of fluids and foods high in fiber.

    c. Increase caffeine intake.

    d. Avoid organic meats.

38. Effects of anticholinergics are to: *Select all that apply.*

    a. constrict pupils.

    b. increase heart rate.

    c. decrease salivation.

    d. increase GI motility.

    e. decrease muscle rigidity.

    f. relax bladder detrusor muscle.

39. The side effects/adverse effects of atropine include: *Select all that apply.*

    a. diarrhea.

    b. flushing.

    c. headache.

    d. dry mouth.

    e. blurred vision.

    f. urinary frequency.

Critical Thinking Exercises

Use a separate sheet of paper for your answers.

G.P., age 62, complains of frequent lower abdominal cramps. She has intermittent diarrhea and constipation. The clinical problem is irritable bowel syndrome. G.P. was prescribed dicyclomine hydrochloride (Bentyl) 20 mg, t.i.d.

1. What type of drug is dicyclomine hydrochloride? What other drug is similar to dicyclomine?

2. Is the dose within the suggested therapeutic range?

3. What are the contraindications for use of dicyclomine?

4. What are three side effects of this drug?

G.P.'s next-door neighbor, F.M., has been diagnosed recently with Parkinson's disease. In treating her early parkinsonism, she was prescribed trihexyphenidyl (Artane) 1 mg/day for 1 week, and then the dose was increased over several weeks to 6 mg/day. Trihexyphenidyl is available as:

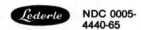

(Lederle) NDC 0005-4440-65

Artane®
Trihexyphenidyl
Hydrochloride
Elixir

This package not for household dispensing.
EACH TEASPOONFUL (5 mL) CONTAINS:
Trihexyphenidyl HCl 2 mg
Alcohol 5%
Preservatives:
Methylparaben 0.08%
Propylparaben 0.02%
AVERAGE DOSAGE:
3 to 5 teaspoonfuls (15-25 mL) daily for maintenance.
See Accompanying Literature.
CAUTION: Federal law prohibits dispensing without prescription.
Store at Controlled Room Temperature 15-30°C (59-86°F).
DO NOT FREEZE
Dispense in tight containers as defined in the USP.
Control No.   Exp. Date

22819 D5
LEDERLE LABORATORIES DIVISION
American Cyanamid Company
Pearl River, NY 10965 Made in U.S.A.

1 Pint (473 mL)

5. Is the daily dose of trihexyphenidyl within the safe therapeutic range?

6. How many milliliters should F.M. receive per day?

7. What type of drug is trihexyphenidyl, and how are its actions similar or opposite to those of dicyclomine?

19 Central Nervous System Stimulants

Study Questions

Define the following:

1. Attention deficit hyperactivity disorder

2. Narcolepsy

3. Dependence

4. Tolerance

5. Hyperkinesis

Complete the following:

6. Long-term use of amphetamines can produce _____ dependence.

7. Narcolepsy is characterized by falling asleep during (early morning/normal waking/evening) hours. (Circle correct answer.)

8. Amphetamine-like stimulants are frequently prescribed for children with _____.

9. Amphetamines (are/are not) recommended for use as appetite suppressants. (Circle correct answer.)

10. The action of amphetamine-like drugs is enhanced by drugs such as _____, and is decreased by _____ and _____.

11. Diamphetamine (Benzedrine) may cause CNS (depression/stimulation) and cardiac _____. (Circle correct answer.)

12. Caffeine and theophylline belong to the _____ group.

13. More than _____ mg of caffeine affects the CNS and heart.

14. CNS stimulants (do/do not) pass into the breast milk. (Circle correct answer.)

15. List the four conditions for which CNS stimulants are medically approved:

    a.

    b.

    c.

    d.

16. List four nursing implications of administering CNS stimulants:

    a.

    b.

    c.

    d.

17. Describe at least four health teaching considerations for clients taking CNS stimulants:

    a.

    b.

    c.

    d.

NCLEX Review Questions

Select the best response.

18. The drug group that acts on the brain stem and medulla to stimulate respiration is:

    a. triptan.

    b. analeptic.

    c. anorexiant.

    d. amphetamine.

Situation: E.B. is 16 years old and is receiving methylphenidate (Ritalin) for treatment of attention deficit hyperactivity disorder (ADHD). Questions 19 to 22 refer to this situation.

19. ADHD has also been referred to as which of the following?

    a. minimal brain dysfunction

    b. hyperkinesis

    c. hyperkinetic syndrome

    d. all of the above

20. You would tell E.B. that common side effects include all of the following EXCEPT:

    a. euphoria and alertness.

    b. hypertension.

    c. irritability.

    d. orthostatic hypotension.

21. The half-life of Ritalin requires dosing:

    a. daily.

    b. 1-3 times per day.

    c. every 3 hours.

    d. every 12 hours.

22. E.B. develops CNS toxicity. The treatment now includes:

    a. decreasing urine pH.

    b. increasing urine pH.

    c. decreasing fluids.

    d. increasing fluids.

23. The best time to administer amphetamines is:

    a. at bedtime.

    b. 1-2 hours before sleep.

    c. with meals.

    d. 6-8 hours before sleep.

24. Long-term use of amphetamines can result in:

    a. diarrhea.

    b. cardiac dysrhythmias.

    c. urinary retention.

    d. rash.

25. J.W. is 11 years old and is taking anorexiants. Your health teaching should include:

    a. that children under 12 should not take anorexiants.

    b. the need to monitor dose.

    c. that the drug should be taken at regular mealtimes.

    d. that the drug should be taken with limited fluid.

26. Which of the following anorexiants has a high potential for abuse?

    a. phentermine (Adipex-P)

    b. doxapram (Dopram)

    c. benzphetamine (Didrex)

    d. naratriptan (Amerge)

27. Which of the following statements is/are true of Ritalin?

    a. It may increase hypertensive crisis with monoamine anhydrase inhibitors.

    b. It may increase effects of oral anticoagulants.

    c. It may alter effects of insulin.

    d. All of the above are correct.

28. If CNS toxicity from amphetamines is suspected, which of the following aids in the excretion of the drug?

    a. increasing urine pH

    b. decreasing urine pH

    c. increasing fluids

    d. using diuretics

29. CNS stimulants are contraindicated for clients with:

    a. heart disease and renal disease.

    b. heart disease and liver disease.

    c. heart disease and hyperthyroidism.

    d. all of the above.

30. Modafinil (Provigil) is a drug prescribed for treatment of:

    a. narcolepsy.

    b. ADHD.

    c. memory loss.

    d. weight loss.

31. Caffeine is used to treat newborns with: *Select all that apply.*

    a. apnea.

    b. narcolepsy.

    c. respiratory distress.

    d. hyperactive disorder.

32. Side effects/adverse reactions of methylphenidate include: *Select all that apply.*

    a. diarrhea.

    b. weight gain.

    c. bradycardia.

    d. hypotension.

    e. restlessness.

Critical Thinking Exercises

Use a separate sheet of paper for your answers.

You are the new school nurse at Countryside Elementary, which has 1000 students. You note that more than 100 students come to the nurse's office "around midday" to take their medications for ADHD. The majority of them take pemoline and the rest take methylphenidate.

1. What is the recommended time to take these medications in relation to food intake?

2. What are the nursing implications of this timing?

3. What might be some of the reasons for the majority of these students taking pemoline?

4. What assessments are important for these students?

5. What laboratory tests require monitoring?

6. There is an outbreak of respiratory illness at the school. What specific health teaching is appropriate for the children taking these drugs?

7. You start a support group for parents and teachers of these children. What are the most likely topics of concern for this group?

20 Central Nervous System Depressants

Study Questions

Define the following:

1. Balanced anesthesia

2. Dependence

3. NREM sleep

4. REM sleep

5. Sedation

Complete the following:

6. The broad classification of central nervous system (CNS) depressants includes the following seven groups: _____, _____, _____, _____, _____, _____, and _____.

7. The two phases of sleep are _____ and _____.

8. The mildest form of CNS depression is _____.

9. Identify at least four nonpharmacologic ways to promote sleep:

   a.

   b.

   c.

   d.

10. Anesthesia (may/may not) be achieved with high doses of sedative-hypnotics. (Circle correct answer.)

11. Thiopental is used in general anesthesia as an _____ anesthetic.

12. General anesthesia depresses the _____ system, alleviates _____, and causes a loss of _____.

13. The first anesthetic developed was _____.

14. An operation is performed during the _____ stage of anesthesia. The other three stages are _____, _____, and _____.

15. Bupivacaine and tetracaine are drugs commonly used for _____ anesthesia.

16. A major potential adverse effect of spinal anesthesia is _____.

17. The type of spinal anesthesia frequently used for clients in labor is a _____ _____.

18. Muscle relaxants (are/are not) part of balanced anesthesia. (Circle correct answer.)

19. Drugs used to induce sleep in those who have difficulty getting to sleep are _____-acting barbiturates.

20. A popular non-benzodiazepine for the treatment of insomnia is _____.

21. The drug of choice for the management of benzodiazepine overdose is _____.

22. Local anesthetics are divided into two groups: _____ and _____.

23. E.D., a 25-year-old mother of four young children, reports that she takes 150 mg of phenobarbital (Nembutal) every night at bedtime. List four points you would include in E.D.'s health teaching plan related to this practice:

    a.

    b.

    c.

    d.

Match the letter of the description with the common side effect of sedative-hypnotics.

Side Effect		Description
____ 24. hangover	a.	need to increase dosage to get desired effect
____ 25. REM rebound		
____ 26. dependence	b.	suppression of respiratory center in the medulla
____ 27. tolerance		
____ 28. respiratory depression	c.	skin rashes
	d.	residual drowsiness
____ 29. hypersensitivity	e.	results in withdrawal symptoms
	f.	vivid dreams and nightmares

NCLEX Review Questions

Select the best response.

30. Because of a high incidence of sleep disorders, the most frequently prescribed drugs are:
    a. triptans.
    b. analeptics.
    c. anesthetics.
    d. sedative-hypnotics.

31. Which drugs are frequently prescribed to control seizures?
    a. ultra-short-acting barbiturates
    b. short-acting barbiturates
    c. intermediate-acting barbiturates
    d. long-acting barbiturates

Situation: J.B., 48 years old, returns to the unit following surgery; she has had spinal anesthesia. Questions 32 to 35 relate to this situation.

32. To decrease the possibility of a spinal headache, you suggest that J.B.:
    a. be positioned in high-Fowler's position.
    b. be positioned flat in bed.
    c. increase fluid intake.
    d. b and c

33. The reason for the client's position after spinal anesthesia:
    a. is to decrease leakage of spinal fluid.
    b. is to increase leakage of spinal fluid.
    c. has no relation to leakage of spinal fluid.
    d. is to maintain the body in good alignment.

34. On the night of postoperative day 4, J.B. requests a sleeping pill. Which of the following barbiturates may be used when the client has difficulty falling asleep and nonpharmacologic measures have not been effective?
    a. secobarbital
    b. amobarbital
    c. butabarbital
    d. aprobarbital

35. Lidocaine is frequently used for:
    a. spinal anesthesia.
    b. local anesthesia.
    c. intravenous anesthesia.
    d. general anesthesia.

36. The primary ingredients of OTC sleep medications are:
    a. barbiturates.
    b. benzodiazepines.
    c. tranquilizers.
    d. antihistamines.

37. Which of the following drugs is considered safer than barbiturates in the elderly?
    a. estazolam (ProSom)
    b. temazepam (Restoril)
    c. triazolam (Halcion)
    d. all of the above

38. The advantage(s) of balanced anesthesia include(s):
    a. slow induction of anesthesia.
    b. reduction of drugs to maintain desired state of anesthesia.
    c. maximum adverse effects postoperatively.
    d. all of the above.

39. Local anesthesia is indicated for which of the following? *Select all that apply.*
    a. dental procedures
    b. diagnostic procedures
    c. suturing a skin laceration
    d. long-duration surgery at a localized area
    e. blocking nerves above spinal anesthetic insertion

40. Balanced anesthesia is comprised of which of the following? *Select all that apply.*
    a. inhaled gas
    b. muscle relaxant
    c. long-acting barbiturate
    d. hypnotic the night before
    e. narcotic analgesic and anticholinergic about 1 hour preoperatively

41. Possible complications as a result of spinal anesthesia include which of the following? *Select all that apply.*
    a. headache
    b. drowsiness
    c. hypertension
    d. dysrhythmias
    e. respiratory distress

Critical Thinking Exercises

Use a separate sheet of paper for your answers.

B.Z. visits the clinic complaining of "trouble sleeping." He states, "I'm afraid to take anything because I may sleep through the alarm clock set for work."

1. Identify three factors that would be part of your nursing assessment of B.Z.

2. The health care provider has ordered a hypnotic, Nembutal. List two characteristics of an ideal hypnotic.

3. In addition, hypnotic therapy should be short term to prevent _____ and _____ .

4. Was Nembutal a drug of choice for this client? Give your rationale.

5. What are the onset and duration of action of this drug?

6. What would you include in your health teaching for this client?

21 | Anticonvulsants

Study Questions

Define the following:

1. Idiopathic

2. Status epilepticus

3. Tonic-clonic (grand mal) seizures

4. Absence (petit mal) seizures

5. Hydantoins

Complete the following:

6. Epilepsy occurs in approximately
   _____% of the population.

7. To diagnose epilepsy, results of a/an
   _____ are useful.

8. Fifty percent of all epilepsy is considered to
   be primary or _____.

9. The international classification of seizures
   describes the two categories of seizures as
   _____ and _____.

10. Anticonvulsant drugs suppress abnormal
    electrical impulses, thus _____ the
    seizure, but they (do/do not) eliminate the
    cause. *(Circle correct answer.)*

11. Anticonvulsants (are/are not) used for all
    types of seizures. *(Circle correct answer.)*

12. Identify at least three types of anticonvul-
    sants used in the treatment of epilepsy:
    _____, _____, and
    _____.

13. The first anticonvulsant used to treat
    seizures was _____, discovered in
    1938, and today the most commonly used
    drug for this condition.

14. It is strongly recommended that the client
    check with the health care provider before
    taking _____ preparations.

15. Administration of phenytoin via the (oral/
    intramuscular/intravenous) route is not
    recommended because of its erratic
    absorption rate. *(Circle correct answer.)*

16. List four nursing implications/interventions
    related to the administration of anticonvul-
    sants:

    a.

    b.

    c.

    d.

17. Identify three purposes of community groups and associations for individuals taking anticonvulsants:

    a.

    b.

    c.

NCLEX Review Questions

Select the best response.

18. The drug of choice for seizure disorders that have not responded to other anticonvulsant drug therapy is:

    a. diazepam.

    b. valproic acid.

    c. ethosuximide.

    d. carbamazepine.

19. Which of the following statements is true about anticonvulsants?

    a. Phenytoin has been linked to cardiac defects.

    b. Valproic acid is associated with cleft palate.

    c. Anticonvulsants are vitamin K agonists.

    d. Trimethadione is recommended.

20. Vigabatrin is an anticonvulsant with qualities including which of the following?

    a. inhibits enzyme that destroys GABA

    b. adult dose is 1-4 g/day in divided doses

    c. used to treat complex partial seizures

    d. all of the above

Situation: J.A., 24 years old, has a seizure disorder and is going to start taking phenytoin, the drug of choice, to control her seizure activity. Questions 21 to 30 relate to this situation.

21. J.A. will initially receive IV phenytoin, which should be administered at a maximum rate of:

    a. 0.5 mg/minute.

    b. 5 mg/minute.

    c. 50 mg/minute.

    d. 500 mg/minute.

22. After several days of IV medication, J.A.'s medication is changed to the oral form. Oral doses of phenytoin are generally scheduled:

    a. once daily.

    b. 2-3 times daily.

    c. every 4 hours.

    d. every 12 hours.

23. When J.A. begins taking the oral medication, the nurse should know that the dose will most likely be:

    a. low.

    b. high.

    c. changed daily.

    d. blood level based.

24. J.A. asks how long she will need these medications. The nurse's answer is based on the understanding that:

    a. the medications are taken for a lifetime.

    b. the medications are taken until the client is seizure-free.

    c. seizures are unpredictable, and therefore so is the drug regimen.

    d. seizure disorders are cured by medications.

25. For maintenance control of seizures in the adult, the usual dose of phenytoin is:

    a. 100 mg daily.

    b. 100 mg t.i.d.

    c. 300 mg t.i.d.

    d. 3 g daily.

26. Serum phenytoin levels should be monitored to determine if the blood serum level is within the therapeutic range, thus avoiding toxic levels. The therapeutic range of phenytoin is:

   a. less than 5 mcg/ml.

   b. 10-20 mcg/ml.

   c. 20-40 mcg/ml.

   d. 40-50 mcg/ml.

27. You are knowledgeable about drug interactions with phenytoin. Which of the following drugs are NOT known to alter the action of phenytoin?

   a. antacids and calcium preparations

   b. antineoplastics

   c. sulfonamides

   d. laxatives

28. In the event that J.A. experiences a seizure, you would document all of the following EXCEPT the:

   a. type of movements.

   b. time the movements started and ended.

   c. ability to stop the movements.

   d. progression of movements.

29. You observe that J.A. is receiving adequate nutrition. Phenytoin may cause all of the following EXCEPT:

   a. anorexia.

   b. nausea.

   c. diaphoresis.

   d. vomiting.

30. List at least four additional items to be included in J.A.'s health teaching plan:

   a.

   b.

   c.

   d.

Situation: E.K. has been taking phenytoin for 20 years. He has not reported any seizure activity while taking the maintenance dose. Questions 31 and 32 relate to this situation.

31. You would assess the client for which common side effect of the drug?

   a. gingival hyperplasia

   b. polyuria

   c. weight gain

   d. irritability

32. As a result of E.K.'s long-term use of phenytoin, which laboratory test results would be monitored?

   a. potassium (K)

   b. complete blood count (CBC)

   c. platelets

   d. blood sugar

33. Trimethadione and succinimides are effective drug therapy for:

   a. grand mal seizures.

   b. mixed seizures.

   c. petit mal seizures.

   d. status epilepticus.

34. Diazepam is the drug of choice for the treatment of:

   a. grand mal seizures.

   b. mixed seizures.

   c. petit mal seizures.

   d. status epilepticus.

35. Phenytoin is effective in the treatment of:

   a. grand mal seizures.

   b. mixed seizures.

   c. petite mal seizures.

   d. status epilepticus.

36. Zonisamide (Zonegran) is contraindicated if the client is allergic/sensitive to which of the following?

   a. cephalosporins

   b. sulfonamides

   c. aminoglycosides

   d. fluoroquinolones

37. Which of the following is/are true about seizures and anticonvulsant use during pregnancy? *Select all that apply.*

    a. Seizures increase 25% in epileptic women.

    b. Many anticonvulsants have teratogenic properties.

    c. Anticonvulsant use increases loss of folic acid.

    d. Anticonvulsants increase the effects of vitamin K.

    e. Valproic acid causes major malformations in 40-80% of infants of pregnant females.

38. You assess the client for side effects of phenytoin, which may include: *Select all that apply.*

    a. nausea.

    b. vomiting.

    c. diarrhea.

    d. headache.

    e. nystagmus.

    f. gingival hyperplasia.

39. Your health teaching plan for the client taking phenytoin would include which of the following? *Select all that apply.*

    a. Restrict fluids while taking phenytoin.

    b. Urine may be a harmless pink or reddish brown color.

    c. Alcoholic beverages are not recommended.

    d. Drug may have a teratogenic effect on a fetus.

    e. Avoid aspirin while taking phenytoin.

Critical Thinking Exercises

Use a separate sheet of paper for your answers.

Many clients in your clinic have epilepsy. M.B. is a 44-year-old executive secretary who has been taking anticonvulsants for more than 25 years. Review of her records indicates she has missed several of her regularly scheduled appointments. You discuss this with her and her response is, "I know all about the disease and the drugs."

1. What is the main variable in determining the dosage of anticonvulsants? Provide your rationale.

2. On what basis is the drug dosage adjusted?

3. Describe the implications for the client when the serum level is below, within, and above the therapeutic range.

4. M.B. has been taking ethotoin, the newest hydantoin. What are the advantages of this drug?

5. Why are drug interactions common with hydantoins?

6. What is the serum therapeutic range for ethotoin?

7. M.B.'s ethotoin serum level is 32 mcg/ml. What nursing interventions are indicated?

8. What specific health teaching is appropriate for M.B.?

22 Drugs for Neurologic Disorders: Parkinsonism and Alzheimer's Disease

Study Questions

Define the following:

1. Acetylcholinesterase inhibitor

2. Bradykinesia

3. Dopamine agonist

4. Dystonic movement

5. Pseudoparkinsonism

Complete the following:

6. The two neurotransmitters within the neurons of the striatum of the brain that have opposing effects are _____ and _____.

7. Which of the neurotransmitters is deficient in parkinsonism? _____

8. The drug prescribed to treat parkinsonism by replacing the neurotransmitter is _____.

9. The substance that inhibits the enzyme dopa decarboxylase and allows more levodopa to reach the brain is _____.

10. An example of an acetylcholinesterase inhibitor is _____.

11. Acetylcholinesterase inhibitors _____ transmission at the cholinergic synapses, both peripheral and central.

12. The drug _____ prolongs action of levodopa and can decrease "on-off" fluctuations in clients with parkinsonism.

13. Entacapone (Comtan) is the newest FDA-approved COMT inhibitor that does not affect _____ function.

14. FDA-approved anticholinergic drugs are _____ and _____.

15. List four nursing implications for administering drugs to treat clients with parkinsonism:

    a.

    b.

    c.

    d.

NCLEX Review Questions

Select the best response.

Situation: C.H., a 51-year-old client, has parkinsonism and is receiving carbidopa-levodopa. Questions 16 to 23 refer to this situation.

16. The usual maintenance dose of carbidopa-levodopa is:
    a. 0.3-0.6 g/day.
    b. 1-3 g/day.
    c. 3-6 g/day.
    d. 6-9 g/day.

17. The nurse monitors C.H. for all of the following side effects of the drug EXCEPT:
    a. gastrointestinal disturbances.
    b. dyskinesia.
    c. fever.
    d. orthostatic hypotension.

18. The nurse's health teaching plan for C.H. would include which of the following?
    a. Take medications before meals.
    b. Urine will darken with exposure to air.
    c. Take vitamin B_6.
    d. All of the above

19. The nurse would recommend that C.H. avoid which of the following foods?
    a. leafy green and yellow vegetables
    b. beans and cereals
    c. cheese
    d. citrus fruits

20. Which drug is most likely to be combined with levodopa to decrease the side effects and the drug's action?
    a. amantadine
    b. carbidopa
    c. Cogentin
    d. Artane

21. Which of the following statements is NOT true?
    a. Entacapone turns urine yellow/orange.
    b. Tolcapone turns urine bright yellow.
    c. Entacapone and tolcapone intensify adverse reactions to levodopa.
    d. Entacapone and tolcapone shorten the effects of levodopa.

22. Two common side effects of acetylcholinesterase inhibitors are: *Select all that apply.*
    a. rhinitis.
    b. depression.
    c. constipation.
    d. weight gain.
    e. increased appetite.

23. The nurse is knowledgeable about drug and food interactions with levodopa. Which of the following types of drugs and foods are known to alter the action of levodopa? *Select all that apply.*
    a. antacids
    b. vitamin B_6
    c. phenytoin
    d. cimetidine
    e. monoamine oxidase inhibitors

24. Anticholinergics are contraindicated for clients with which of the following? *Select all that apply.*
    a. shingles
    b. glaucoma
    c. GI obstruction
    d. urinary frequency
    e. prostatic hypertrophy

Critical Thinking Exercises

Use a separate sheet of paper for your answers.

D.G., 76 years old, was diagnosed as having parkinsonism 6 years ago, for which he took levodopa 750 mg, t.i.d. Because of side effects, levodopa was discontinued and carbidopa-levodopa was started.

1. What are three characteristic symptoms of parkinsonism?

    a.

    b.

    c.

2.   How does parkinsonism differ from myasthenia gravis?

3.   How effective is levodopa in alleviating symptoms of parkinsonism? Explain.

4.   What are some of the side effects D.G. may have encountered while taking levodopa?

5.   Why is carbidopa-levodopa more effective and desirable for treatment of parkinsonism than levodopa only?

6.   When would an anticholinergic antiparkinsonism drug be used for parkinsonism? Is D.G. a candidate for this group of drugs? Explain.

7.   What type of drug is amantadine, and when is it used for parkinsonism?

8.   What are the similarities of amantadine, bromocriptine, and pergolide?

9.   What are four client teaching strategies that the nurse may include in D.G.'s care?

     a.

     b.

     c.

     d.

23 Drugs for Neuromuscular Disorders: Myasthenia Gravis, Multiple Sclerosis, and Muscle Spasms

Study Questions

Define the following:

1. Acetylcholinesterase inhibitor

2. Cholinergic crisis

3. Dopamine agonist

4. Muscle relaxant

5. Myasthenic crisis

6. Myoneural junction

Complete the following:

7. The drug used to diagnose myasthenia gravis (MG) is _____.

8. Multiple sclerosis (MS) is characterized by multiple lesions that form plaques on the _____.

9. Muscle relaxants relieve spasms and pain associated with _____ injuries and _____ debilitating disorders.

10. The drug that is most effective in reducing spasticity in clients with MS is _____.

11. Muscle relaxants are usually contraindicated during _____.

12. What was the first acetylcholinesterase inhibitor used to control MG? _____

13. List four nursing interventions for administering drugs to clients with MG:

    a.

    b.

    c.

    d.

14. List four points to be included in a health teaching plan for clients taking muscle relaxants:

    a.

    b.

    c.

    d.

15. When clients who have myasthenia gravis do not respond to acetylcholinesterase inhibitors, _____ drugs may be required.

16. _____ is a symptom of acetylcholinesterase inhibitor overdosing, as well as underdosing.

NCLEX Review Questions

Select the best response.

Situation: M.W., age 62, is receiving treatment for myasthenia gravis with an acetylcholinesterase inhibitor. Questions 17 to 19 refer to this situation.

17. The nurse assesses M.W. for the common side effects of the drug, including:
    a. gastrointestinal disturbances.
    b. miosis.
    c. increased salivation.
    d. all of the above.

18. The nurse observes changes in M.W. She is drooling, and she has increased tearing and sweating. M.W. is experiencing a/an:
    a. cholinergic crisis.
    b. myasthenic crisis.
    c. vascular spasm.
    d. anaphylactic reaction.

19. The antidote for the episode that M.W. is experiencing is:
    a. edrophonium.
    b. atropine.
    c. Valium.
    d. pyridostigmine.

Situation: S.Q., age 32, was recently diagnosed with MS. S.Q. has muscle weakness in the right extremity and complains of diplopia. S.Q. was given 80 units of adrenocorticotropic hormone (ACTH) in 500 ml of D_5 W per day for 5 days. Questions 20 to 22 relate to this situation.

20. MS is difficult to diagnose. A diagnostic test useful in identifying MS and new lesions is:
    a. magnetic resonance imaging (MRI).
    b. computed tomography (CT).
    c. x-ray.
    d. angiography.

21. ACTH is used to:
    a. increase blood flow.
    b. increase exacerbations.
    c. increase demyelinating axons.
    d. decrease the acute inflammatory process.

22. The nurse should instruct S.Q. to avoid all of the following drugs EXCEPT:
    a. histamine$_2$ blockers.
    b. beta blockers.
    c. cephalosporins.
    d. certain nonsteroidal antiinflammatory drugs (NSAIDs).

Situation: T.R. has had MS for several years, during which he has had many remissions and exacerbations. He has been prescribed Imuran and Betaseron. Questions 23 and 24 relate to this situation.

23. Biologic response modifiers (BRMs) and immunosuppressant drugs are prescribed for all of the following purposes EXCEPT to:
    a. reduce spasticity.
    b. increase muscular movement.
    c. decrease steroid (glucocorticoid) use.
    d. form new neurons and axons.

24. T.R. had an acute attack of MS. The following drugs may be used to alleviate the acute attack with the exception of:
    a. immunosuppressant (cyclophosphamide).
    b. ACTH.
    c. glucocorticoid (prednisone).
    d. 6α-methylprednisolone.

25. The actions of centrally acting muscle relaxants include which of the following?
    a. decrease pain and do not affect range of motion
    b. decrease pain and increase range of motion
    c. increase range of motion and do not affect pain
    d. decrease pain and decrease range of motion

26. Side effects related to peripherally acting muscle relaxants include: *Select all that apply.*

    a. nausea.

    b. diplopia.

    c. drowsiness.

    d. bradycardia.

    e. hypertension.

27. Which of the following is a centrally acting muscle relaxant? *Select all that apply.*

    a. baclofen (Lioresal)

    b. orphenadrine (Norflex)

    c. ambenonium (Mytelase)

    d. meprobamate (Miltown)

    e. cyclobenzaprine (Flexeril)

28. Which of the following causes drug dependence? *Select all that apply.*

    a. carisoprodol (Soma)

    b. metaxalone (Skelaxin)

    c. cyclobenzaprine (Flexeril)

    d. methocarbamol (Robaxin)

    e. chlorzoxazone (Paraflex)

Critical Thinking Exercises

Use a separate sheet of paper for your answers.

G.D., 21 years old, has muscle spasms following a spinal cord injury. He is receiving carisoprodol (Soma) to relax his muscles.

1. Differentiate between the actions of drugs used to manage skeletal muscle spasticity and drugs used to treat muscle spasms.

2. Identify two appropriate nursing diagnoses for G.D.

3. Which medications should not be taken concurrently with carisoprodol?

4. What are four client teaching strategies that the nurse may include in G.D.'s care?

    a.

    b.

    c.

    d.

24 Antiinflammatory Drugs

Study Questions

Define the following:

1. DMARDs

2. Immunosuppressives

3. NSAIDs

4. Prostaglandins

5. Uricosuric

Complete the following:

6. Inflammation is a response to tissue
   _____ and _____.

7. Inflammation and infection are terms that
   (should/should not) be used interchangeably.
   (Circle correct answer.)

8. The five cardinal signs of inflammation are
   _____, _____,
   _____, _____, and
   _____.

9. The oldest antiinflammatory drug is
   _____.

10. Leukocyte infiltration of the inflamed tissue
    occurs during the _____ phase of
    inflammation.

11. The half-life of each NSAID (does/does not)
    differ greatly. *(Circle correct answer.)*

12. When using NSAIDs for inflammation, the
    dosage is generally _____ than for
    pain relief.

13. The half-life of corticosteroids is greater than
    _____ hours.

14. Compare the action of immunomodulators
    with that of NSAIDs. _____

15. Available:

N 3 0378-0377-01 1
250 mg

Each tablet contains:
Naproxen, USP .... 250 mg

NDC 0378-0377-01

MYLAN®

NAPROXEN
TABLETS, USP
250 mg

100 TABLETS

CAUTION: Federal law
prohibits dispensing
without prescription.

Dispense in a tight,
light-resistant container
as defined in the USP
using a child-resistant closure.

STORE AT CONTROLLED
ROOM TEMPERATURE
15°-30°C (59°-86°F).
PROTECT FROM LIGHT.

Usual Dosage: See insert.

Mylan Pharmaceuticals Inc.
Morgantown, WV 26505

RM0377A2

N 3 0378-0451-01 8
500 mg

Each tablet contains:
Naproxen, USP .... 500 mg

NDC 0378-0451-01

MYLAN®

NAPROXEN
TABLETS, USP
500 mg

100 TABLETS

CAUTION: Federal law
prohibits dispensing
without prescription.

Dispense in a tight,
light-resistant container
as defined in the USP
using a child-resistant closure.

STORE AT CONTROLLED
ROOM TEMPERATURE
15°-30°C (59°-86°F).
PROTECT FROM LIGHT.

Usual Dosage: See insert.

Mylan Pharmaceuticals Inc.
Morgantown, WV 26505

RM0451A2

B.J. has been prescribed naproxen 500 mg b.i.d. for moderate arthritic pain. What is the correct number of tablets to give B.J. per dose? Per 24 hours?

16. Which tablet concentration is preferred? Provide a rationale.

17. B.J. asks if he can take this medication on an empty stomach. What correct instructions would you give B.J.?

NCLEX Review Questions

Select the best response.

18. The vascular phase of inflammation is associated with:
    a. vasoconstriction and fluid influx to the interstitial space.
    b. vasodilation with increased capillary permeability.
    c. leukocyte and protein infiltration to inflamed tissue.
    d. vasoconstriction with leukocyte infiltration to inflamed tissue.

19. The following are among the eight groups of NSAIDs, with which exception?
    a. macrolides
    b. fenamates
    c. indoles
    d. oxicams

20. Which of the following is NOT a property of antiinflammatory agents?
    a. analgesic
    b. antipyretic
    c. anticoagulant
    d. antihypertensive

21. A common side effect of NSAIDs is:
    a. tachycardia.
    b. hypotension.
    c. GI distress.
    d. polyuria.

22. The mechanism of action of nonsteroidal antiinflammatory drugs includes:
    a. enhancement of the inflammatory process.
    b. inhibition of synthesis of prostaglandins.
    c. inhibition of phagocytic activity.
    d. decrease in red and white blood cells.

23. The client is taking large doses of aspirin for an arthritic condition. The nurse needs to know all the following information EXCEPT that:
    a. tinnitus is a common symptom of early toxicity.
    b. the half-life of aspirin in large doses is approximately 15-30 hours.
    c. aspirin can lower blood sugar in clients with diabetes, causing hypoglycemia.
    d. aspirin taken at mealtime or with food will reduce GI distress.

24. The analgesic drug to give a child with a virus or flu is:
    a. aspirin.
    b. acetaminophen.
    c. ibuprofen.
    d. Indocin.

25. The medication for a child with a virus should be one that prevents:
    a. gastric distress.
    b. clot formation.
    c. osteoarthritis.
    d. Reye's syndrome.

Situation: J.W. is taking ibuprofen. Questions 26 to 30 relate to this situation.

26. Ibuprofen is a rapid-acting NSAID that inhibits prostaglandin synthesis. This agent/drug is classified as a/an:
    a. para-aminophenol derivative.
    b. indole/indene derivative.
    c. propionic acid derivative.
    d. anthranilic acid derivative.

27. Ibuprofen is generally scheduled to be taken:
    a. daily.
    b. 2-3 times per day.
    c. 3-4 times per day.
    d. every 2 hours.

28. The usual adult dose of ibuprofen is:
    a. 30-80 mg.
    b. 300-800 mg.
    c. 2 g.
    d. 4 g.

29. Ibuprofen (Motrin, Advil, Nuprin) is a frequently taken antiinflammatory, analgesic, and antipyretic agent. Which of the following is true about ibuprofen?
    a. It causes less GI upset than other NSAIDs.
    b. It should be taken between meals with water.
    c. It has a long half-life of 20 to 30 hours.
    d. It has severe side effects, including hypertension, deafness, and renal insufficiency.

30. J.W.'s health teaching plan would include all of the following EXCEPT:
    a. explaining common side effects.
    b. suggesting a decreased fluid intake.
    c. avoiding use of ibuprofen 1 to 2 days before menstruation.
    d. not to take concurrently with aspirin.

31. Piroxicam (Feldene) is a NSAID. Its advantage over other agents is which of the following?
    a. well-tolerated
    b. low incidence of toxic problems
    c. long half-life
    d. fast-acting

32. Nursing strategies related to administering NSAIDs include all of the following EXCEPT:
    a. reporting epigastric distress.
    b. advising the client that alcohol can be taken with NSAIDs.
    c. observing for tarry stools, bleeding gums, and bruising, while taking NSAIDs for an extended time.
    d. advising those with heavy menstrual flow to take NSAIDs 1-2 days before menstruation and not during heavy flow.

33. What characteristics are associated with celecoxib (Celebrex)?
    a. not to be used for cardiac precautions like ASA
    b. avoid during third trimester of pregnancy
    c. relieves pain and inflammation without causing GI distress
    d. all of the above

34. Clients receiving gold therapy for advanced arthritic conditions may receive a corticosteroid as part of the early multiple-dosage regimen. The client may ask about the reason for the combination of a steroid and a DMARD. Your best reply would be that the:
    a. health care provider usually combines these drugs.
    b. combination of drugs improves the outcome.
    c. gold takes time to achieve its effects; the steroid assists immediately in the alleviation of arthritic symptoms.
    d. combination of drugs causes an absence of symptoms.

35. The antigout drug colchicine acts by:
    a. inhibiting migration of leukocytes to the inflamed area.
    b. inhibiting the final steps of uric acid biosynthesis.
    c. blocking reabsorption of uric acid excretion.
    d. reabsorbing uric acid from distal tubules of the kidney.

36. Uricosuric agents such as probenecid (Benemid) are used in the treatment of gout. Benemid promotes:
    a. retention of urate crystals in the body.
    b. uric acid excretion via the kidney.
    c. reabsorption of urates from the kidney.
    d. uric acid excretion via the sweat glands.

37. Side effects of Benemid include:
    a. sore gums and headache.
    b. flushed skin and oliguria.
    c. constipation and edema.
    d. blurred vision and urinary retention.

38. A client is taking corticosteroids for an arthritic condition. The nurse would include which of the following in a health teaching plan?
    a. Corticosteroids are used to control arthritic flare-ups in severe cases.
    b. Corticosteroids have a short half-life and are taken several times a day.
    c. Corticosteroid dosage must be tapered when discontinuing therapy.
    d. a and c only

39. When discontinuing steroid therapy, the dosage should be tapered over a period of how many days?
    a. 1-3
    b. 4-6
    c. 5-10
    d. >10

40. Which of the following statements are true regarding ketorolac? *Select all that apply.*
    a. can be administered orally
    b. has an efficacy equal to morphine
    c. can be administered intramuscularly
    d. can be administered intravenously
    e. may be given only 5 days or less
    f. has a usual adult dose of 15 mg IM q6h

41. Client teaching for those receiving gold therapy includes which of the following? *Select all that apply.*
    a. Desired clinical effect may take 3 to 4 months.
    b. Adherence to scheduled lab tests is essential.
    c. Meticulous dental hygiene is required.
    d. Measures to control constipation are needed.
    e. Report metallic taste or pruritus to health care provider.

42. Client teaching related to antigout drugs includes which of the following? *Select all that apply.*
    a. Take large doses of vitamin C.
    b. Increase fluid intake.
    c. Avoid alcohol and caffeine.
    d. Avoid foods high in purine.
    e. Take medication with food.

Critical Thinking Exercises

Use a separate sheet of paper for your answers.

M.B., 37 years old, comes to the clinic for treatment of an inflammatory condition. She reports taking 975 mg of aspirin q4h for the past week.

1. What is the usual adult dosage of aspirin? What recommendations are indicated for this client?

2. What is the serum therapeutic range for aspirin? What is the toxicity level?

3. What laboratory tests are influenced by aspirin?

4. What is the mode of action of aspirin?

M.B. also complains of anorexia and stomach pains and wonders, "What else is wrong with me?"

5. How should the nurse respond?

6. Identify at least three adverse reactions to aspirin.

    a.

    b.

    c.

7. Identify at least four health teaching points for this client.

    a.

    b.

    c.

    d.

25 Nonopioid and Opioid Analgesics

Study Questions

Define the following:

1. Abstinence syndrome

2. Opioid agonist-antagonist

3. Opioid agonist

4. Opioid antagonist

It is important to identify the type of pain a client is experiencing and to know what group of drugs is most effective in providing relief. Match the type of pain with the letter of the appropriate drug group.

Type of Pain		Drug Group
____ 5.	moderate acute pain	a. nonopioid and comfort measures
____ 6.	chronic pain	b. NSAIDs
____ 7.	deep pain	c. combination of opioid and nonopioid
____ 8.	mild superficial pain	d. opioid
____ 9.	somatic pain	e. nonopioid
		f. antipyretics
		g. antihistamines

Complete the following:

10. Most _____ will lower an elevated body temperature.

11. NSAIDs from the _____ _____ group, such as ibuprofen, fenoprofen, and suprofen, have an analgesic effect.

12. Aspirin is contraindicated for a client with a (viral/bacterial) infection. *(Circle correct answer.)*

13. Aspirin and NSAIDs relieve pain by inhibiting the synthesis of _____.

14. These drugs should be taken with _____, at _____, or with a full _____ to reduce gastric irritation.

15. The most serious result of an overdose of acetaminophen (Tylenol) that extends beyond several days is _____.

16. Acetaminophen (is/is not) the drug of choice to treat an inflammatory process. *(Circle correct answer.)*

17. Identify four areas of nursing intervention or areas for health teaching for clients taking nonopioid analgesics:

    a.

    b.

    c.

    d.

18. Opioids act primarily on the _____ and nonopioid analgesics act on the _____ at the pain receptor sites.

19. In addition to suppressing pain impulses, opioids also suppress _____ and _____.

20. In addition to pain relief, many opioids have _____ and _____ effects.

21. Opioids are contraindicated for use in clients with _____ and _____.

22. Identify two areas for client teaching related to analgesics/opioids:

    a.

    b.

23. For clients taking meperidine, drugs belonging to the _____ category are contraindicated.

24. Your client taking meperidine reports blurred vision. You know this is a _____ and would report this finding to the _____.

25. List three side effects of opioids with specific nursing interventions for each:

Side Effect	Nursing Interventions
a.	
b.	
c.	

26. Pentazocine, an opioid agonist-antagonist, is classified as a Schedule _____ drug.

NCLEX Review Questions

Select the best response.

Situation: E.A., age 53, has just returned to the unit from the OR for the placement of a pin to stabilize her fractured hip. For the first 48 hours postoperatively, meperidine (Demerol) is ordered for pain control. Questions 27 to 31 refer to this situation.

27. The usual adult dose of meperidine postoperatively is:
    a. 50 mg q3h.
    b. 50-100 mg q4h PRN.
    c. 25-100 mg q6h.
    d. 50-100 mg daily PRN.

28. During the time E.A. is taking meperidine, frequent monitoring of _____ is required.
    a. urine output
    b. temperature
    c. pulse
    d. blood pressure

29. The nurse assesses for toxic effects of the drug. Which of the following effects is an adverse reaction?
    a. tachycardia
    b. constipation
    c. urinary retention
    d. constricted pupils

30. Which nursing assessment would be least important when monitoring a client receiving meperidine?
    a.   fluid intake
    b.   bowel sounds
    c.   urinary output
    d.   vital signs

31. The teaching plans for E.A. would include:
    a.   not to use alcohol and central nervous system (CNS) depressants while taking meperidine.
    b.   to report side effects.
    c.   prevention of constipation.
    d.   all of the above.

32. Based on your knowledge of analgesia, which factor is most relevant to the relief of chronic pain?
    a.   administration of drugs at client's request
    b.   use of injectable drugs
    c.   opioid analgesics
    d.   use of drugs with long half-lives

33. The opioid antagonist used to treat an overdose of a morphine-like substance is:
    a.   pentazocine (Talwin).
    b.   ibuprofen (Motrin).
    c.   naloxone (Narcan).
    d.   probenecid (Benemid).

34. Mixed opioid agonist-antagonists were developed in hopes of decreasing:
    a.   pain.
    b.   renal failure.
    c.   opioid abuse.
    d.   respiratory depression.

35. Withdrawal symptoms usually occur _____ hours after the last opioid dose.
    a.   6-12
    b.   24-48
    c.   48-72
    d.   72-96

36. Methadone treatment programs can be effective in helping the opioid-addicted person withdraw. Which of the following is the recommended maintenance dose of methadone?
    a.   100-150 mg/day
    b.   40-120 mg/day
    c.   10-35 mg/day
    d.   2-10 mg/day

37. The benefits of methadone over other opioids is (are):
    a.   less dependency.
    b.   shorter half-life.
    c.   daily dosing.
    d.   a and c only.

38. Elderly clients frequently require a reduction in opioid dosage to avoid severe side effects. Reasons for this include which of the following?
    a.   decreased excretion of drug
    b.   decreased metabolism of drug
    c.   polypharmacy
    d.   all of the above

39. Which of the following drugs tends to be more toxic in elderly clients than middle-age clients?
    a.   Vicodin
    b.   morphine
    c.   Demerol
    d.   all of the above

40. It may be difficult to assess pain in children. Pain management is more apt to be successful if the nurse does which of the following?
    a.   uses age-appropriate communication skills
    b.   uses "ouch scale"
    c.   discusses child's response with parents
    d.   all of the above

41. Drug-food interactions with acetaminophen include which of the following?
    a.   increase effect with caffeine and diflunisal
    b.   increase effect with oral contraceptives
    c.   increase effect of alcohol
    d.   decrease effect of antibiotics

42. Side effects of opioid analgesics/agonists include: *Select all that apply.*

   a. sedation.

   b. constipation.

   c. hypertension.

   d. urinary frequency.

   e. nausea and vomiting.

   f. respiratory depression.

43. Which of the following is true regarding naloxone? *Select all that apply.*

   a. Is used to treat an overdose.

   b. Is only administered intravenously.

   c. May be given every 1 minute to a maximum of 10 mg.

   d. Has a higher affinity to opiate receptor sites than opioids.

   e. Is approved for use in neonates to reverse respiratory depression.

Critical Thinking Exercises

Use a separate sheet of paper for your answers.

E.K., 55 years old, is brought to the emergency department complaining of severe chest pain of 30 minutes duration that began after a tense business meeting and was unrelieved by nitroglycerin. The nurse does a thorough assessment. The health care provider orders include morphine sulfate 10 mg for the severe pain.

Morphine sulfate is available as follows:

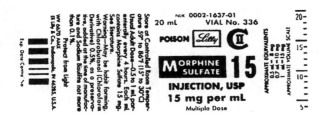

1. What quantity of the drug should be administered? What is the preferred route of administration?

2. Is the dose within the acceptable range?

3. What precautions must be observed when administering this medication?

Three hours later, E.K. is resting more comfortably in high-Fowler's position and complains, "I'm not able to pass my water." You also note that his blood pressure has dropped to 120/40 mm Hg. Laboratory test results are pending.

4. What is the most likely cause of urinary retention?

5. Are you concerned about his blood pressure? Give rationale.

6. What effects does morphine sulfate have on laboratory tests associated with acute myocardial infarction?

7. What would you include in your health teaching for E.K.?

26 Antipsychotics and Anxiolytics

Study Questions

Define the following:

1. Acute dystonia

2. Akathisia

3. Anxiolytics

4. Neuroleptic

5. Psychosis

6. Schizophrenia

7. Tardive dyskinesia

Complete the following:

8. Antipsychotic drugs were developed to improve the _____ and _____ of clients with psychotic symptoms resulting from an imbalance in the neurotransmitter _____.

9. Typical antipsychotics are subdivided into phenothiazines and nonphenothiazines. Nonphenothiazines are divided into one of four classes: _____, _____, _____, and _____.

10. The atypical antipsychotics do not cause _____ side effects.

11. The most common side effect of all antipsychotics is _____.

12. Antipsychotics may lead to side effects that include _____ and _____.

13. Phenothiazines (increase/decrease) the seizure threshold; adjustment of anticonvulsants may be required. *(Circle correct answer.)*

14. Anxiolytics (are/are not) usually given for secondary anxiety. *(Circle correct answer.)*

15. Long-term use of anxiolytics is not recommended because _____ may develop within a short time.

16. The action of anxiolytics resembles that of _____, not antipsychotics.

17. Symptoms of a severe anxiety attack include _____, _____, _____, and _____.

18. Nonpharmacologic measures to decrease anxiety include _____, _____, and _____.

19. An anxiolytic, _____, has fewer side effects than other drugs in this group; it is not clinically effective until 1 to 2 weeks after continuous use.

20. Hydroxyzine hydrochloride (Atarax, Vistaril) and diphenhydramine hydrochloride (Benadryl) can cause drowsiness and have a sedative effect. Though they are not anxiolytic drugs, they may be used for short-term relief of anxiety. These drugs are classified as_____.

21. List five side effects of benzodiazepines with specific nursing interventions for each:

Side Effect	Nursing Interventions

a.

b.

c.

d.

e.

Match the following drugs with their drug classification.

Drug Classification		Drug
_____ 22.	clozapine (Clozaril)	a. phenothiazines
_____ 23.	chlorpromazine (Thorazine)	b. non-phenothi-azines
_____ 24.	fluphenazine (Prolixin)	c. atypical antipsychotics
_____ 25.	droperidol (Inapsine)	
_____ 26.	haloperidol (Haldol)	
_____ 27.	risperidone (Risperdal)	

NCLEX Review Questions

Select the best response.

28. Antipsychotic drugs are useful in the management of:
    a. anxiety and neurosis.
    b. psychotic illnesses.
    c. depression and lifting of mood.
    d. psychosomatic disorders.

29. A full effective therapeutic response to antipsychotics usually takes:
    a. 24 hours.
    b. 3 days.
    c. 1 week.
    d. 3-6 weeks.

30. Client education for use of these drugs is important. The nursing actions for these individuals include advising client and significant others that:
    a. a therapeutic response to the medication is expected in a few days.
    b. the drug should be taken as prescribed and to consult the health care provider before discontinuing use.
    c. taking alcohol or barbiturates with the drug is acceptable.
    d. rapid change in position from supine to standing may cause vertigo.

31. Typical or traditional antipsychotics may cause extrapyramidal symptoms (EPS) or pseudoparkinsonism. Which of the following symptoms is NOT caused by EPS?
    a. stooped posture with mask-like facies
    b. shuffling gait
    c. downward eye movement
    d. sucking and smacking movements of the lips

32. Clients taking high-potency typical antipsychotics may develop adverse extrapyramidal reactions, such as:
    a. paralysis of the extremities.
    b. akathisia.
    c. disorientation.
    d. talking excessively.

33. The most severe adverse extrapyramidal reaction is:
    a. acute dystonia.
    b. akathisia.
    c. tardive dyskinesia.
    d. pseudoparkinsonism.

34. Anticholinergic agents are used to decrease these extrapyramidal symptoms. Examples include:
    a. benztropine (Cogentin) and trihexyphenidyl (Artane).
    b. atropine and bethanechol (Urecholine).
    c. doxepin (Sinequan) and nortriptyline (Aventyl).
    d. diazepam (Valium) and alprazolam (Xanax).

Situation: D.S. has been diagnosed with schizophrenia. The health care provider prescribed fluphenazine (Prolixin). Questions 35 to 38 relate to this situation.

35. Fluphenazine (Prolixin) is classified as a(n):
    a. aliphatic phenothiazine.
    b. piperazine phenothiazine.
    c. piperidine phenothiazine.
    d. thioxanthene.

36. Fluphenazine (Prolixin) commonly produces effects of:
    a. bradycardia.
    b. extrapyramidal symptoms.
    c. oliguria.
    d. diarrhea.

37. The nurse is aware that an overdose of fluphenazine would require which of the following treatments?
    a. activated charcoal administration
    b. limitation of fluid
    c. cholinergics
    d. beta-adrenergic blockers

38. Antipsychotic dosage for older adults should be:
    a. the same as an adult dose.
    b. 10% less than an adult dose.
    c. 25% to 50% less than an adult dose.
    d. avoided by clients who are older than 70 years.

39. Haloperidol (Haldol) is frequently used as an antipsychotic. The nurse should know that it:
    a. has a sedative effect on agitated, combative persons.
    b. is the drug of choice for older clients with liver disease.
    c. will not cause extrapyramidal symptoms.
    d. can be used by clients with narrow-angle glaucoma.

40. A client is taking Haldol 5 mg t.i.d. and complains of nearly falling down when he gets out of bed. The client is most likely experiencing:
    a. anticholinergic reaction.
    b. tardive dyskinesia.
    c. orthostatic hypotension.
    d. tachycardia.

41. The category for atypical antispychotics is:
    a. phenothiazines.
    b. serotonin/dopamine antagonists.
    c. butyrophenones.
    d. thioxanthenes.

42. The atypical antipsychotics, marketed in the United States since 1990, have a weak affinity for the D_2 receptors; thus these agents cause:
    a. an increase in EPS.
    b. fewer EPS.
    c. an absence of EPS.
    d. no effect on EPS.

43. Atypical antipsychotics have a stronger affinity to:
    a. D_1 receptors.
    b. D_2 receptors; they block serotonin receptors.
    c. D_3 receptors.
    d. D_4 receptors; they block serotonin receptors.

44. Antipsychotic drugs are NOT used to treat:
    a. catatonia.
    b. depression.
    c. schizophrenia.
    d. violent behavior.

45. Serotonin antagonists, atypical antipsychotics, are effective for treating which type(s) of schizophrenia?
    a. positive symptoms
    b. negative symptoms
    c. both positive and negative symptoms
    d. anxiety

46. The anxiolytic alprazolam (Xanax) is from which drug group?
    a. antihistamines
    b. azapirones
    c. benzodiazepines
    d. propanediol

47. Dependency can occur when taking benzodiazepines over extended periods. Withdrawal symptoms, which can occur when benzodiazepines are abruptly stopped, include:
    a. gastrointestinal discomfort.
    b. drowsiness.
    c. increased thirst.
    d. irritability and nervousness.

Situation: J.T. has anxiety over the recent terrorist attacks. The health care provider prescribed diazepam (Valium) 5 mg, b.i.d. Questions 48 to 51 relate to this situation.

48. Valium is classified as a(n):
    a. phenothiazine.
    b. benzodiazepine.
    c. antihistamine.
    d. serotonin antagonist.

49. J.T. asks what "b.i.d." means. Your response would be which of the following?
    a. "Once a day."
    b. "Twice a day."
    c. "Three times a day."
    d. "Four times a day."

50. J.T. should be told NOT to take Valium with:
    a. vitamins, because they increase the effects of Valium to toxic levels.
    b. antacids, because they increase serum Valium levels.
    c. alcohol, because it can cause CNS depression and respiratory distress.
    d. an antihypertensive agent, because J.T.'s blood pressure could be increased.

51. Contraindications for taking fluphenazine include which of the following? *Select all that apply.*
    a. blood dyscrasias
    b. hepatic dysfunction
    c. neuromuscular pain
    d. subcortical brain damage
    e. narrow-angle glaucoma

52. Lorazepam is an anxiolytic drug; however, it may be prescribed for other clinical problems. For which of the following may it be prescribed? *Select all that apply.*
    a. anxiety
    b. status epilepticus
    c. preoperative sedation
    d. manage schizophrenia
    e. depression and delusions

Critical Thinking Exercises

Use a separate sheet of paper for your answers.

Clozapine (Clozaril) was the first atypical antipsychotic that has been effective in treating clients with severe schizophrenia. B.B. had been taking mesoridazine besylate (Serentil), which has been ineffective in treating his withdrawal behavior and his lack of interest in himself and his surroundings. B.B. was prescribed clozapine (Clozaril) 50 mg per day for the initial doses. If tolerated, the dosage would increase to 100 mg, t.i.d.

1. For treating B.B.'s symptoms, how does clozapine differ from mesoridazine?

2. What is the most severe side effect of clozapine? With long-term use, how should this be managed?

3. Would B.B.'s daily doses of clozapine be within the normal therapeutic range?

4. B.B. asked if it is okay to miss one of the daily doses, which he may forget to take. What should your response be?

5. What drug-drug interactions should be considered when clozapine is taken?

6. What assessment and teaching strategies should be implemented for B.B.?

27 Antidepressants and Mood Stabilizers

Study Questions

Complete the following word search. Clues are given in questions 1-7. Circle your responses.

```
P   M   T   R   O   V   S   K   L   N   Q   M   B   C   E   I   B
J   A   N   T   I   D   E   P   R   E   S   S   A   N   T   S   W
P   O   X   R   J   T   W   Z   N   A   C   U   Y   K   H   F   L
K   I   W   I   Q   P   U   A   R   I   H   O   E   Y   I   R   W
Q   S   E   C   J   U   T   A   I   E   M   V   O   D   N   Z   S
R   X   C   Y   I   P   L   N   E   N   I   U   B   M   Z   A   I
T   W   R   C   I   O   J   P   X   T   Z   B   V   R   O   P   M
P   H   D   L   P   Y   M   N   C   R   S   B   I   E   W   F   H
R   O   U   I   I   N   M   A   N   I   C   A   P   C   Q   J   W
V   T   B   C   I   S   E   M   N   X   Z   P   O   T   A   W   E
F   R   P   S   S   R   I   S   I   W   T   J   O   B   M   I   A
```

1. Swing-type moods

2. Abbreviation for selective serotonin reuptake inhibitors

3. Abbreviation for monoamine oxidase inhibitors

4. A sense of euphoria

5. Groups of drugs used to treat depression

6. A depression that has a sudden onset

7. Blocks the uptake of norepinephrine and serotonin in the brain

Complete the following:

8. The three groups of antidepressants are
_____, _____ , and
_____.

9. The clinical response to tricyclic antidepressants (TCAs) is expected after _____ weeks of drug therapy.

10. TCAs are usually administered at _____ to minimize problems caused by the sedative action.

11. Second-generation antidepressants are called _____.

12. The uses for SSRIs include _____ and _____.

13. Clients who do not respond to TCAs or second-generation antidepressants are commonly prescribed _____.

14. Monoamine oxidase inhibitors (MAOIs) and TCAs (should/should not) be taken together. (Circle correct answer.)

15. Examples of MAOIs include _____, _____ , and _____.

Match the following drugs with their drug classification.

Drug		Drug Classification
_____ 16.	mirtazapine (Remeron)	a. atypical antidepressants
_____ 17.	reboxetine (Vestra)	b. SSRIs
_____ 18.	citalopram (Celexa)	c. MAOIs
_____ 19.	amitriptyline (Elavil)	d. tricyclic antidepressants
_____ 20.	tranylcypromine (Parnate)	
_____ 21.	paroxetine (Paxil)	

Complete the drug chart for sertraline hydrochloride:

Selective Serotonin Reuptake Inhibitor (SSRI)

Drug Name Sertraline HCl (Zoloft) **Pregnancy Category:**	**Dosage:**	**Assessment and Planning**	**Nursing Process**
Contraindications:	**Drug-Lab-Food Interactions:**		
Pharmacokinetics: *Absorption:* *Distribution:* **PB:** *Metabolism:* **t½:** *Excretion:*	**Pharmacodynamics:** *PO:* Onset: Peak: Duration:	**Interventions**	
Therapeutic Effects/Uses: **Mode of Action:**		**Evaluation**	
Side Effects:	**Adverse Reactions:** **Life-Threatening:**		

NCLEX Review Questions

Select the best response.

22. Which is the drug of choice for treatment of enuresis in children?
    a. fluvoxamine (Luvox)
    b. sertraline (Zoloft)
    c. citalopram (Celexa)
    d. imipramine (Tofranil)

Situation: P.H. is taking an MAOI for chronic anxiety and fear. Questions 23 to 30 relate to this situation.

23. P.H. begins taking phenelzine (Nardil). This medication is generally scheduled to be taken:
    a. once daily.
    b. 2-3 times daily.
    c. every 4 hours.
    d. every other day.

24. The usual adult dose of Nardil is:
    a. 5 mg q.i.d.
    b. 1 mg t.i.d.
    c. 15 mg t.i.d.
    d. 15 mg daily.

25. Assessment is essential with clients taking MAOIs. Frequent monitoring of which of the following is required?
    a. blood pressure
    b. pulse
    c. urine output
    d. hemoglobin

26. The nurse assesses P.H. for side effects of the drug. Which of the following is NOT a side effect of MAOIs?
    a. restlessness
    b. insomnia
    c. orthostatic hypotension
    d. urinary retention

27. If P.H. were to ingest drugs and/or foods that interact, which of the following is likely to occur?
    a. anaphylaxis
    b. orthostatic hypotension
    c. hypertensive crisis
    d. hallucinations

28. P.H. is having difficulty selecting foods from his menu. Tyramine-rich foods to be avoided include:
    a. cheese, chocolate, and raisins.
    b. sausage, beer, and whole-grain breads.
    c. yogurt, eggs, and bananas.
    d. spinach, liver, and milk.

29. The two herbs that may be used for management of mild depression with health care provider's approval are:
    a. ephedra and garlic.
    b. St. John's wort and ginkgo.
    c. feverfew and ginger.
    d. garlic and goldenseal.

30. Before surgery, the use of many herbal products should be discontinued:
    a. 24 hours before surgery.
    b. 5 days before surgery.
    c. 1 to 2 weeks before surgery.
    d. 1 month before surgery.

31. The SSRIs tend to be more popular than TCAs because they have fewer side effects. SSRIs:
    a. cause less sedation and fewer hypotensive effects.
    b. cause less hypotension and fewer circulatory changes.
    c. cause less GI distress and fewer hypotensive effects.
    d. cause less sexual dysfunction and moderate sedation.

32. Many subcategories are listed as "atypical antidepressants." Which of the following groups is NOT classified as an atypical antidepressant?
    a. NDRIs
    b. serotonin antagonists
    c. SNRIs
    d. SSRIs

Situation: R.T. is an acutely manic client prescribed lithium for the first time. Questions 33 to 37 relate to this situation.

33. Nursing interventions associated with lithium carbonate in the management of bipolar disorders include all of the following EXCEPT:
    a. blood levels are drawn monthly to ensure a blood level between 0.8 and 1.5 mEq/L.
    b. understanding that the drug is most effective in the depressive phase.
    c. monitoring for thirst, weight gain, and increased urination.
    d. emphasizing the importance of taking the medication as ordered.

34. Specific nursing interventions with R.T. would include monitoring all of the following EXCEPT:
    a. daily weight.
    b. serum lithium level.
    c. daily ECG.
    d. intake and output.

35. Understanding R.T.'s need for hydration, you encourage him to have at least _____ ml (cc) of fluid daily.
    a. 1000
    b. 2000
    c. 3000
    d. 4000

36. After taking lithium carbonate 1200 mg/day for 5 days, R.T. remains agitated and hyperactive. Today's plasma level was 0.8 mEq/L, and R.T. complains of feeling slowed down and having increased thirst. Your analysis is that the client is:
    a. still manic, with some serious signs of toxicity.
    b. toxic.
    c. still manic without serious signs of toxicity.
    d. a nonresponder.

37. Health teaching for R.T. includes all of the following EXCEPT:
    a. if the medication is stopped, the depressive symptoms will reappear.
    b. avoid caffeine products that may aggravate manic phase.
    c. take medication with food.
    d. encourage client to wear/carry an ID tag indicating the drug taken.

38. You are knowledgeable about drug and/or food interactions with phenelzine (Nardil). Which of the following types of drugs/foods are known to interact with Nardil? *Select all that apply.*
    a. beer
    b. pork
    c. cheese
    d. citrus fruits
    e. many cold medications

39. Potential side effects/adverse reactions for a client taking fluoxetine (Prozac) include: *Select all that apply.*
    a. tremors
    b. seizures
    c. insomnia
    d. headache
    e. dysrhythmias

Critical Thinking Exercises

Use a separate sheet of paper for your answers.

R.C., a 65-year-old executive with the local newspaper company, has recently moved to the area. He tells you he is taking Prozac 80 mg at night because of insomnia, lack of energy, and the death of his son in a motor vehicle accident 2 months ago. You do a thorough nursing assessment.

1. Describe what assessments are indicated for R.C.

2. Is the dose of Prozac appropriate for R.C.? Give your rationale. What modifications, if any, might you suggest to the health care provider?

3. It usually takes weeks to see the clinical effects of this drug.

4. Based on the limited information provided, does R.C. have primary or secondary depression? Provide your rationale.

5. Describe community resources that might be appropriate for R.C.

6. Identify at least six specific areas to be included in health teaching for R.C.

    a.

    b.

    c.

    d.

    e.

    f.

28 Penicillins and Cephalosporins

Study Questions

Define the following:

1. Acquired resistance

2. Antibacterials

3. Antimicrobials

4. Bactericidal

5. Bacteriostatic

6. Broad-spectrum antibiotic

7. Immunoglobulins

8. Nosocomial infections

9. Superinfection

Complete the following:

10. Bacteriostatic drugs such as tetracycline (inhibit/kill) the growth of bacteria. *(Circle correct answer.)*

11. Bactericidal drugs such as penicillin (inhibit/kill) bacteria. *(Circle correct answer.)*

12. The four mechanisms of action of antibacterial drugs are:

    a.

    b.

    c.

    d.

13. Antibacterials with a longer half-life usually maintain a (greater/lesser) concentration at the binding site. *(Circle correct answer.)*

14. Most antibiotics (are/are not) highly protein-bound. *(Circle correct answer.)*

15. The steady state of an antibacterial drug occurs after the _____ to _____ half-life.

16. An antibacterial drug is eliminated from the body after the_____half-life.

17. Bacterial resistance may be natural or caused by previous exposure to the drug. The latter is known as _____ resistance.

18. Infections acquired while the client is hospitalized are known as _____ infections.

19. The three major adverse effects related to antibacterial drugs are:

    a.

    b.

    c.

20. The organism continues to grow when the bacteria are (sensitive/resistant) to the drug. *(Circle correct answer.)*

21. The minimum effective concentration (MEC) depends on the following four processes:

    a.

    b.

    c.

    d.

22. When minimum bactericidal concentration (MBC) is needed, a greater concentration of the drug is required, so the client should be monitored for _____.

23. A continuous infusion regimen is recommended for severe infections because of the need for_____ drug concentration and _____ exposure.

24. List at least four factors related to the host's defense mechanisms:

    a.

    b.

    c.

    d.

25. List at least six nursing interventions related to the administration of penicillin: _____, _____, _____, _____, _____, and _____.

26. List at least four areas to include in teaching for clients taking penicillin:

    a.

    b.

    c.

    d.

27. Second-generation cephalosporins have the same effectiveness as first-generation cephalosporins with the addition of organisms such as _____ and _____.

28. Third-generation cephalosporins extend effectiveness to gram-negative bacteria such as_____ and _____.

29. Most cephalosporins are administered by the _____and _____ routes.

NCLEX Review Questions

Select the best response.

30. Drugs with similar actions, such as penicillins and cephalosporins, can result in:
    a. cross-resistance.
    b. inherent resistance.
    c. nosocomial infections.
    d. bacteriostatic effect.

31. A condition that occurs when the normal flora is disturbed during antibiotic therapy is known as:
    a. organ toxicity.
    b. superinfection.
    c. hypersensitivity.
    d. allergic reaction.

32. All of the following statements are true about the pharmacokinetics of penicillin derivatives amoxicillin and cloxacillin EXCEPT:

    a. amoxicillin is 20% protein-bound and cloxacillin is about 90% protein-bound.

    b. both drugs have short half-lives.

    c. amoxicillin is excreted in the urine and cloxacillin is excreted in bile and urine.

    d. both drugs are absorbed well from the GI tract.

33. Allergic effects occur in what percentage of persons receiving penicillin compounds?

    a. 1%-4%

    b. 5%-10%

    c. 11%-15%

    d. >15%

34. A drug interaction occurs with cephalosporins and which of the following?

    a. alcohol

    b. anticonvulsants

    c. antacids

    d. antihypertensives

35. Aztreonam (Azactam) is effective against which of the following?

    a. *Haemophilus influenzae*

    b. *Escherichia coli*

    c. *Proteus* spp.

    d. *Pseudomonas* spp.

36. When probenecid is administered with cefazolin (Ancef) or cefamandole (Mandol), which of the following results?

    a. Hypersensitivity is common.

    b. Glucosuria occurs.

    c. Drug action is decreased.

    d. Drug action is increased.

Situation: S.W., age 40, is suffering from an *E. coli* infection. She is unable to swallow pills, so an oral suspension of cephalexin 250 mg is ordered. Questions 37 to 43 refer to this situation.

37. S.W. is taking cephalexin (Keflex). This medication is generally scheduled to be taken:

    a. q2h.

    b. q4h.

    c. q6h.

    d. q12h.

38. The usual dose of Keflex is:

    a. 250-500 mg q6h.

    b. 250 mg-1 g q6h.

    c. 1-2 g q6h.

    d. 2-3 g q6h.

39. Available:

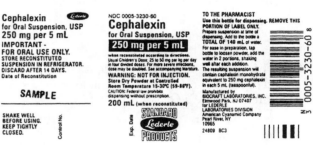

How many ml of the drug should S.W. receive per dose, and per 24 hours?

40. Which of the following drugs/foods are known to change the action of Keflex?

    a. laxatives

    b. antacids

    c. alcohol

    d. uricosurics

41. The health teaching plan for S.W. would include all of the following EXCEPT:

    a. taking total amount of prescribed antibiotic.

    b. resting.

    c. finishing antibiotics from a previous prescription.

    d. being alert for signs and symptoms of superinfection.

42. The drug that may be used as a substitute for penicillin is:

    a.   erythromycin.

    b.   amoxicillin.

    c.   cephalosporin.

    d.   tetracycline.

43. The broad-spectrum penicillins may decrease the effectiveness of which of the following?

    a.   antacids

    b.   oral contraceptives

    c.   anticonvulsants

    d.   cholinergics

44. Quinupristin/dalfopristin (Synercid) is marketed for IV use against life-threatening infection caused by which of the following?

    a.   vancomycin-resistant *Enterococcus faecium*

    b.   *Streptococcus* spp.

    c.   *Escherichia coli*

    d.   *Proteus mirabilis*

45. The nurse should assess a client taking a cephalosporin for which of the following side effects? *Select all that apply.*

    a.   Nausea

    b.   Vomiting

    c.   Tinnitus

    d.   Diarrhea

    e.   Itching

46. Specific nursing interventions for a client taking ceftazidime (Fortaz) would include which of the following? *Select all that apply.*

    a.   taking culture for C & S (culture and sensitivity)

    b.   administering IV dose over 20 minutes every day

    c.   assessing for allergic reaction

    d.   monitoring urinary output

    e.   restricting fluids

Critical Thinking Exercises

Use a separate sheet of paper for your answers.

J.L., 25 years old, is hospitalized for treatment of a severe penicillin G–resistant *Staphylococcus aureus* infection. He is receiving nafcillin parenterally.

1. What is nafcillin's drug classification?

2. What is the usual adult dose for this drug?

3. What are the preferred routes of administration?

4. Available:

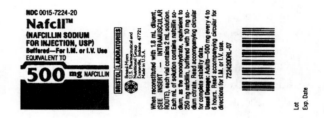

    How many ml are required to administer 500 mg IM of the drug?

5. What drug should be readily available in the event of severe allergic reaction?

6. What are the differences between the penicillin groups?

7. List four nursing interventions related to the administration of the drug to J.L.

    a.

    b.

    c.

    d.

29 Macrolides, Tetracyclines, Aminoglycosides, and Fluoroquinolones

Study Questions

Define the following:

1. Bacteriostatic

2. Bactericidal

3. Pathogen

4. Superinfection

Complete the following:

5. Vancomycin is a (bactericidal/bacteriostatic) drug. (*Circle correct answer.*)

6. The drug frequently prescribed for clients with hypersensitivity to penicillin is _____.

7. The newest classification of antibiotics that is structurally related to macrolides is _____.

8. Azithromycin acts by inhibition of the steps of _____ synthesis.

9. List four nursing interventions related to administration of fluoroquinolones:

   a.

   b.

   c.

   d.

10. A drug usually effective against drug-resistant *Staphylococcus aureus* in clients with penicillin allergy is _____.

11. Two adverse reactions of vancomycin are _____ and _____.

12. It is necessary to draw serum peak and trough levels for vancomycin to minimize _____ effects.

13. A newer aminoglycoside with a decreased occurrence of toxicity is _____. Its pregnancy category is _____.

14. Serious adverse reactions to aminoglycosides include _____ and _____.

15. List four specific nursing interventions for administration of aminoglycosides:

    a.

    b.

    c.

    d.

16. Fluoroquinolones are (bactericidal/bacterio-static). *(Circle correct answer.)*

17. Fluoroquinolones are used for treatment of serious infections such as _____.

18. Spectinomycin (Trobicin) is the single IM dose treatment for _____.

19. Aztreonam (Azactam) is effective against the organism _____.

NCLEX Review Questions

Select the best response.

20. Which of the following is NOT a fluoroquinolone with daily dosing?
    a. levofloxacin (Levaquin)
    b. ofloxacin (Floxin)
    c. sparfloxacin (Zagam)
    d. trovafloxacin (Trovan)

Situation: J.T. is taking tetracycline for a respiratory tract infection. Questions 21 to 27 refer to this situation.

21. The usual dose of tetracycline is:
    a. 250-500 mg q6h.
    b. 250-500 mg q4h.
    c. 500 mg-1 g q4h.
    d. 1-2 g q4h.

22. A laboratory test influenced by tetracycline is:
    a. blood urea nitrogen.
    b. serum calcium level.
    c. prothrombin time.
    d. white blood cell count.

23. For best results, it is recommended that tetracycline be taken:
    a. with meals.
    b. with extra fluids.
    c. on an empty stomach.
    d. one-half hour after meals.

24. The health teaching plan for J.T. would NOT include which of the following?
    a. Outdated tetracycline breaks down into toxic by-products and must be discarded.
    b. Observe for superinfection.
    c. Avoid tetracycline during pregnancy.
    d. Anticipate urinary urgency.

25. Available:

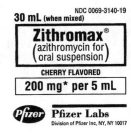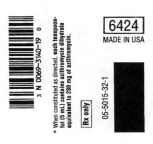

J.T.'s health care provider has ordered Zithromax (azithromycin) for his mild-moderate strep infection. How many milliliters of this suspension are required for the first dose and for each of the daily doses for the next 4 days?

26. The nurse knows that food (increases/ decreases) absorption of the drug by 50%. (Circle correct answer.) Therefore what instructions would you give J.T.?

27. The nurse assesses a client who is taking gentamicin (Garamycin) for side effects/ adverse reactions including: *Select all that apply.*

    a. nausea.

    b. ototoxicity.

    c. constipation.

    d. photosensitivity.

    e. thrombocytopenia.

28. The nurse knows that which of the following drugs modify the action of tetracycline? *Select all that apply.*

    a. iron

    b. antacids

    c. warfarin

    d. milk products

    e. beta blockers

29. Specific nursing interventions for the 34-year-old female client taking tetracycline include: *Select all that apply.*

    a. restricting fluids.

    b. storing the drug away from light.

    c. monitoring laboratory test results.

    d. obtaining a specimen for culture and sensitivity.

    e. advising the client to use additional contraceptives when taking this drug.

Critical Thinking Exercises

Use a separate sheet of paper for your answers.

A.B. comes to the health care provider complaining of a productive cough, fever, and flu-like symptoms. Ciprofloxacin (Cipro) is prescribed.

1. Is Cipro a reasonable choice of drug? Give your rationale. What specific nursing assessments are indicated?

2. What are the usual adult dosages for mild/ moderate and severe infections?

3. Under what circumstances is this drug used with caution?

4. What laboratory tests require monitoring?

5. List three specific nursing interventions related to the administration of fluoroquinolones.

    a.

    b.

    c.

6. List three recommendations for client teaching for A.B.

    a.

    b.

    c.

30 Sulfonamides

Study Questions

Define the following:

1. Cross-sensitivity

2. Photosensitivity

3. Synergistic effect

Complete the following word search. Clues are given in questions 4-11. Circle your responses.

```
P  E  N  I  C  I  L  L  I  N  T  F  T  Q  I
F  O  L  I  C  A  C  I  D  K  U  I  P  C  U
L  K  Z  Q  I  S  Y  E  N  D  I  K  I  I  H
M  R  I  B  O  S  S  B  S  Z  T  T  B  N  L
M  I  E  U  S  S  R  R  E  O  A  N  R  C  G
C  R  R  V  O  A  A  D  N  T  I  I  T  R  N
A  P  C  P  I  P  C  S  S  Z  I  M  S  E  O
F  P  V  W  O  L  I  O  X  G  T  D  P  A  L
X  Q  B  A  U  H  I  T  S  L  Q  J  A  S  Y
F  W  S  P  L  R  T  T  V  E  S  H  Y  E  M
C  J  X  G  E  U  U  E  O  X  N  W  Z  M  A
W  S  X  T  G  X  A  Q  M  N  D  Y  W  Z  F
F  E  C  K  P  M  F  L  N  I  E  U  L  U  L
X  A  N  H  Q  C  C  W  U  G  R  R  Q  Y  U
B  C  B  Q  P  I  B  E  N  Z  O  T  A  D  S
```

4. Sulfonamides inhibit bacterial synthesis of
   _____.

5. Clinical use of sulfonamides has decreased
   because of the availability and effectiveness
   of _____.

6. The new antibacterial drug that has a
   synergistic effect with sulfonamides is
   _____.

7. Sulfonamides (are/are not) effective against
   viruses and fungi. *(Circle correct answer.)*

8. Anaphylaxis (is/is not) common with the use of sulfonamides. *(Circle correct answer.)*

9. Sulfonamide drugs are metabolized in the _____ and excreted by the _____.

10. Sulfonamides are (bacteriostatic/bactericidal). *(Circle correct answer.)*

11. The use of warfarin with sulfonamides (increases/decreases) the anticoagulant effect. *(Circle correct answer.)*

NCLEX Review Questions

Select the best response.

12. A sulfonamide derivative for the treatment of second- and third-degree burns is:
    a. sulfamethizole (Sulfasol).
    b. sulfasalazine (Azulfidine).
    c. sulfacetamide sodium (Isopto Cetamide).
    d. mafenide acetate (Sulfamylon).

13. The drug used to treat seborrheic dermatitis is:
    a. sulfacetamide sodium (Isopto Cetamide).
    b. mafenide acetate (Sulfamylon).
    c. sulfisoxazole (Gantrisin).
    d. sulfadiazine (Microsulfon)

Situation: P.J., 45 years old, is admitted for treatment of a severe urinary tract infection. His current medications include Septra (trimethoprim/ sulfamethoxazole) and digoxin. Questions 14 to 17 refer to this situation.

14. The usual adult dose of Septra (also ordered for P.J.) is which of the following?
    a. 160 mg TMP/800 mg SMZ q6h
    b. 160 mg TMP/800 mg SMZ q12h
    c. 40 mg TMP/60 mg SMZ q6h
    d. 40 mg TMP/60 mg SMZ q12h

15. Available:
Septra tablets: each scored tablet contains 80 mg of trimethoprim and 400 mg of sulfamethoxazole. How many tablets should P.J. take for each dose and per 24 hours?

16. The nurse would:
    a. administer medications and extra fluids.
    b. monitor urinary output.
    c. observe for allergic response.
    d. do all of the above.

17. Displacement of the sulfonamides from the protein-binding sites results in:
    a. increased levels of free drug in the blood.
    b. decreased levels of free drug in the blood.
    c. no change in free drug levels in the blood.
    d. synergistic effect of the drug.

18. Which of the following possible side effects/ adverse reactions of trimethoprim/ sulfamethoxazole should the nurse advise the client of? *Select all that apply.*
    a. anorexia
    b. constipation
    c. crystalluria
    d. photosensitivity
    e. decreased WBCs and platelets

19. Which of the following is/are true regarding sulfonamides? *Select all that apply.*
    a. Are considered safe in newborns.
    b. Increase anticoagulant effect of warfarin.
    c. Stevens-Johnson syndrome is an adverse reaction.
    d. May lead to decreased serum creatinine levels.
    e. Increase hypoglycemic effect with sulfonylureas.

Critical Thinking Exercises

Use a separate sheet of paper for your answers.

Y.M., 11 years old, complains of "pain when I go to the bathroom." Gantrisin is prescribed with a loading dose of 3.75 grams. Y.M. weighs 110 pounds.

1.   What is the recommended dose? Is Y.M.'s loading dose within safe parameters?

2.   Why is this drug so effective in treating urinary tract infections?

3.   List three nursing interventions related to the administration of sulfonamides.

      a.

      b.

      c.

4.   List four areas for client teaching related to the drug.

      a.

      b.

      c.

      d.

5.   Explain why it is advisable that Y.M. increase her fluid intake.

31 Antituberculars, Antifungals, Peptides, and Metronidazole

Study Questions

Define the following:

1. First-line drugs

2. Opportunistic infections

3. Peptides

4. Prophylaxis

5. Second-line drugs

Complete the following:

6. The first and also current drug prescribed to treat tuberculosis is _____.

7. Single-drug therapy for tuberculosis (is/is not) more effective than multiple-drug therapy. *(Circle correct answer.)*

8. First-line drugs are (less/more) effective and less toxic than second-line drugs in treating tuberculosis. *(Circle correct answer.)*

9. Vitamin _____ is frequently given with isoniazid.

10. Prophylactic doses of isoniazid are given to family members of a person newly diagnosed with tuberculosis for a period of _____ to _____ months.

11. Second-line tuberculosis drugs may be used in combination with first-line drugs in clients with _____ tuberculosis.

12. The drug of choice to prevent disseminated *Mycobacterium avium* complex (MAC) disease in clients with advanced HIV infection is _____.

13. List four groups of antifungal drugs:

    a.

    b.

    c.

    d.

14. Systemic fungal infections usually involve the _____ or _____.

15. Fungi are normal flora of the following four organs/cavities: _____, _____, _____, and _____.

16. To treat severe systemic fungal infections, the drug of choice is _____, administered in low doses via the _____ route.

17. Excretion of amphotericin B (is/is not) affected by renal disease. *(Circle correct answer.)*

18. The action of nystatin (increases/decreases) the permeability of the fungal cell membrane. *(Circle correct answer.)*

19. Two common oral antifungal agents are _____ and _____.

20. Many early polymyxins were discontinued as a result of toxicity causing _____ and _____; lab values for _____ and _____ require monitoring.

21. Polymyxins are (bactericidal/bacteriostatic). *(Circle correct answer.)*

22. Polymyxins are effective against most (gram-negative/gram-positive) bacteria. *(Circle correct answer.)*

23. The preferred route of administration for polymyxins is _____.

24. When a polymyxin is discontinued, neurotoxicity (is/is not) usually reversible. *(Circle correct answer.)*

25. List at least three specific nursing interventions related to the administration of INH:

    a.

    b.

    c.

26. List five conditions that metronidazole is prescribed to treat:

    a.

    b.

    c.

    d.

    e.

NCLEX Review Questions

Select the best response.

27. A serious adverse effect of isoniazid is:
    a. ototoxicity.
    b. crystalluria.
    c. palpitations.
    d. hepatotoxicity.

28. A contraindication for prophylactic treatment of tuberculosis is:
    a. alcoholism.
    b. parkinsonism.
    c. concurrent warfarin.
    d. concurrent theophylline.

Situation: R.T. is a 21-year-old male admitted with gastroenteritis. He is receiving colistin-S. Questions 29 to 31 refer to this situation.

29. The usual dose of colistin-S is:
    a. 5-15 mg/kg/day.
    b. 3-5 mg/kg/day.
    c. 40,000 units/day.
    d. 60,000-100,000 units/day.

30. Colistin-S is excreted via which of the following?
    a. lungs
    b. feces
    c. urine
    d. liver

31. R.T. is now receiving the medication intramuscularly. Special considerations include:
    a. using the Z-track technique.
    b. using an 18-gauge needle.
    c. adding 1% lidocaine to the medication.
    d. using the vastus lateralis site.

Situation: B.T., 69 years old, is taking isoniazid (INH). Questions 32 to 36 refer to this situation.

32. During the admission interview, you should obtain which of the following?
    a. history of TB
    b. last PPD, chest x-ray, and results
    c. drug allergies
    d. all of the above

33. The usual dose of INH for active treatment is:
    a.   1-4 mg/kg/day.
    b.   5-10 mg/kg/day.
    c.   11-15 mg/kg/day.
    d.   16-20 mg/kg/day.

34. When the client is taking INH, frequent monitoring of which of the following is required?
    a.   liver enzymes
    b.   WBCs
    c.   creatinine
    d.   BUN

35. Which of the following drugs/foods change the action of INH?
    a.   laxatives
    b.   cheese
    c.   antacids
    d.   digoxin

36. Health teaching for B.T. would include all of the following EXCEPT:
    a.   possible need to take vitamin B$_6$ to avoid peripheral neuritis.
    b.   increase fluid intake; avoid alcohol.
    c.   urine and saliva may be red-orange.
    d.   monitor weight daily.

37. Which of the following is/are true about the drug rifapentine?
    a.   newest drug for treating tuberculosis
    b.   has twice-weekly dosing
    c.   taken with another antitubercular drug to avoid resistance
    d.   all of the above

Situation: B.G., age 67, is being treated for histoplasmosis. Questions 38 to 42 relate to this situation.

38. B.G. is receiving amphotericin B. This medication is generally administered:
    a.   rectally.
    b.   topically.
    c.   intramuscularly.
    d.   intravenously.

39. The usual dose of amphotericin B is:
    a.   0.25-1 mg/kg/day.
    b.   1-2 mg/kg/day.
    c.   2-3 mg/kg/day.
    d.   3-4 mg/kg/day.

40. During the time B.G. is receiving this drug, frequent monitoring of which of the following is required?
    a.   WBCs
    b.   BUN
    c.   platelets
    d.   eosinophils

41. The health teaching plan for B.G. would include all of the following EXCEPT to:
    a.   avoid operating hazardous equipment.
    b.   report weakness.
    c.   obtain lab testing as ordered.
    d.   consume no alcohol.

42. Metronidazole is primarily used for treatment of disorders caused by organisms in which of the following?
    a.   respiratory tract
    b.   urinary tract
    c.   GI tract
    d.   peripheral nervous system

43. In combination with other agents, metronidazole is commonly used to treat *Helicobacter pylori* associated with recurrent:
    a.   peptic ulcers.
    b.   urinary retention.
    c.   adenomas.
    d.   gastroesophageal reflux disease (GERD).

44. Side effects of metronidazole may include:
    a.   urinary retention.
    b.   photophobia.
    c.   abdominal cramps and diarrhea.
    d.   headache and depression.

45. Available:

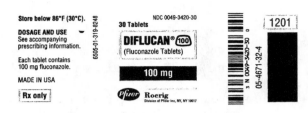

M.M.'s prescription is for a maintenance dose of fluconazole (Diflucan), 150 mg/day. How many tablets should M.M. take per dose?

46. Which of the following must be frequently monitored for the client taking fluconazole? *Select all that apply.*

    a. AST

    b. ALT

    c. BUN

    d. pulse

    e. blood pressure

47. Side effects/adverse reactions of peptides include which of the following? *Select all that apply.*

    a. dizziness

    b. hypertension

    c. neurotoxicity

    d. nephrotoxicity

    e. tingling/numbness of the extremities

48. Side effects/adverse reactions of amphotericin B include which of the following? *Select all that apply.*

    a. flushing

    b. hypotension

    c. hypertension

    d. hypokalemia

    e. thrombophlebitis

Critical Thinking Exercises

Use a separate sheet of paper for your answers.

C.J., a 22-year-old female, has come to the health maintenance organization (HMO) complaining of "white spots in my mouth." She has been taking multiple antibiotics during the past month for a severe lower respiratory tract infection. Mycostatin is ordered, 250,000 units oral swish and swallow q.i.d.

Available:

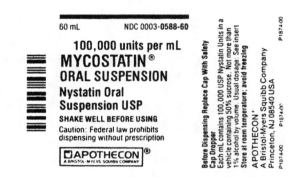

1. Is C.J.'s dose within the recommended adult dose range?

2. What is the most likely cause of these "white spots"?

3. What is the most likely causative organism?

4. What are specific instructions related to the correct administration of this drug?

5. List at least four general areas for health teaching related to antifungal drugs:

    a.

    b.

    c.

    d.

6. Compare and contrast nystatin and amphotericin B.

32 Antivirals, Antimalarials, and Anthelmintics

Study Questions

Define the following:

1. Erythrocytic phase

2. Opportunistic infection

3. Tissue phase

Complete the following word search. Clues are given in questions 4-8. Circle your responses.

```
S R A L L E C I R A V K R H H
D U E A U I S Z Q K W E E O E
I A R N C O Y K J A W R D T R
D Y C I A V R K B O P A S C P
A B P E V L M I L E X U E Y E
N K R Y V O T S S P V U S T S
O D C S W T L S R U J U G I Z
S L P W C I I A H I D M G C O
I P S L S M U Z G E F K L I S
N A R C P T J A Q E P A W X T
E A K L V T M O G U M A W O E
H X E C X K O S H W O O T T R
M X X I E L M J X U V K T I J
I R E P L I C A T I O N B Y C
R I M A N T I D I N E H C L C
```

4. Antiviral drugs prevent _____ of the virus.

5. AZT (is/is not) the only FDA-approved antiviral drug for treating persons with AIDS. *(Circle correct answer.)*

6. Antiviral drug development has been (slower/faster) than antibacterial drug development in part because of _____ of some antivirals. *(Circle correct answer.)*

7. A new drug to treat influenza A is _____. When a client is taking this drug, two organ functions that require monitoring are _____ and _____.

8. The drug vidarabine, introduced as an antineoplastic for the treatment of leukemia, is now known to have effects against which four organisms? _____, _____, _____, and _____.

9. Amantadine hydrochloride (Symmetrel) and rimantadine hydrochloride (Flumadine) were used to treat type _____ influenza.

10. Chills, fever, and sweating are symptoms of the _____ phase of malaria.

11. The pork roundworm can cause _____, which is diagnosed by a _____.

NCLEX Review Questions

Select the best response.

12. A serious adverse effect of ganciclovir (Cytovene) used for treatment of cytomegalovirus is:

    a.   ototoxicity.

    b.   granulocytosis.

    c.   thrombocytopenia.

    d.   electrocardiogram changes.

13. The most common site for helminthiasis is in the:

    a.   liver.

    b.   blood.

    c.   intestines.

    d.   urinary tract.

Situation: M.I., 17 years old, is receiving treatment for herpes simplex 1. Acyclovir sodium 200 mg q2h is prescribed. Questions 14 to 17 refer to this situation.

Available:

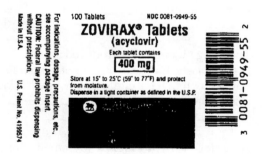

14. Is the prescribed dose within safe parameters? How many tablets should M.I. take at each dose?

15. Acyclovir is effective against the herpes virus. It was first introduced as an:

    a.   antiviral.

    b.   antineoplastic.

    c.   antimalarial.

    d.   antidepressant.

16. A drug interaction occurs between acyclovir and which of the following drugs?

    a.   primaquine

    b.   amantadine

    c.   probenecid

    d.   flucytosine

17. Which of the following drugs are effective in combating herpes simplex viruses (HSV-1, HSV-2)?

    a.   famciclovir (Famvir)

    b.   ganciclovir sodium (Cytovene)

    c.   valacyclovir (Valtrex)

    d.   all of the above

18. Which of the following is/are true about Relenza and Tamiflu?

    a.   promote activity of neuraminidase

    b.   are a substitute for flu shots

    c.   should be taken within 48 hours of flu symptoms

    d.   all of the above

19. Today, malaria is a common disease caused by:

    a.   a fungus.

    b.   a virus.

    c.   bacteria.

    d.   protozoa.

20. The drug of choice for treatment of chloroquine-resistant malaria is:

    a.   a combination of antimalarials.

    b.   quinidine.

    c.   Aralen.

    d.   primaquine.

21. Chloroquine affects all of the following laboratory test results EXCEPT:
    a.   BUN.
    b.   RBCs.
    c.   hemoglobin.
    d.   hematocrit.

22. The client taking chloroquine needs to know about which of the following possible side effects?
    a.   anorexia
    b.   fatigue
    c.   pruritus
    d.   all of the above

23. Nursing interventions during antimalarial drug therapy include:
    a.   monitoring urinary output and liver function.
    b.   assessing hearing; drugs may be ototoxic.
    c.   assessing for visual changes; chloroquine may cause retinopathy.
    d.   all of the above.

24. What is the recommended schedule for taking chloroquine in preparation for a visit to a country infested with malaria?
    a.   during the visit
    b.   during the visit and after the visit
    c.   before the visit and during the visit
    d.   before, during, and after the visit

25. Assessment of clients for treatment with anthelmintics includes which of the following?
    a.   history of food intake
    b.   collection of stool specimen
    c.   determining if other household members have same signs and symptoms
    d.   all of the above

26. Which of the following drugs is commonly used in the treatment of giant roundworms and pinworms?
    a.   bithionol (Actamer)
    b.   pyrantel pamoate (Antiminth)
    c.   mebendazole (Vermox)
    d.   oxamniquine (Vansil)

27. Long-term therapy with anthelmintics is required with all of the following drugs EXCEPT:
    a.   niclosamide.
    b.   mebendazole.
    c.   piperazine.
    d.   thiabendazole.

28. Client teaching for anthelmintics includes:
    a.   the importance of washing hands after toileting and before eating.
    b.   showering rather than bathing.
    c.   changing towels, underwear, and bed clothes daily.
    d.   all of the above.

29. When teaching the client taking acyclovir (Zovirax) about the side effects/adverse reactions that are associated with this drug, which of the following should the nurse include? *Select all that apply.*
    a.   nausea
    b.   headache
    c.   lethargy
    d.   decreased BUN
    e.   increased AST

30. Chloroquine (Aralen) increases the effects of which of the following drugs? *Select all that apply.*
    a.   digoxin
    b.   antacids
    c.   anticoagulants
    d.   anticonvulsants
    e.   neuromuscular blockers

31. Neurologic problems related to anthelmintics include which of the following? *Select all that apply.*
    a.   dizziness
    b.   headache
    c.   weakness
    d.   drowsiness
    e.   urinary retention

Critical Thinking Exercises

Use a separate sheet of paper for your answers.

K.B., age 35, has been attending the HIV clinic for several years. One of his medications is didanosine (Videx).

1. This drug belongs to which class of antivirals?

2. What are specific instructions for when to take this medication?

3. Which laboratory test results require monitoring when a client is taking Videx?

4. What adverse reactions should clients report to the health care provider?

5. Describe recommended oral hygiene. Give your rationale.

33 Drugs for Urinary Tract Disorders

Study Questions

Define the following:

1. Bacteriostatic

2. Bactericidal

3. Urinary analgesics

4. Urinary antiseptics/antiinfectives

5. Urinary antispasmodics

6. Urinary stimulants

Complete the following:

7. The therapeutic action of urinary antiseptics occurs in the renal _____ and _____.

8. Urine cultures should be done (before/after) starting drug treatment. (Circle correct answer.)

9. *Pseudomonas aeruginosa* is resistant to the drug _____.

10. Cranberry juice (decreases/increases) urine pH. *(Circle correct answer.)*

11. Inform clients that the drug nitrofurantoin changes the color of urine to _____ and it also may stain the _____.

12. Health teaching includes that the color of urine changes to red-orange when taking the drug _____.

13. Drug dosage of quinolones should be (decreased/increased) in clients with renal dysfunction. *(Circle correct answer.)*

14. Parasympathomimetics are used to stimulate _____.

15. Urinary antispasmodics are (recommended/contraindicated) for use in clients with urinary obstruction. *(Circle correct answer.)*

16. To be an effective antiseptic, the urine pH should be below _____.

17. The urinary stimulant drug that is frequently prescribed is _____.

18. One of the drugs of choice for uncomplicated urinary tract infections is the sulfonamide _____.

19. A drug, taken as a single dose, for the treatment of uncomplicated urinary tract infections in women is _____.

20. List four nursing interventions related to administering drugs for urinary tract disorders:

    a.

    b.

    c.

    d.

NCLEX Review Questions

Select the best response.

21. Methenamine (Mandelamine) should not be used with sulfonamides because of the risk of:
    a. bleeding.
    b. crystalluria.
    c. chest pain.
    d. intestinal distention.

22. All of the following substances can be taken to decrease urine pH EXCEPT:
    a. ammonium chloride.
    b. cranberry juice.
    c. potassium chloride.
    d. ascorbic acid.

Situation: L.P. is 53 years old and is receiving nalidixic acid (NegGram) for a chronic urinary tract infection. Questions 23 to 25 relate to this situation.

23. The dose of NegGram for long-term use is:
    a. 1 g daily.
    b. 1 g b.i.d.
    c. 1 g t.i.d.
    d. 1 g q.i.d.

24. Your health teaching plan for L.P. would include all of the following EXCEPT:
    a. urine may turn orange.
    b. protection against photosensitivity is necessary when taking this medication.
    c. increase fluid intake.
    d. avoid operating hazardous machinery.

25. Common urinary antiseptic drug-drug interactions include all of the following EXCEPT that:
    a. nalidixic acid increases effects of warfarin.
    b. antacids increase nitrofurantoin absorption.
    c. antiseptics cause false-positive Clinitest results.
    d. sodium bicarbonate inhibits action of methenamine.

26. Clients taking nitrofurantoin should report which of the following to the health care provider?
    a. chest pain
    b. fever
    c. cough
    d. all of the above

27. A specific adverse effect from nitrofurantoin is:
    a. superinfection.
    b. peripheral neuropathy.
    c. anorexia.
    d. drowsiness.

28. Urinary analgesics are used to relieve all of the following EXCEPT:
    a. burning sensation.
    b. frequency.
    c. urgency.
    d. retention.

29. A commonly prescribed urinary analgesic is:
    a. phenazopyridine hydrochloride (Pyridium).
    b. trimethoprim (Trimpex).
    c. flavoxate (Urispas).
    d. bethanechol (Urecholine).

30. Nursing interventions associated with administering urinary analgesics include all of the following EXCEPT:
    a. administering drug with food or milk.
    b. instructing that chewable tablets are to be chewed.
    c. observing for side effects.
    d. monitoring blood pressure.

31. Urinary tract spasms are commonly treated with which of the following drugs?
    a. trimethoprim (Trimpex)
    b. phenazopyridine hydrochloride (Pyridium)
    c. flavoxate (Urispas)
    d. bethanechol (Urecholine)

32. The drug used to control an overactive bladder and contraindicated in clients with narrow-angle glaucoma is which of the following?
    a. tolterodine tartrate (Detrol)
    b. bethanechol chloride (Urecholine)
    c. flavoxate hydrochloride (Urispas)
    d. phenazopyridine hydrochloride (Pyridium)

33. The groups of urinary antiseptics include which of the following?
    a. aztreonam
    b. phenothiazide
    c. methenamine
    d. quinolones
    e. nitrofurantoin

34. Your assessment of a client for side effects of a fluoroquinolone would include which of the following?
    a. headache and rash
    b. syncope and visual disturbance
    c. chest pain and fever
    d. peripheral neuritis
    e. photosensitivity

35. Clients taking bethanechol should report which of the following to the health care provider?
    a. abdominal discomfort
    b. headache
    c. increased salivation
    d. urgency
    e. abdominal cramps

Critical Thinking Exercises

Use a separate sheet of paper for your answers.

J.B., 11 years old, is taking a urinary antispasmodic for treatment of an injury to his urinary tract causing spasms of the smooth muscle. Ditropan 5 mg, t.i.d., has been prescribed.

1. What drug classification is Ditropan?

2. What is the recommended dosage range for J.B.? Describe nursing responsibilities, if any.

3. What are the side effects of this drug to include in client teaching?

4. What are the contraindications for the use of this drug? Is this an appropriate drug for J.B. based on the information provided?

5. What are the drug-food and drug-laboratory effects of this drug?

6. Compare the side effects of Ditropan and Pro-Banthine.

34 HIV- and AIDS-Related Drugs

Study Questions

Define the following:

1. Antibody

2. Antigen

3. Antiretroviral

4. HAART

5. Postexposure prophylaxis

Match the descriptors with the letter of the class of agents.

Descriptor		Class of Agents
____6.	block protease	a. nucleoside analogues
____7.	act by inhibiting HIV reverse transcriptase	b. nonnucleoside analogues
____8.	suppress virions in infected cell populations	c. protease inhibitors
____9.	infection of new cells	

Complete the following:

10. Identify at least six areas for assessment of clients with HIV or AIDS:

    a.

    b.

    c.

    d.

    e.

    f.

11. List at least four potential nursing diagnoses for the client with AIDS:

    a.

    b.

    c.

    d.

12. List at least six specific nursing interventions related to antiretroviral agents:

    a.

    b.

    c.

    d.

    e.

    f.

13. A health teaching plan for a client with HIV would likely include the following six factors:

    a.

    b.

    c.

    d.

    e.

    f.

NCLEX Review Questions

Select the best response.

14. A leading AIDS indicator is:
    a. *Pneumocystis carinii* pneumonia.
    b. CD4 counts of less than 200 cells/mm^3.
    c. Kaposi's sarcoma.
    d. *Mycobacterium avium* complex.

15. Potential benefits of early initiation of antiretroviral therapy in the asymptomatic HIV-infected client include all of the following EXCEPT:
    a. control of viral replication.
    b. decreased risk of drug toxicity.
    c. earlier development of drug resistance.
    d. prevention of progressive immunodeficiency.

16. Potential risks of early initiation of antiretroviral therapy in clients with asymptomatic HIV infection include all of the following EXCEPT:
    a. unknown long-term toxicity.
    b. reduction in quality of life from adverse effects.
    c. earlier development of drug resistance.
    d. decreased risk of selection of resistant virus.

17. The goal of combination antiretroviral therapy is to:
    a. increase the CD4 count, decrease the viral load, and have the client clinically well.
    b. decrease the viral load and decrease the CD4 count.
    c. replace the memory cells within the immune system.
    d. decrease the CD4 count and increase the viral load.

18. The decision to treat asymptomatic individuals with detectable HIV RNA in plasma should include which of the following?
    1. client's age and support
    2. amount of time since diagnosis
    3. client's willingness to accept therapy
    4. probability of adherence to therapy
    a. 1, 2
    b. 1, 2, 3, 4
    c. 1, 3, 4
    d. 3, 4

19. Combination therapy (HAART):
    a. targets enzymes in the HIV life cycle.
    b. offers a cure to AIDS-defined patients.
    c. offers a cure to pediatric patients.
    d. provides prophylaxis/treatment of major secondary infections.

Situation: Questions 20 to 24 relate to J.C., who is taking zidovudine.

20. Zidovudine received FDA approval in which of the following years?
    a. 1987
    b. 1991
    c. 1994
    d. 1996

21. Zidovudine is generally scheduled to be taken at which of the following frequencies?
    a. daily
    b. q12h
    c. q4-6h
    d. q1-3h

22. The usual adult dose of zidovudine is which of the following?
    a. 300 mg b.i.d.
    b. 200 mg q12h
    c. 300 mg daily
    d. 1.5 mg/kg q3h

23. During the time that J.C. is taking zidovudine, frequent monitoring of which of the following is/are required?
    a. CBC
    b. renal function
    c. hepatic function
    d. all of the above

24. You assess J.C. for the side effects of zidovudine, which may include all of the following EXCEPT:
    a. numbness and pain in lower extremities.
    b. headache.
    c. seizures.
    d. difficulty swallowing.

Situation: Questions 25 to 29 relate to Z.B., who is taking efavirenz.

25. Efavirenz received FDA approval in which of the following years?
    a. 2000
    b. 1998
    c. 1996
    d. 1994

26. Z.B. is taking efavirenz, which is generally initially scheduled to be taken at which of the following intervals?
    a. 14-day lead-in, give one 600 mg tablet daily, then one 600 mg tablet twice a day in combination with other antiretroviral agents
    b. 600 mg q12h
    c. 600 mg q8h
    d. 600 mg q24h

27. The usual adult dose of efavirenz is which of the following?
    a. 600 mg q12h
    b. 600 mg q8h
    c. 300 mg q12h
    d. none of the above

28. During the time that Z.B. is taking efavirenz, periodic monitoring of which of the following is/are required?
    a. CBC and platelets
    b. hepatic function
    c. renal function
    d. none of the above

29. You assess Z.B. for the side effects of efavirenz, which may include all of the following EXCEPT:
    a. CNS effects.
    b. diarrhea.
    c. difficulty swallowing.
    d. rash.

Situation: Questions 30 to 34 relate to lopinavir.

30. Lopinavir received FDA approval in which of the following years?
   a.   1998
   b.   1999
   c.   2000
   d.   2001

31. Lopinavir is generally scheduled to be taken at which of the following intervals?
   a.   daily
   b.   twice a day
   c.   three times a day
   d.   four times a day

32. The usual adult dose of lopinavir is which of the following?
   a.   600 mg twice a day
   b.   800 mg/day in 2 divided doses
   c.   1200 mg/day
   d.   400 mg q8h

33. Frequent monitoring of which of the following (is/are) required while taking lopinavir?
   a.   liver function
   b.   triglycerides
   c.   cholesterol
   d.   all of the above

34. Which of the following is NOT a class of medications undergoing clinical trials for HIV/AIDS?
   a.   maturation inhibitors
   b.   leukotrine receptor antagonists
   c.   integrase inhibitors
   d.   CCR5 entry inhibitors

35. Prophylaxis for *Mycobacterium avium* complex might include all EXCEPT which of the following?
   a.   Bactrim DS one po daily
   b.   azithromycin 1200 mg po every week
   c.   rifabutin 300 mg po daily
   d.   clarithromycin 500 mg po b.i.d.

36. First choice of drugs for prophylaxis for PCP is:
   a.   dapsone 50 mg po b.i.d.
   b.   atovaquone 750 mg po b.i.d.
   c.   Bactrim DS 1 tablet po daily.
   d.   aerosolized pentamidine by mouth.

37. Postexposure prophylaxis includes all of the following EXCEPT 4 weeks (28 days) of:
   a.   ritonavir and ddI.
   b.   ZDV + 3TC and nelfinavir.
   c.   ZDV + 3TC and indinavir.
   d.   both zidovudine and lamivudine.

38. In the pregnant client, zidovudine monotherapy is begun at how many weeks of gestation?
   a.   6
   b.   10
   c.   12
   d.   14

39. The dose of prophylactic zidovudine for the pregnant client is which of the following?
   a.   100 mg five times a day
   b.   300 mg two times a day
   c.   200 mg three times a day
   d.   200 mg five times a day

40. The side effects of lopinavir may include the following: *Select all that apply.*
   a.   vomiting
   b.   urinary retention
   c.   diarrhea
   d.   nausea

41. The following nursing interventions increase adherence to the therapeutic regimen: *Select all that apply.*
   a.   pill organizers
   b.   pill counting
   c.   timers/beepers
   d.   scheduled pill holidays

35 Vaccines

Study Questions

Define the following:

1. Anaphylaxis

2. Seroconversion

3. Toxoids

4. Antibodies

5. Antigen

NCLEX Review Questions

Select the best response.

6. Vaccines made from the inactivated disease-causing substances produced by some micoorganisms are called:
   a. toxoids.
   b. recombinant subunit vaccines.
   c. conjugate vaccines.
   d. attenuated vaccines.

7. Acquired passive immunity is important in all but one of the following situations:
   a. when time does not permit active vaccination alone
   b. when the exposed individual is at high risk for complications of the disease
   c. in newborns
   d. when a person suffers from an immune system deficiency that renders that person unable to produce an effective immune response

8. The process in which antibodies are received by an individual, used for protection against a particular pathogen, and acquired from another source best describes:
   a. active immunity.
   b. most childhood immunizations.
   c. toxoids.
   d. passive immunity.

9. Acquisition of detectable levels of antibodies in the bloodstream best describes:
   a. passive immunity.
   b. acquired natural immunity.
   c. immunization.
   d. seroconversion.

10. Following administration, most vaccines:
    a. stimulate an immune response.
    b. cause an allergic reaction.
    c. are perceived by the body as antibodies.
    d. produce mild disease.

11. Immunity that usually persists for the remainder of the individual's life is:

    a. humoral.

    b. passive natural.

    c. active natural.

    d. passive acquired.

12. A child's first vaccine is usually administered:

    a. by mouth.

    b. at 2 months of age.

    c. at birth.

    d. at 4 months of age.

13. Newborns naturally have passive immunity as a result of:

    a. frequent colds and flu "bugs."

    b. additives in commercially-prepared formula.

    c. immunizations administered before discharge from the newborn nursery.

    d. transfer of maternal antibodies across the placenta.

14. Rubella is commonly known as:

    a. smallpox.

    b. German measles.

    c. hard measles.

    d. rubeola.

15. Susceptible individuals 13 years of age or older receive 2 doses of varicella vaccine spaced _____ apart.

    a. at least 4 weeks

    b. 3 months

    c. 6 months

    d. 1 month

16. In the event of an adverse reaction to a vaccine, a health care provider reports details of the event to:

    a. his/her immediate supervisor.

    b. the Vaccine Adverse Events Reporting System (VAERS).

    c. the vaccine manufacturer.

    d. the Centers for Disease Control and Prevention (CDC).

17. The following vaccine is not administered to individuals 7 years of age or older:

    a. varicella

    b. MMR

    c. Td

    d. DTaP

18. The following vaccines are administered to adults 65 years of age and older:

    a. Td, pneumococcal (PPV), influenza, zoster

    b. human papillomavirus (HPV), Td, influenza, pneumococcal (PPV)

    c. rotavirus, Td, influenza

    d. Tdap, pneumococal (PPV), influenza, zoster

19. The type of immunity conferred by tetanus-diphtheria (Td) vaccine would best be described as:

    a. active.

    b. passive.

    c. natural.

    d. inactive.

20. Examples of live, attenuated vaccines include:

    a. measles-mumps-rubella (MMR) and *Haemophilus influenzae* type B (Hib).

    b. varicella and Td.

    c. MMR and varicella.

    d. influenza and hepatitis B.

21. Symptoms of influenza include:

    a. vomiting and diarrhea.

    b. abdominal pain and cough.

    c. fever and diarrhea.

    d. fever, myalgias, and cough.

22. A physically and medically neglected 15-month-old child has recently been placed in foster care. The foster parents present with this child today for immunization update. They have no idea what, if any, vaccines he has previously received. Today the nurse would most likely administer:

    a. no vaccines because it is assumed he is up-to-date.

    b. DTaP #4, Hib #4, and MMR #1.

    c. DTaP, Hib, hepatitis A, hepatitis B, MMR, IPV, pneumococcal (PCV), and varicella.

    d. DTaP, Hib, hepatitis B, and MMR. Have the child return in 2 weeks for hepatitis A, IPV, pneumococcal (PCV), and varicella.

23. When measles-mumps-rubella vaccine is not given the same day as varicella vaccine, the minimum interval between administration should be:

    a. 7 days.

    b. 14 days.

    c. 21 days.

    d. 28 days.

Situation: Andy, a 4-month-old boy, was seen in the emergency department of the local hospital 3 days ago and was diagnosed with a cold and an ear infection. He is taking amoxicillin, an antibiotic, as prescribed for his ear infection and is generally improved. Questions 24 to 28 refer to this situation.

24. Andy's mother is concerned that he should not receive vaccines today because of his illness and medication use. Which of the following is the BEST response to this mother's concern?

    a. You empathize with her concern but suggest that neither a mild acute illness nor antibiotic usage is a contraindication to immunizing her son today.

    b. You agree that Andy should not receive immunizations today and suggest that his mom return in 2 weeks after he has completed the amoxicillin.

    c. The cold is a contraindication to immunizing Andy today, but the medication he is taking is not.

    d. Amoxicillin is a contraindication to immunizing Andy today, but his cold is not.

25. Andy's immunization record shows he received hepatitis B vaccine on day 2 of life. At 2 months of age, he received hepatitis B, DTaP, Hib, pneumococcal (PCV), rotavirus, and IPV vaccines. If you elected to immunize him today, what vaccines would you administer?

    a. pneumococcal and influenza

    b. hepatitis B, DTaP, Hib, rotavirus, and IPV

    c. DTaP, Hib, and influenza

    d. DTaP, Hib, pneumococcal (PCV), rotavirus, and IPV

26. Andy's mother reports that after his first dose of DTaP he experienced some redness and tenderness at the injection site in his left thigh. With this in mind, you would administer:

    a. DTaP again as these are common side effects, not contraindications.

    b. DT in the right thigh.

    c. DTaP subcutaneously instead of intramuscularly to prevent muscle soreness.

    d. half the usual dose of DTaP to reduce the likelihood of a reaction.

27. Following today's visit, you would recommend that Andy return for immunizations:

    a. in 2 weeks after he has recovered from his cold and ear infection.

    b. at 9 months of age.

    c. at 6 months of age.

    d. at 12 months of age.

28. Before leaving the clinic today, the nurse appropriately provides Andy's mother with: *Select the best response.*

    a. Vaccine Information Statements (VISs) for all vaccines administered.

    b. an immunization record.

    c. a report of adverse reaction form.

    d. an appointment card for the next immunization clinic visit.

29. A source of health and immunization information for nurses assisting clients before foreign travel is:

    a. the U.S. embassy in the destination country.

    b. the Centers for Disease Control and Prevention.

    c. the client's travel agent.

    d. not necessary because there are no special immunization needs for travelers.

30. In the case of an anaphylactic reaction to a vaccine, which of the following should the nurse have readily available?

    a. epinephrine

    b. acetaminophen

    c. pseudoephedrine

    d. diphenhydramine

31. It is a federal law to provide a client who is to receive vaccines with:

    a. an immunization record.

    b. no more than four immunizations on any given day.

    c. Vaccine Information Statements (VISs).

    d. no more than two immunizations at any given visit.

32. The three viruses combined in the MMR vaccine include: *Select all that apply.*

    a. rubella.

    b. roseola.

    c. measles.

    d. mumps.

Critical Thinking Exercises

Use a separate sheet of paper for your answers.

A 70-year-old man presents to the clinic on Halloween after having stepped on a nail. He has suffered a puncture wound to the sole of his right foot. He wonders whether he needs a "lock jaw" shot. He says he has not had any shots since he was in the Army for a 4-year stint "straight out of high school." He is taking atenolol for hypertension but otherwise does not "go to the doctor much." He has no known medication allergies.

1. What is another name for "lock jaw"?

2. What are the symptoms of tetanus?

3. What vaccine would routinely be administered in this circumstance?

4. What is the route of administration for the above vaccine?

5. Given this man's age and the time of year, name the two vaccines for which he might also be eligible.

6. What are contraindications to the administration of influenza vaccine?

36 Anticancer Drugs

Study Questions

Define the following:

1. Adjuvant chemotherapy

2. Apoptosis

3. Combination chemotherapy

4. Cell-cycle nonspecific (CCNS) chemotherapy

5. Cell-cycle specific (CCS) chemotherapy

6. Cytoprotectants

7. Dose-dense chemotherapy

8. Multidrug resistance

9. Protocol

10. Vesicant

Match the chemotherapy drugs/terms in Column A with the MOST appropriate term in Column B.

Column A	Column B
____11. angiogenesis inhibitors	a. associated with hemorrhagic cystitis
____12. aromatase inhibitors	b. leucovorin rescue
____13. cyclophosphamide (Cytoxan)	c. stomatitis is early sign of toxicity
____14. doxorubicin (Adriamycin)	d. associated with cardiotoxicity
____15. dose-dense chemotherapy	e. associated with neurotoxicity
____16. fluorouracil (5-FU; Adrucil)	f. powder-free gloves, mask, impermeable gown
____17. hormonal agents	g. not true chemotherapy agents
____18. methotrexate (Trexall)	h. prevents growth of new blood vessels
____19. ways to reduce exposure to chemotherapy	i. intervals between doses of chemotherapy shortened
____20. vincristine (Oncovin)	j. block conversion of androgens to estrogen

NCLEX Review Questions

Select the best response.

21. Which of the following is TRUE with regard to combination chemotherapy?
    a. It has better response rates than single-agent chemotherapy.
    b. It is always more effective than surgery or radiation.
    c. It is never given with other treatment modalities (e.g., surgery).
    d. Survival time is decreased as compared to single-agent chemotherapy.

22. You are teaching a community group about factors that influence the development of cancer in humans. Which of the following would you include in your teaching?
    a. Aflatoxin is associated with cancer of the lung.
    b. Benzene is associated with cancer of the tongue.
    c. Epstein-Barr virus is associated with cancer of the stomach.
    d. Human papillomavirus is associated with cancer of the cervix.

23. Your client has been diagnosed with cancer and will be treated with chemotherapy. Which of the following pieces of information should you provide to your client with regard to tumor size and chemotherapy effectiveness?
    a. Chemotherapy is most effective against large, slow-growing tumors.
    b. Chemotherapy is most effective against small tumors with a high growth fraction.
    c. Chemotherapy is most effective against large tumors with a high growth fraction.
    d. Chemotherapy is most effective against large tumors with a low growth fraction.

24. Your client is to receive chemotherapy for the treatment of his cancer. You should be aware of which of the following concerning the side effects of chemotherapy?
    a. Side effects are minimal because chemotherapy drugs are highly selective.
    b. Side effects are minimal because chemotherapy does not affect normal cells.
    c. Side effects of chemotherapy are caused by toxicities to normal cells.
    d. Side effects of chemotherapy are usually permanent.

25. Your male client has advanced cancer that has spread to other areas of his body. He is scheduled to receive palliative chemotherapy. The purpose of palliative chemotherapy is to:
    a. control the cancer.
    b. cure the cancer.
    c. improve quality of life.
    d. slow the growth of the cancer.

26. Your client is scheduled to receive chemotherapy that will cause a low white blood cell count. Which of the following nursing actions would you plan to carry out?
    a. Assess for a change in temperature.
    b. Assess for an increase in diarrhea.
    c. Assess for evidence of petechiae.
    d. Assess for taste changes.

27. Your client has low platelet counts secondary to the administration of chemotherapy. Which of the following nursing actions would be MOST appropriate?
    a. Assess for diarrhea and provide small, frequent meals.
    b. Assess intake and output and help the client conserve energy.
    c. Assess for localized infections and monitor breath sounds.
    d. Assess for occult bleeding and apply pressure to injection sites.

28. You are the nurse caring for a client who is experiencing diarrhea secondary to chemotherapy. Which of the following would you include in teaching your client about chemotherapy-related diarrhea?

    a. Eat only very hot or very cold foods.

    b. Increase intake of fresh fruits and vegetables.

    c. Increase intake of high-fiber foods.

    d. Limit caffeine intake.

29. An oncology client is to receive cyclophospha-mide (Cytoxan) as part of his chemotherapy protocol. You note on his medical record that the client is taking digoxin (Lanoxin) each morning to treat atrial fibrillation. The nurse should be aware that cyclophosphamide:

    a. decreases digoxin levels.

    b. has no effect on digoxin levels.

    c. increases digoxin levels.

    d. is never given to a client receiving digoxin.

30. A client in the outpatient oncology clinic is receiving fluorouracil (5-FU; Adrucil) as part of his treatment for colon cancer. The physician prescribes metronidazole (Flagyl) to treat trichomoniasis. You would question the physician because you know that:

    a. 5-FU may decrease the effectiveness of metronidazole.

    b. 5-FU may increase the toxicity of metronidazole.

    c. metronidazole may decrease the effectiveness of 5-FU.

    d. metronidazole may increase 5-FU toxicity.

31. Your client is to receive doxorubicin (Adriamycin) as part of her chemotherapy protocol. Which of the following would be the MOST important for the nurse to assess before administration of Adriamycin?

    a. cardiac status

    b. liver function

    c. lung sounds

    d. mental status

32. Your client is receiving cyclophosphamide (Cytoxan), doxorubicin (Adriamycin), and methotrexate (Trexall) (CAM) for the treatment of prostate cancer. During morning rounds he complains of feeling short of breath. Your physical assessment reveals crackles in both lungs. These symptoms are MOST LIKELY to be caused by:

    a. Adriamycin.

    b. cyclophosphamide.

    c. methotrexate.

    d. client anxiety.

33. Your client is to receive fluorouracil (5-FU; Adrucil) as part of his treatment protocol for colon cancer. When teaching your client about this drug, you would be sure to tell him that the nadir in the blood counts usually occurs:

    a. 1 to 4 days after administration.

    b. 5 to 9 days after administration.

    c. 10 to 14 days after administration.

    d. 15 to 19 days after administration.

34. Your client has reached the nadir of his blood counts secondary to chemotherapy. Which one of the following nursing diagnoses would be the MOST appropriate?

    a. *risk for cardiac failure*

    b. *risk for dehydration*

    c. *risk for infection*

    d. *risk for malnutrition*

35. Which of the following nursing outcomes would be MOST appropriate as part of your planning for a client scheduled to receive cyclophosphamide (Cytoxan)?

    a. Client will be free of symptoms of stomatitis.

    b. Client will maintain cardiac output.

    c. Client will limit exposure to sunlight.

    d. Client will maintain blood counts in the desired range.

36. Your client is to receive cyclophosphamide (Cytoxan) as part of his cancer treatment. Which of the following nursing interventions should you expect to complete?

   a. Assess for signs of hematuria, urinary frequency, or dysuria.

   b. Decrease fluids to reduce the risk of urate deposition or calculus formation.

   c. Hydrate the client with IV fluids only after administration of cyclophosphamide.

   d. Medicate with an antiemetic only after the client complains of nausea.

37. You are teaching your 29-year-old female client about cyclophosphamide (Cytoxan), which will be given as part of her treatment protocol for cancer. Which of the following should be included in your teaching?

   a. Hair loss has never been reported with the use of cyclophosphamide.

   b. Menstrual irregularities and sterility are not expected with this drug.

   c. No special isolation procedures are needed when receiving this chemotherapy.

   d. Pregnancy should be prevented during treatment with cyclophosphamide.

38. You are administering IV fluorouracil (5-FU; Adrucil) to a client in the outpatient oncology clinic. Which of the following nursing interventions would be MOST appropriate?

   a. 5-FU is a vesicant, so assess for tissue necrosis at the IV site.

   b. Apply heat to the IV site if extravasation occurs.

   c. Assess for hyperpigmentation along the vein in which the drug is given.

   d. Encourage mouth rinses once every 8 hours during chemotherapy.

39. A client receiving cyclophosphamide (Cytoxan), epirubicin (Ellence), and fluorouracil (5-FU; Adrucil) (CEF) has experienced severe nausea, vomiting, and diarrhea over the past week. He has lost 5.5 pounds. Which of the following nursing diagnoses would be MOST appropriate?

   a. *knowledge deficit related to chemotherapeutic regimen*

   b. *pain, secondary to diarrhea*

   c. *risk for altered nutrition*

   d. *risk for infection, secondary to low WBC counts*

40. You are teaching a client about doxorubicin (Adriamycin), which she will receive as part of her treatment for breast cancer. Which of the following statements, made by your client, indicates that she needs ADDITIONAL teaching?

   a. "Adriamycin is a severe vesicant."

   b. "My blood counts will be checked."

   c. "My cardiac status will be closely monitored."

   d. "This drug may make my urine turn blue."

41. You are administering doxorubicin (Adriamycin) to a client in the outpatient oncology clinic. You would be sure to include which of the following in your client teaching?

   a. Blood counts will most likely remain normal.

   b. Complete alopecia rarely occurs with this drug.

   c. Report any shortness of breath, palpitations, or edema to your doctor.

   d. Tissue necrosis usually occurs 2 to 3 days after administration.

42. You are administering doxorubicin (Adriamycin) to a client diagnosed with cancer. Which of the following should you keep in mind with regard to tissue necrosis associated with this drug?

    a. Tissue necrosis may occur 3 to 4 weeks after administration.

    b. Tissue necrosis occurs immediately after administration.

    c. Tissue necrosis occurs 2 to 4 days after administration.

    d. Tissue necrosis rarely occurs with this drug.

43. One week ago in the outpatient oncology clinic your client received his first cycle of chemotherapy consisting of cyclophospha-mide (Cytoxan), doxorubicin (Adriamycin), and fluorouracil (5-FU; Adrucil) (CAF). He returns to the clinic today for follow-up. Which of the following nursing interventions would be MOST appropriate at this time?

    a. Culture the IV site and send a specimen to the laboratory for analysis.

    b. Monitor blood counts and laboratory values.

    c. Offer analgesics for pain and evaluate effectiveness.

    d. Teach the client about good skin care.

44. You are preparing IV vinblastine (Velban), bleomycin (Blenoxane), and cisplatin (Platinol) (VBP) for administration to a client on your nursing unit. Which of the following precautions should the nurse take when hanging chemotherapy?

    a. Wear a clean cotton gown.

    b. Wear shoe covers.

    c. Wear a hair net.

    d. Wear powder-free gloves.

45. Your male client is being discharged after receiving IV chemotherapy. Which of the following statements, made by the client, indicates a need for ADDITIONAL teaching?

    a. "Chemotherapy is excreted in my bodily fluids."

    b. "I will not need to know how to check my temperature."

    c. "My wife should wear gloves when emptying my urinal."

    d. "The chemotherapy will remain in my body for 2 to 3 days."

46. You are preparing to administer chemo-therapy, which can cause severe nausea and vomiting, to a client in the outpatient clinic. Which of the following nursing actions would be MOST appropriate?

    a. Give an antiemetic before administering the chemotherapy.

    b. Withhold any antiemetic drugs until the client complains of nausea.

    c. Give an antiemetic only after the client has vomited.

    d. Offer the client a glass of ginger ale to prevent nausea.

47. A client is admitted to the hospital 1 week after receiving teniposide (VP-16) in the outpatient oncology clinic. On physical assessment the nurse notes the presence of petechiae, ecchymoses, and bleeding gums. Which of the following nursing diagnoses would be MOST appropriate?

    a. *risk for fatigue*

    b. *risk for infection*

    c. *risk for bleeding*

    d. *risk for falls*

48. Your client with breast cancer is scheduled to receive anastrozole (Arimidex), an aromatase inhibitor. Which of the following statements would you include as part of your client teaching?

    a. Aromatase inhibitors block the peripheral conversion of androgens to estrogens.

    b. Aromatase inhibitors are used to treat tumors that are not hormonally sensitive.

    c. Aromatase inhibitors are used only in premenopausal women with breast cancer.

    d. Aromatase inhibitors are used only in postmenopausal women with breast cancer.

49. A client is scheduled to receive vincristine (Oncovin) as part of treatment for his cancer. The medication record for the client indicates that he is receiving phenytoin (Dilantin) to control a seizure disorder. The nurse would monitor the client carefully because:

    a. phenytoin increases the side effects of vincristine.

    b. phenytoin decreases the side effects of vincristine.

    c. vincristine increases phenytoin effects.

    d. vincristine decreases phenytoin effects.

50. A client is scheduled to receive vincristine as part of her treatment for non-Hodgkin's lymphoma. She reports that she takes bromelain (pineapple exact) at home to prevent constipation. The nurse is aware that the combination of vincristine (Oncovin) and bromelain may increase the client's risk for which of the following?

    a. diarrhea

    b. constipation

    c. bone marrow depression

    d. hair loss

51. A client in the outpatient oncology clinic complains of fatigue secondary to her cancer therapy. Which of the following would be the MOST appropriate nursing intervention?

    a. Assess for other things that might be contributing to her fatigue (e.g., pain, sleep disturbances).

    b. Plan a high-protein, high-calorie diet with the client.

    c. Suggest that the client participate in daily strenuous exercise.

    d. Tell the client to sleep as much as possible during the day if she cannot sleep at night.

52. A cancer client in the outpatient oncology clinic has developed mucositis secondary to cancer therapy. Which of the following statements, made by the client, would indicate that she needs ADDITIONAL teaching about mucositis?

    a. "I will rinse my mouth out frequently with normal saline."

    b. "I will try using ice pops or ice chips to help relieve mouth pain."

    c. "I will use a mouthwash that has an alcohol base."

    d. "I will use a soft toothbrush."

53. Your client presents with neutropenia secondary to cancer therapy. Which one of the following nursing diagnoses would be the MOST appropriate?

    a. *risk for cardiac failure*

    b. *risk for dehydration*

    c. *risk for infection*

    d. *risk for malnutrition*

54. Refer to Prototype Drug Chart 36-4 in the text to answer the following question.

    A client is receiving vincristine (Oncovin) as part of his chemotherapy protocol. During therapy, the client complains of severe abdominal pain, nausea, and vomiting. The client's medical record indicates that he has not had a bowel movement in 3 days. Auscultation of the abdomen reveals an absence of bowel sounds. The nurse knows that these are characteristic signs for which of the following LIFE-THREATENING side effects of vincristine administration?

    a. extravasation

    b. intestinal necrosis

    c. hyponatremia

    d. hyperuricemia

55. Which of the following have been identified as causes of multidrug resistance to chemotherapy? *Select all that apply.*

    a. Cancer cells that are not killed may mutate and become resistant to chemotherapy.

    b. Some cancer cells may be naturally resistant to chemotherapy.

    c. Cell cycle non-specific chemotherapy drugs.

    d. Gene amplification can cause overproduction of proteins that make chemotherapy less effective.

    e. Cancer cells develop the ability to repair damage caused by chemotherapy.

    f. Some cancer cells pump chemotherapy agents out of the cell and decrease the effectiveness of chemotherapy.

56. Review information found in Table 36-4 in the text to answer the following question.

    A client is experiencing mucositis (stomatitis) secondary to receiving chemotherapy. Which of the following symptomatic treatments would be appropriate? *Select all that apply.*

    a. Encourage frequent mouth rinses.

    b. Provide antiemetics.

    c. Apply topical anesthetics.

    d. Encourage stress reduction.

    e. Administer antibiotics.

    f. Administer antifungal medication.

    g. Use saliva substitutes.

    h. Consider sperm banking.

    i. Provide pain medication.

    j. Avoid invasive procedures.

37 Targeted Therapies to Treat Cancer

Study Questions

Define the following:

1. Growth factor

2. Cell signalling cascades

3. Tyrosine kinase

4. Ligand binding

5. Receptor

6. Angiogenesis

7. Targeted therapy

8. Monoclonal antibody

NCLEX Review Questions

Select the best response.

9. In cancer tumor cells the EGFR-TK signal is inappropriately turned on, leading to:
   a. proliferation.
   b. invasion.
   c. angiogenesis.
   d. metastasis.

10. During the first dose of trastuzumab (Herceptin), the client complains of shortness of breath and pruritus. The nurse should:
    a. decrease the infusion rate by 50% and notify the physician.
    b. stop the infusion and manage the reaction.
    c. review the pretreatment MUGA scan.
    d. disconnect the IV and attach a 0.22 micron filter.

11. The rationale for administering bevacizumab in a client with metastatic colon cancer is to:
    a. enhance the client's immune response.
    b. modulate an inflammatory response.
    c. increase apoptosis.
    d. inhibit formation of blood supply.

12. A client with NHL will be receiving treatment with CHOP and rituximab. While doing initial client teaching the nurse explains that premedications will be given to decrease the incidence of hypersensitivity reaction to:
    a. cyclophosphamide.
    b. doxorubicin.
    c. vincristine.
    d. rituximab.

13. Iressa most frequently causes which of the following toxicities:

    a.   acneiform rash

    b.   diarrhea

    c.   myelosuppression

    d.   nausea and vomiting

14. An oncology client is to begin treatment for NSCLC with administration of gefitinib. You note on his medical record that the client is also taking warfarin daily for atrial fibrillation. The nurse should be aware that gefitinib:

    a.   increases the effects of warfarin.

    b.   may reach toxic levels when given concurrently with warfarin.

    c.   is never given to a client taking anticoagulants.

    d.   may require a dose increase when taken with warfarin.

15. A client in the outpatient oncology clinic is receiving sunitinib as part of his treatment for GIST. The physician prescribes metronidazole to treat trichomoniasis. You would question the physician because you know that:

    a.   sunitinib may decrease the effectiveness of metronidazole.

    b.   sunitinib may lead to toxic levels of metronidazole.

    c.   metronidazole may decrease the effectiveness of sunitinib.

    d.   metronidazole may potentiate sunitinib toxicity.

16. Your client is beginning therapy with the EGFR erlotinib (Tarceva) for NSCLC. Which of the following would be the MOST important for the nurse to assess before beginning this targeted agent?

    a.   cardiac status

    b.   liver function

    c.   lung sounds

    d.   mental status

17. A client is admitted to the hospital 1 week after receiving teniposide (VP-16) in the outpatient oncology clinic. On physical assessment the nurse notes the presence of petechiae, ecchymosis, and bleeding gums. Which of the following nursing diagnoses would be MOST appropriate?

    a.   *risk for fatigue*

    b.   *risk for infection*

    c.   *risk for bleeding*

    d.   *risk for falls*

18. Which of the following nursing outcomes would be most appropriate as part of your planning for a client about to begin therapy with the oral MKI sorafenib?

    a.   Client will be free of symptoms of stomatitis.

    b.   Client will be free of cardiac dysfunction.

    c.   Client will maintain skin integrity.

    d.   Client will maintain adequate fluid balance.

19. Which of the following nursing outcomes would be MOST appropriate as part of your planning for a client scheduled to begin treatment with imatinib (Gleevec)?

    a.   Client will maintain adequate nutrition and hydration status.

    b.   Client will maintain cardiac output.

    c.   Client will maintain blood counts in the desired range.

    d.   Client will maintain renal function.

38 Biologic Response Modifiers

Define the following:

1. Nadir

2. Absolute neutrophil count (ANC)

3. Thrombocytopenia

4. Interferons

5. Myelosuppression

6. Epidermal growth factor receptor (EGFR)

7. Human epidermal growth factor receptor 2 (HER2)

8. Regulation

9. Targeted therapy

10. Vascular epithelial growth factor (VEGF)

11. Pegylation

12. Keratinocyte-growth factor

13. Granulocyte-macrophage colony–stimulating factor (GM-CSF)

14. Interferons (IFNs)

15. Colony-stimulating factors (CSFs)

16. Erythrocyte stimulating agents (ESAs)

17. Epidermal growth factor receptor (EGFR)

18. Interleukins

19. Hybridoma technology

20. Granulocyte colony–stimulating factor (G-CSF)

Match the description in Column II with the appropriate term in Column I.

Column I		Column II
____ 21.	colony-stimulating factors (CSFs)	a. glycoprotein that regulates the production of neutrophils within the bone marrow
____ 22.	erythropoietin	b. proteins that stimulate growth and maturation of bone marrow stem cells
____ 23.	granulocyte colony–stimulating factor (G-CSF)	
____ 24.	granulocyte-macrophage colony–stimulating factor (GM-CSF)	c. glycoprotein produced by kidneys in response to hypoxia
____ 25.	Neumega (oprelvekin)	d. supports survival, clonal expression, and differentiation of hematopoietic progenitor cells
		e. indicated for prevention of severe thrombocytopenia

Complete the following:

26. E.K. is receiving G-CSF for an ANC of 300/mm^3. The client's platelet count is 5000/mm^3. Will G-CSF increase this count? Why or why not?

27. Describe the nursing interventions for clients receiving EPO three times per week with a hemoglobin of 21 g/dl and a hematocrit of 42%.

28. List three differences between G-CSF and GM-CSF:

a.

b.

c.

NCLEX Review Questions

Select the best response.

29. The primary functions of BRMs include all of the following EXCEPT:
    a. enhance host immunologic function.
    b. destroy tumor activities.
    c. improve liver functioning.
    d. promote differentiation of stem cells.

30. Your client is receiving G-CSF therapy. You assess for a consistent client reaction of:
    a. bone pain.
    b. urinary retention.
    c. flu-like syndrome.
    d. rash.

31. Your client is receiving GM-CSF therapy. As the nurse, you know that attention is focused on which system both during and after these infusions?
    a. cardiac system
    b. respiratory system
    c. central nervous system
    d. musculoskeletal system

32. Special preparation and administration of EPO is recommended, including all of the following EXCEPT:
    a. inject less than 3 ml volume/injection.
    b. do not re-enter the vial.
    c. discard unused portion; no preservatives.
    d. warm vial to room temperature.

Situation: F.F., 64 years old, has hairy cell leukemia that is being treated with the IFN alfa Roferon. Questions 33 to 39 relate to this situation.

33. The dose-limiting side effect is:
    a. malaise.
    b. chills.
    c. fever.
    d. fatigue.

34. F.F. reports all of the following gastrointestinal side effects. Which side effect is considered the dose-limiting toxicity for the gastrointestinal system?

    a. taste alteration

    b. anorexia

    c. xerostomia

    d. diarrhea

35. F.F. also reports neurologic side effects. The most appropriate response to F.F.'s questions would be that:

    a. these side effects rarely occur.

    b. they are reversible after the drug is stopped.

    c. they are not reversible.

    d. the worst effect is the mild confusion.

36. The best time to administer a BRM is:

    a. at bedtime.

    b. 2 hours after meals.

    c. with meals.

    d. 1 hour before meals.

37. To assess renal and hepatic effects of the drugs, the following laboratory studies are monitored: *Select all that apply.*

    a. BUN

    b. creatinine

    c. transaminase

    d. bilirubin

38. Dermatologic effects of the alfa IFNs include the following: *Select all that apply.*

    a. vesicle formation

    b. alopecia

    c. irritation at injection site

    d. pruritus

39. Health teaching for F.F. and significant others would include the following: *Select all that apply.*

    a. that most BRM side effects disappear within 72–96 hours after discontinuation of therapy

    b. provision for return demonstration of drug administration techniques

    c. reporting weight gain

    d. providing information on the effect of BRM-related fatigue on ADLs, including sexuality

40. GM-CSF should be administered to clients with which of the following conditions? *Select all that apply.*

    a. ANC <500/mm^3

    b. autologous BMT recipient

    c. allogenic BMT recipient

    d. 2 weeks post high-dose chemotherapy administration

Critical Thinking Exercises

Use a separate sheet of paper for your answers.

J.G. is a 67-year-old client diagnosed with metastatic renal cell carcinoma. His medical oncologist has prescribed interleukin-2 (IL-2). J.G. weighs 150 pounds, and he will receive 600,000 International Units/kg (0.037 mg/kg) intravenously every 8 hours for 5 days (total of 14 doses of IL-2). He will have a 9-day rest after the initial 14 doses and then receive another 14 doses. Pretreatment laboratory work includes CBC, serum electrolytes, and renal and liver function tests. Client education will focus on review of treatment schedule, side effect profile, and postinfusion management.

1. What mg dose of IL-2 should J.G. receive?

2. In addition to his cancer, J.G. has congestive heart failure (CHF). How should this underlying condition affect nursing care?

3. J.G. calls his oncology nurse 3 days after receiving the last dose of IL-2. He is complaining of dizziness, pruritus, and urinary retention. What should the nurse advise?

4. Eight days after receiving IL-2, J.G. experiences confusion and lethargy. Are these symptoms related to the IL-2? How should the client be treated?

39 Drugs for Upper Respiratory Disorders

Study Questions

Define the following:

1. Antihistamines

2. Antitussives

3. Decongestants

4. Expectorants

5. Rebound nasal congestion

Complete the following word search. Clues are given in questions 6-11. Circle your responses.

```
L  Q  A  D  P  R  U  O  F  O  T  O  W  T  A
A  N  Q  C  L  Z  I  Z  D  B  O  P  P  R  S
R  Q  K  S  U  X  Z  N  O  S  L  Z  E  T  E
Y  S  R  G  K  T  H  A  P  P  D  N  A  M  D
N  I  R  A  L  S  E  P  H  E  O  W  O  G  A
G  T  H  Y  D  T  A  R  T  T  F  N  D  J  T
I  I  A  I  P  T  B  C  H  Q  O  C  P  G  I
T  S  U  P  E  W  I  F  Y  I  J  E  P  A  O
I  U  P  K  F  R  V  S  C  R  N  E  J  K  N
S  N  I  K  T  L  U  B  B  J  A  I  I  Z  H
R  I  U  S  D  M  G  W  P  B  U  N  T  Q  L
I  S  N  P  K  V  G  N  U  G  H  G  I  I  N
L  O  E  L  F  L  E  F  M  R  U  X  V  R  S
C  C  O  M  M  O  N  C  O  L  D  G  B  K  U
N  C  E  Q  S  I  T  I  L  L  I  S  N  O  T
```

6. Upper respiratory tract infections include the following five conditions: _____, _____, _____, _____, and _____.

7. The most common cause of upper respiratory infections (URIs) is _____.

8. On average, adults have _____ to _____ colds per year.

9. When the H_1 receptor is stimulated, smooth muscle lining the nasal cavity is _____.

10. Second-generation antihistamines differ from first-generation antihistamines because they do not cause _____.

11. Clients taking antihistamines need to be monitored for signs and symptoms of _____ dysfunction.

12. After constant use of a nasal spray, _____ congestion is likely to occur.

13. Do NOT use nasal sprays for children less than _____ years of age.

14. The drug group that acts on the cough control center in the medulla is _____.

15. A nondrug expectorant available to everyone is _____.

16. In emergency situations such as anaphylaxis, antihistamines (are/are not) helpful. *(Circle correct answer.)*

17. Drug therapy for acute laryngitis has (minimal/optimal) impact on the condition. *(Circle correct answer.)*

18. List four health teaching points for individuals with the common cold:

    a.

    b.

    c.

    d.

NCLEX Review Questions

Select the best response.

19. Antihistamines, another group of drugs used for the relief of cold symptoms, have _____ properties that result in decreased secretions.
    a. cholinergic
    b. anticholinergic
    c. analgesic
    d. antitussive

20. Compared to first-generation antihistamines, second-generation antihistamines have a lower incidence of which of the following?
    a. vomiting
    b. tinnitus
    c. drowsiness
    d. headache

21. The FDA has ordered removal of all cold remedies containing which of the following drugs?
    a. propranolol
    b. dextromethorphan
    c. guaifenesin
    d. phenylpropanolamine

Situation: R.T., age 20, is experiencing acute rhinitis, and diphenhydramine (Benadryl) has been prescribed. Questions 22 to 26 refer to this situation.

22. The recommended dose of Benadryl is:
    a. 25-50 mg q4-6h.
    b. 25-50 mg daily.
    c. 50-100 mg q4-6h.
    d. 100 mg daily.

23. Benadryl also has which of the following effects?
    a. antihypertensive
    b. anticoagulant
    c. antitussive
    d. anticonvulsant

24. Benadryl, a/an _____ blocker, competes with histamine for the receptor site.
    a. H_1
    b. H_2
    c. B_1
    d. B_2

25. Since R.T. is breast-feeding her daughter, you would advise her that:
    a. large amounts of the drug pass into milk; breast-feeding is not recommended.
    b. the drug does not affect breast-feeding.
    c. small amounts of the drug pass into breast milk; breast-feeding is not recommended.
    d. breast-feeding is not recommended.

26. R.T.'s health teaching plan would include the side effects of Benadryl. Which of the following is NOT a side effect?
    a. drowsiness
    b. disturbed coordination
    c. urinary retention
    d. tinnitus

27. The advantage of systemic decongestants over nasal sprays and drops is that they:
    a. are less costly.
    b. provide longer relief.
    c. have fewer side effects.
    d. are preferred by elders.

28. An expectorant that is frequently an ingredient in cold remedies is:
    a. guaifenesin.
    b. ephedrine.
    c. hydrocodone.
    d. promethazine.

29. Nursing interventions for the common cold include:
    a. monitoring vital signs.
    b. observing color of bronchial secretions; antibiotics may be needed.
    c. monitoring reaction; codeine preparations for cough suppression can lead to physical dependence.
    d. all of the above.

30. The groups of drugs used to treat cold symptoms include which of the following? *Select all that apply.*
    a. decongestants
    b. antitussives
    c. expectorants
    d. indoles
    e. antihistamines.

31. Decongestants are contraindicated for clients with which of the following? *Select all that apply.*
    a. hyperthyroidism
    b. cardiac disease
    c. obesity
    d. diabetes mellitus
    e. hypertension

32. Which of the following is important to include in teaching a client who is taking medications for a common cold? Teach the client: *Select all that apply.*
    a. to use 4 puffs of nasal spray for a full 10 days.
    b. to read labels for OTC drugs for any interactions with current medications.
    c. that antibiotics are also needed to fight a common cold virus.
    d. not to drive during initial use of a cold remedy containing an antihistamine.
    e. to take cold remedies with a decongestant for a better night's sleep.

Critical Thinking Exercises

Use a separate sheet of paper for your answers.

S.Y. is 80 years old and complains, "My head is all filled up. I need something to open it up." A decongestant, Afrin, is ordered. S.Y. reports having numerous medications in the bathroom cabinet.

1. What is the recommended dose and schedule for administration of this drug?

2. What is the recommended length of time for use?

3. What possible side effects would you discuss with the client? Are they expected to increase or decrease with use of the drug?

4. Describe rebound nasal congestion. What preventive measures would you advise?

5. What are the dietary restrictions, if any?

6. What would you advise S.Y. about the use of OTC cold preparations?

40 Drugs for Lower Respiratory Disorders

Study Questions

Define the following:

1. Bronchodilator

2. Bronchospasm

3. Glucocorticoids

4. Mucolytic

Complete the following:

5. The substance responsible for maintaining bronchodilation is _____.

6. In acute bronchospasm caused by anaphylaxis, the drug administered subcutaneously to promote bronchodilation and elevate the blood pressure is _____.

7. The first line of defense in an acute asthmatic attack are the drugs categorized as _____.

8. Isuprel, one of the first drugs to treat bronchospasm, is a (selective/nonselective) beta$_2$ agonist. *(Circle correct answer.)*

9. Sympathomimetics cause dilation of the bronchioles by increasing _____.

10. Theophylline (increases/decreases) the risk of digitalis toxicity. *(Circle correct answer.)*

11. When theophylline and beta$_2$-adrenergic agonists are given together, a _____ effect can occur.

12. The half-life of theophylline is (shorter/longer) for smokers than for nonsmokers. *(Circle correct answer.)*

13. Aminophylline, theophylline, and caffeine are _____ derivatives used to treat _____.

14. The drug commonly prescribed to treat unresponsive asthma is _____.

15. Cromolyn (Intal) is used as _____ treatment for bronchial asthma. It acts by inhibiting the release of _____.

16. A serious side effect of cromolyn is _____.

17. The newer drugs for asthma are more selective for _____ receptors.

18. The leukotriene receptor antagonist considered safe for use in children 6 years and older is _____.

19. The preferred time of day for the administration of Singulair is _____.

20. The usual dose of Singulair for an adult is _____ and for a child is _____ administered without food.

21. A group of drugs used to liquefy and loosen thick mucous secretions is _____.

22. With infection resulting from retained mucous secretions, a/an _____ may be prescribed.

NCLEX Review Questions

Select the best response.

Situation: E.B., 54 years old, is receiving treatment for chronic obstructive pulmonary disease (COPD). Questions 23 to 25 refer to this situation.

23. E.B.'s medication is delivered via a metered-dose inhaler. Related health teaching would include which one of the following?
    a. Test the inhaler first to see if the spray works.
    b. Shake the inhaler well just before use.
    c. Refrigerate the inhaler.
    d. Hold the inhaler upside down.

24. Which of the following is NOT true about inhaler drug dose?
    a. lower than an oral dose
    b. higher than an oral dose
    c. fewer side effects than an oral dose
    d. onset of action more rapid than that of an oral dose

25. Remind E.B. to wait _____ minute(s) after using a bronchodilator before using the glucocorticoid preparation.
    a. 1
    b. 3
    c. 5
    d. 10

Situation: M.M. is brought to the emergency department with an acute asthmatic attack. Questions 26 to 33 refer to this situation.

26. M.M. was given an IV loading dose of aminophylline. He is now receiving oral Theo-Dur. This medication is generally scheduled to be taken:
    a. q2h.
    b. q3-4h.
    c. q6-12h.
    d. daily.

27. The usual adult dose of Theo-Dur is:
    a. 100-200 mg q8-12h.
    b. 200-300 mg q8-12h.
    c. 300-400 mg q8-12h.
    d. 400-500 mg q8-12h.

28. The nurse knows that it is essential to keep the serum theophylline level within which of the following ranges?
    a. 10-20 mcg/ml
    b. 20-30 mcg/ml
    c. 30-40 mcg/ml
    d. 40-50 mcg/ml

29. Which one of the following side effects is NOT associated with Theo-Dur?
    a. tachycardia
    b. insomnia and restlessness
    c. cardiac dysrhythmias
    d. urinary retention

30. Dietary influences for M.M. include all of the following EXCEPT:
    a. increased metabolism with low-carbohydrate diet.
    b. decreased elimination with high-carbohydrate diet.
    c. increased elimination with high-carbohydrate diet.
    d. increased metabolism with high-protein diet.

31. Which one of the following is NOT a contraindication for the use of Theo-Dur?
    a. hypertension
    b. severe cardiac dysrhythmias
    c. peptic ulcer disease
    d. uncontrolled seizure disorder

32. Specific nursing interventions for Theo-Dur include all of the following EXCEPT:
    a. provide hydration.
    b. monitor vital signs.
    c. observe for confusion.
    d. weigh daily.

33. M.M.'s health teaching plan includes avoidance of all of the following EXCEPT:
    a. smoking.
    b. fluid intake.
    c. OTC products.
    d. caffeine products.

34. Which one of the following is NOT a side effect of long-term use of glucocorticoids?
    a. hypoglycemia
    b. impaired immune response
    c. fluid retention
    d. hyperglycemia

35. The anticholinergic drug _____ has few systemic effects and is administered by aerosol.
    a. Amcort
    b. Aristocort
    c. Atrovent
    d. Theo-Dur

36. Drug selection and dosage for older adults with an asthmatic condition need to be considered. The use of large, continuous doses of a beta$_2$-adrenergic agonist may cause which side effect in the older adult?
    a. urinary retention
    b. bronchoconstriction
    c. constipation
    d. tachycardia

37. Which of the following herbs should be avoided by clients taking theophylline products?
    a. feverfew
    b. ephedra
    c. ginkgo
    d. garlic

38. When the client who has COPD has questions about using the inhaler, which of the following should the nurse include in a review of inhaler administration? *Select all that apply.*
    a. Keep lips secure around mouthpiece and inhale while pushing top of canister once.
    b. Hold breath for a few seconds, remove mouthpiece, and exhale slowly.
    c. Wait 5 minutes and repeat the procedure if a second inhalation is required.
    d. Cleanse all washable parts of inhaler equipment daily.
    e. Teach client to monitor heart rate.

39. Health teaching for the client who has COPD also includes that frequent use of bronchodilators may lead to which of the following? *Select all that apply.*
    a. bradycardia
    b. nervousness
    c. tremors
    d. insomnia
    e. palpitations

40. Which of the following are known to have a drug interaction with Theo-Dur? *Select all that apply.*
    a. beta-blockers
    b. digitalis
    c. stool softeners
    d. lithium
    e. phenytoin

Critical Thinking Exercises

Use a separate sheet of paper for your answers.

Sarah, age 15, has severe asthma. She is being treated with theophylline and an inhaled glucocorticoid.

1. Are inhaled glucocorticoids the treatment of choice for severe asthmatic attacks? Explain.

2. When should theophylline be taken in relation to food?

3. What are the possible side effects associated with oral inhalers? What may prevent or diminish these side effects?

4. Steroid use for prolonged periods is likely to cause which side effects?

5. List at least three nursing interventions associated with bronchodilators.

    a.

    b.

    c.

6. List at least three points to be included in Sarah's health teaching.

    a.

    b.

    c.

41 Cardiac Glycosides, Antianginals, and Antidysrhythmics

Study Questions

Crossword puzzle: Use the definition to determine the pharmacologic/physiologic term.

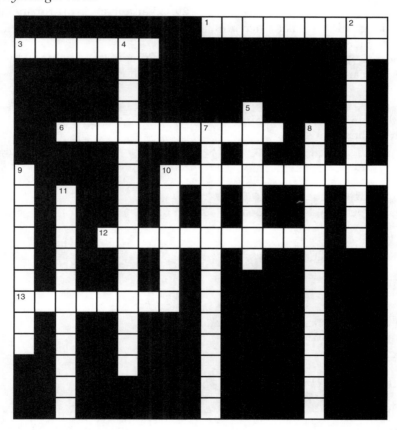

Across

1. Peripheral vascular resistance
3. Amount of blood in the ventricle at the end of diastole
6. Pulse rate below 60 beats/min
10. Increased carbon dioxide in the blood
12. Low serum potassium level
13. Lack of blood supply to the (heart) muscle

Down

2. Drug category used to treat angina pectoris
4. Drug group used to treat disturbed heart rhythm
5. Drug group used to control angina pain by relaxing coronary vessels
7. Myocardium at rest
8. Myocardial contraction
9. Cardiac _____ causes cardiac muscles to contract more efficiently
10. Lack of oxygen to body tissues
11. Pulse rate above 100 beats/min

Complete the following:

14. Heart failure occurs when the myocardium (strengthens/weakens) and (shrinks/enlarges), which causes the heart to lose its ability to pump blood through the heart and circulatory system. *(Circle correct answers.)*

15. With heart failure there is a/an (increase/decrease) in preload and afterload. *(Circle correct answer.)*

16. Another name for heart failure is _____ failure.

17. Cardiac glycosides are also called _____ _____ .

18. The action of antianginal drugs is to increase blood flow and to (increase/decrease) oxygen supply or to (increase/decrease) oxygen demand by the myocardium. *(Circle correct answers.)*

19. Name three of the four effects of digitalis preparations on the heart muscle (myocardium): _____, _____, and _____ .

20. Beta blockers and calcium channel blockers (decrease/increase) the workload of the heart. *(Circle correct answer.)*

21. Nitroglycerin (NTG) is not swallowed because _____, thereby decreasing it effectiveness.

22. NTG sublingually acts within _____ minutes. Administration may be repeated _____ times.

23. The most common side effect of NTG is _____ .

24. The drug group that may be used as an antianginal, antidysrhythmic, and antihypertensive is _____ .

25. A calcium channel blocker that is effective in the long-term treatment of angina and has the side effect of bradycardia is _____ .

26. Beta blockers and calcium channel blockers should not be discontinued without health care provider approval. Withdrawal symptoms may include _____ and _____ .

27. Classic angina occurs when the client is _____ .

28. Unstable angina (preinfarction) has the following pattern of occurrence: _____ .

29. Variant angina (Prinzmetal's angina) occurs when the client _____ .

30. Prinzmetal's angina is due to _____ of the vessels.

31. The major systemic effect of nitrates is _____ .

32. List four nonpharmacologic means to decrease anginal attacks:

    a.

    b.

    c.

    d.

33. Cardiac dysrhythmias can result from (hypoxia/hyperoxia) and (hypocapnia/hypercapnia). *(Circle correct answers.)*

34. Examples of antidysrhythmics include
_____, _____, and
_____.

35. Clients taking antidysrhythmics should avoid
_____ and _____.

Matching
The nurse should obtain a history of herbs the client is taking. This is especially true for clients taking digoxin. Match the herbs with their effects on digoxin.

Herb		**Effect on Digoxin**
____ 36.	St. John's wort	a. increased risk of digitalis toxicity
____ 37.	ephedra	b. decreased digoxin absorption
____ 38.	Metamucil	c. decreased effects of digoxin
____ 39.	aloe	d. falsely elevated digoxin levels
____ 40.	goldenseal	
____ 41.	ginseng	

NCLEX Review Questions

Select the best response.

42. Digitalis preparations are effective for treating:
    a. bowel obstruction.
    b. congestive heart failure (CHF).
    c. thrombophlebitis.
    d. urinary tract infection.

43. Phosphodiesterase inhibitors are used to treat CHF by inhibiting the enzyme phosphodiesterase. These agents promote:
    a. positive inotropic response.
    b. negative inotropic response.
    c. vasoconstriction.
    d. increased serum sodium and potassium levels.

44. An example of a phosphodiesterase inhibitor is:
    a. digoxin.
    b. isosorbide dinitrate (Isordil).
    c. amlodipine (Norvasc).
    d. inamrinone lactate (Inocor).

45. Dysrhythmia means:
    a. absence of heart rhythm.
    b. disturbed heart rhythm.
    c. heart rhythm greater than 200 beats/min.
    d. functional heart rate.

46. Quinidine was the first antidysrhythmic used to treat cardiac dysrhythmias; however, it has many side effects. Procainamide (Pronestyl, Procanbid), another antidysrhythmic, causes less cardiac depression than quinidine. Both of these drugs are classified as:
    a. beta blockers.
    b. calcium channel blockers.
    c. fast sodium channel blocker IB.
    d. fast sodium channel blocker IA.

47. The effects of quinidine and procainamide are that they:
    a. slow conduction and shorten repolarization.
    b. slow conduction and prolong repolarization.
    c. increase conduction and prolong repolarization.
    d. increase conduction and shorten repolarization.

48. Propranolol (Inderal) is a:
    a. nonselective beta blocker.
    b. cardioselective beta blocker.
    c. calcium channel blocker.
    d. fast sodium blocker.

49. An antidysrhythmic drug used during life-threatening situations to convert ventricular fibrillation to normal sinus rhythm when lidocaine and procainamide are ineffective is:
    a. phenytoin (Dilantin).
    b. tocainide.
    c. atropine.
    d. bretylium.

50. The action of antidysrhythmics includes all of the following EXCEPT:
    a. block adrenergic stimulation of the heart.
    b. increase myocardial contractility.
    c. decrease myocardial contractility.
    d. increase recovery time of the myocardium.

51. The antidysrhythmic drug lidocaine (Xylocaine) is used primarily for the treatment of:
    a. bradycardia.
    b. ventricular dysrhythmias.
    c. atrial dysrhythmias.
    d. heart block.

52. A common problem with the use of verapamil is:
    a. tachycardia.
    b. bradycardia.
    c. headache.
    d. nausea.

53. The most potent calcium blocker is:
    a. nicardipine (Cardene).
    b. diltiazem (Cardizem).
    c. verapamil (Calan).
    d. nifedipine (Procardia).

54. Clients taking calcium blockers need to have which of the following laboratory values monitored?
    a. BUN
    b. creatinine
    c. liver enzymes
    d. urinary output

Situation I: J.H., 80 years old, is taking digoxin daily along with several other medications. Questions 55 to 65 refer to this situation.

55. Atrial natriuretic peptide (ANP) and brain natriuretic peptide (BNP) laboratory tests were ordered to determine if J.H.'s health problem was:
    a. emphysema.
    b. peptic ulcer.
    c. colon cancer.
    d. heart failure.

56. J.H's BNP was 420 pg/ml. His BNP is considered:
    a. within normal/reference range.
    b. slightly elevated.
    c. markedly elevated.
    d. within normal/reference range for his age.

57. Digitalis preparations are effective in treating all of the following conditions EXCEPT:
    a. CHF.
    b. atrial flutter.
    c. emphysema.
    d. atrial fibrillation.

58. The usual maintenance dose of digoxin is:
    a. 0.125-0.5 mg/day.
    b. 0.5-1 mg/day.
    c. 0.04-0.06 mg/day.
    d. 0.4-0.6 mg/day.

59. J.H.'s serum digoxin level should be within the range of:
    a. 0.15-0.5 ng/ml.
    b. 0.5-2 ng/ml.
    c. 2-3.5 ng/ml.
    d. 3.5-4 ng/ml.

60. You assess J.H. for all of the following signs and symptoms of digitalis toxicity EXCEPT:
    a. anorexia.
    b. diarrhea.
    c. bradycardia.
    d. visual disturbances.

61. An antidote for digitalis toxicity is:
    a. protamine.
    b. vitamin K.
    c. digoxin immune Fab.
    d. gamma globulin.

62. The drugs that alter the action of digoxin include all of the following EXCEPT:
    a. furosemide (Lasix).
    b. cortisone.
    c. nitroglycerin.
    d. potassium-wasting diuretics.

63. Specific nursing interventions include taking J.H.'s pulse at the:
    a. radial site for 30 seconds.
    b. radial site for 60 seconds.
    c. apical site for 30 seconds.
    d. apical site for 60 seconds.

64. You would NOT advise J.H. to include which of the following foods in his diet?
    a. fruits
    b. potatoes
    c. fruit juice
    d. sausage

65. J.H.'s teaching plan may NOT include:
    a. take blood pressure daily.
    b. read drug labels carefully.
    c. eat foods high in potassium.
    d. report pulse rate <60 beats/min.

66. Other drugs that may be used to treat heart failure include all of the following EXCEPT:
    a. vasodilators.
    b. angiotensin-converting enzyme (ACE) inhibitors.
    c. beta blockers.
    d. diuretics.

Situation II: B.A. is receiving NTG sublingually for anginal pain. Questions 67 to 72 refer to this situation.

67. You monitor B.A.'s vital signs. Which of the following is associated with antianginal drugs?
    a. hypotension
    b. hypertension
    c. increased heart rate
    d. decreased heart rate

68. You assess B.A. for the most common side effect of NTG, which is:
    a. faintness.
    b. dizziness.
    c. headache.
    d. weakness.

69. Health teaching for B.A. includes all of the following EXCEPT:
    a. a biting sensation indicates that the NTG tablet is fresh.
    b. store NTG away from light.
    c. the contents of an opened bottle of NTG remain effective for approximately 6 months.
    d. if pain persists after five tablets, notify the health care provider immediately.

70. Later, a Nitro transdermal patch was prescribed for B.A. How often is the patch applied?
    a. every 6 hours
    b. every 12 hours
    c. every 24 hours
    d. every 48 hours

71. Also prescribed for B.A. was atenolol (Tenormin) 50 mg daily. Atenolol is a/an:
    a. nonselective beta blocker.
    b. cardioselective beta blocker.
    c. calcium channel blocker.
    d. adrenergic stimulant.

72. The nurse evaluates the effects of atenolol on angina by:
    a. asking B.A. if the presence of angina pain has subsided.
    b. checking for the presence of bronchoconstriction because of atenolol.
    c. determining if B.A.'s urinary output has decreased.
    d. monitoring B.A.'s blood pressure for hypertension.

Situation III: S.W. is taking acebutolol (Sectral) 200 mg b.i.d. for irregular heart rate. Questions 73 to 77 refer to this situation.

73. S.W. asks the nurse how often she should take the drug. The nurse replies:
    a. once a day.
    b. twice a day.
    c. three times a day.
    d. every other day.

74. Acebutolol (Sectral) is a:
    a. nonselective beta blocker.
    b. cardioselective beta blocker.
    c. calcium channel blocker.
    d. fast sodium channel blocker.

75. The nurse instructs S.W. that, when stopping Sectral, she should:
    a. notify the doctor within a week after stopping the drug.
    b. ask a friend or family member to loan her a tablet until the drug can be refilled.
    c. not abruptly stop taking Sectral to prevent an adverse reaction.
    d. have the drug refilled no later than a month after taking the last dose.

76. The nurse informs S.W. of all the following side effects of Sectral EXCEPT:
    a. dizziness.
    b. nausea.
    c. possible impotence.
    d. hypertension.

77. A month later the nurse evaluates S.W.'s response to Sectral. The nurse should check all of the following EXCEPT:
    a. vital signs.
    b. presence of side effects.
    c. compliance (whether S.W. is taking the drug as ordered).
    d. urinary output.

78. The nursing interventions related to digoxin administration include the following: *Select all that apply.*
    a. Check the apical pulse rate before administering digoxin.
    b. Check the sodium level before administering digoxin.
    c. Instruct the client to report side effects of digoxin such as pulse rate greater than 100 beats/min.
    d. Advise the client who is taking a potassium-wasting diuretic such as thiazide to eat foods rich in potassium.
    e. Advise the client to avoid taking the herb St. John's wort because it can decrease the absorption of digoxin.

79. The nurse is administering the nitrate drug for angina pectoris. The nursing interventions would include the following: *Select all that apply.*
    a. Instruct the client to swallow the sublingual nitrate during chest pain.
    b. Inform the client that headaches may occur when first taking a nitrate product.
    c. Instruct the client not to ingest alcohol while taking a nitrate drug.
    d. A subQ nitroglycerin 0.4 mg could be taken every 30 minutes during chest pain.
    e. If the chest pain is not alleviated with nitroglycerin tablet after repeating the dose three times, the health care provider should be immediately notified.

80. Cardiac dysrhythmias can result from which of the following: *Select all that apply.*
    a. hypoxia
    b. hypocapnia
    c. electrolyte imbalance
    d. excess catecholamines
    e. vertigo

81. The client is prescribed acebutolol (Sectral) 0.4 g, b.i.d. for the treatment of ventricular dysrhythmias.
    Available: acebutolol 200 mg capsule
    Question: How many capsule(s) would you give per dose?
    Answer: _____

Critical Thinking Exercises

Use a separate sheet of paper for your answers.

J.B., 61 years old, has had several attacks of angina pectoris. J.B. has nitroglycerin gr $\frac{1}{150}$ sublingual tablets to relieve acute attacks, and metoprolol (Lopressor) 25 mg b.i.d. was prescribed. Vital signs: BP 154/88 mm Hg, P 82 beats/min, R 26 breaths/min.

1. From which of the following NTG bottles should J.B. take his medication?

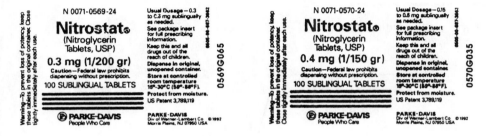

2. What are the nursing interventions for J.B. regarding the use of NTG tablets?

3. Why should J.B.'s vital signs be monitored?

4. What are the similarities and differences of metoprolol tartrate and propranolol hydrochloride? Which drug should a client with asthma take? Why?

5. Metoprolol tartrate and propranolol hydrochloride can be prescribed for what other cardiac conditions?

6. What nonpharmacologic measures should the nurse include in the health teaching for J.B.? J.B.'s antianginal drug was changed to diltiazem 60 mg t.i.d.

7. How does this drug compare to other calcium channel blockers?

8. Is the diltiazem dose within the normal range? What is the maximum daily dose?

42 Diuretics

Study Questions

Indicate which diuretic group acts on the segment of the renal tubule in the figure below:

a.
b.
c.
d.
e.

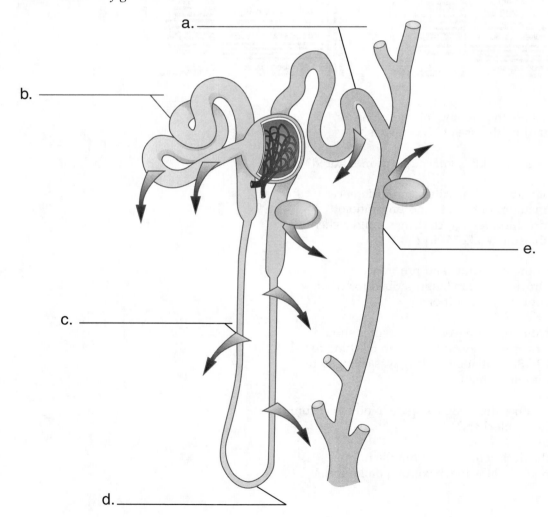

Define the following:

1. Diuresis

2. Hyperglycemia

3. Hyperkalemia

4. Natriuresis

5. Oliguria

6. Osmolality

7. Potassium-wasting diuretics

Complete the following:

8. The two main purposes for the use of diuretics are _____ and _____ .

9. Diuretics act by inhibiting sodium and water (retention/reabsorption) from the kidney (ureters/tubules). *(Circle correct answers.)*

10. Five groups of diuretics are _____, _____, _____, _____, and _____ .

11. Thiazide and loop (high-ceiling) diuretics cause the loss of the cellular electrolyte _____ .

12. The most serious thiazide drug interaction occurs with the digitalis preparation _____. It may result in _____ _____ .

13. Loop diuretics have (little/much) effect on blood sugar. *(Circle correct answer.)*

14. Diuretics that promote potassium retention are called potassium-_____ diuretics.

15. Potassium-sparing diuretics are (weaker/ stronger) than thiazides and loop diuretics. *(Circle correct answer.)*

16. Potassium-sparing diuretics interfere with the sodium-potassium pump that is controlled by the mineralocorticoid hormone _____ .

17. The main side/adverse effect of potassium-sparing diuretics is (hypokalemia/ hyperkalemia). *(Circle correct answer.)*

18. Currently, a combination drug of potassium-wasting and potassium-sparing agents is frequently prescribed, such as _____ .

19. When a combination of diuretics is used, the dosage of each is usually (less/more) than the dose of one drug. *(Circle correct answer.)*

20. Mannitol is the most frequently prescribed _____ diuretic.

21. Carbonic anhydrase inhibitors (decrease/ increase) intraocular pressure in clients with glaucoma. *(Circle correct answer.)*

List the possible abnormal serum chemistry test results associated with thiazides.

Laboratory Test	**Abnormal Results**
22. Potassium	
23. Magnesium	
24. Calcium	
25. Chloride	
26. Bicarbonate	
27. Uric acid	
28. Blood sugar	
29. Blood lipids	

NCLEX Review Questions

Select the best response.

30. Diuretics, as the first line of antihypertensive drugs, are generally ordered for clients with systolic pressures greater than:
   a.   130 mm Hg.
   b.   140 mm Hg.
   c.   150 mm Hg.
   d.   160 mm Hg.

31. Which of the following groups of diuretics is NOT frequently prescribed to treat hypertension and congestive heart failure?
   a.   osmotic
   b.   potassium-sparing
   c.   loop
   d.   thiazides

32. When compared with thiazides, loop (high-ceiling) diuretics:
   a.   are more effective as antihypertensives.
   b.   are more potent as diuretics.
   c.   promote potassium absorption.
   d.   cause calcium reabsorption.

33. Herb-diuretic interaction should be assessed by the nurse. An herb that may increase the blood pressure when it is taken with thiazide diuretics is:
   a.   St. John's wort.
   b.   licorice.
   c.   ginkgo.
   d.   ginger.

34. The pharmacologic action of Aldactone is to:
   a.   increase potassium and sodium excretion.
   b.   promote potassium retention and sodium excretion.
   c.   promote potassium, sodium, and calcium retention.
   d.   promote potassium excretion and sodium retention.

Situation: B.T. had an acute myocardial infarction (AMI) 6 months ago. He was prescribed spironolactone (Aldactone) 25 mg daily to aid in treating an irregular heart rate. Questions 35 to 39 relate to B.T.

35. Spironolactone (Aldactone) is a:
   a.   potassium-wasting diuretic.
   b.   potassium-sparing diuretic.
   c.   osmotic diuretic.
   d.   thiazide diuretic.

36. The purpose of prescribing Aldactone for B.T. is to:
    a. retain more sodium for heart contraction.
    b. excrete potassium to lessen circulatory (serum) potassium level.
    c. retain circulatory (serum) potassium for the heart muscle.
    d. retain calcium for heart contraction.

37. B.T. requests assistance with his diet. Which of the following foods would you NOT recommend?
    a. lean meat
    b. bananas
    c. apples
    d. squash

38. When evaluating the effects of Aldactone, the nurse should check the:
    a. serum potassium level.
    b. complete blood count (CBC).
    c. serum lipoproteins.
    d. blood glucose level.

39. B.T.'s serum potassium level should be monitored periodically. If the serum potassium level is 5.5 mEq/L, what intervention should be considered?
    a. The Aldactone dose should be reduced or stopped and the client instructed to decrease intake of foods rich in potassium.
    b. The Aldactone dose should be continued and the client encouraged to eat fruits, vegetables, and meats.
    c. The Aldactone dose should be increased and the client instructed to decrease foods rich in potassium.
    d. Instruct the client to continue the prescribed Aldactone dose and report any signs or symptoms of hypokalemia.

Situation: M.J. is taking acetazolamide (Diamox) 500 mg daily for the treatment of glaucoma. Questions 40 to 42 relate to this situation.

40. Acetazolamide (Diamox) is prescribed for:
    a. open-angle glaucoma.
    b. narrow-angle glaucoma.
    c. acute glaucoma.
    d. acute heart failure.

41. What type of acid-base imbalance could occur if M.J. is taking high doses of Diamox or with constant use of the drug?
    a. respiratory acidosis
    b. respiratory alkalosis
    c. metabolic alkalosis
    d. metabolic acidosis

42. A mountain climber has been prescribed to take Diamox with her for:
    a. maintaining potassium levels.
    b. preventing high-altitude sickness.
    c. preventing dehydration.
    d. increasing endurance when climbing mountains.

Situation: J.H., 80 years old, is under treatment for hypertension and congestive heart failure. Hydrochlorothiazide (HydroDIURIL) is one of his medications. Questions 43 to 53 refer to this situation.

43. HydroDIURIL is generally scheduled to be taken:
    a. q2h.
    b. q4h.
    c. q6h.
    d. daily.

44. The usual dose of HydroDIURIL is:
    a. 25-100 mg/day.
    b. 100-150 mg/day.
    c. 150-200 mg/day.
    d. 200-250 mg/day.

45. The optimal time to administer diuretics is:
    a.   at bedtime.
    b.   with meals.
    c.   on an empty stomach.
    d.   in the morning.

46. While J.H. is taking HydroDIURIL, monitoring of all of the following laboratory values is required EXCEPT:
    a.   serum calcium.
    b.   uric acid.
    c.   blood sugar.
    d.   alkaline phosphatase.

47. When taking HydroDIURIL, which of the following laboratory values should also be monitored?
    a.   serum cholesterol
    b.   BUN
    c.   low-density lipoprotein
    d.   triglycerides

48. You assess J.H. for side effects, which include all of the following EXCEPT:
    a.   electrolyte imbalances.
    b.   dizziness.
    c.   diarrhea.
    d.   headache.

49. Thiazides can cause all of the following drug-lab interactions EXCEPT:
    a.   enhance action of lithium.
    b.   enhance hypertensive state when used with alcohol.
    c.   potentiate other antihypertensives.
    d.   cause hypokalemia.

50. You would recommend that J.H. include all of the following fruits in his diet EXCEPT:
    a.   oranges.
    b.   dates.
    c.   apples.
    d.   bananas.

51. The health teaching plan for J.H. includes all of the following EXCEPT:
    a.   maintaining nutrition.
    b.   advising the client to arise slowly to a standing position.
    c.   monitoring pulse and respiratory rates.
    d.   weighing daily.

52. Thiazides are contraindicated for use in clients with which of the following?
    a.   emphysema
    b.   arteriosclerotic cardiovascular disease
    c.   renal failure
    d.   liver failure

53. As a nurse, you would encourage clients taking a loop (high-ceiling) diuretic to including the following foods in their diet: *Select all that apply.*
    a.   fresh and dry fruits
    b.   ice cream
    c.   potato skins
    d.   peanut butter
    e.   bread

54. Nursing intervention(s) for clients who are hypertensive and receiving a thiazide diuretic would include: *Select all that apply.*
    a.   Assess extremities for pitted edema.
    b.   Monitor lung sounds.
    c.   Monitor laboratory results.
    d.   Encourage fluids.
    e.   Monitor vital signs.

55. The client is hyptertensive and receiving hydrochlorothiazide 75 mg per day.

    Available:

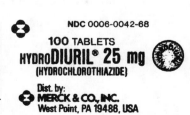

    USUAL ADULT DOSAGE: 2 to 4 tablets daily. See accompanying circular. Keep container tightly closed. Protect from light, moisture, freezing. −20°C (−4°F) and store at room temperature, 15-30°C (59-86°F). Dispense in a tight container. CAUTION: Federal (USA) law prohibits dispensing without prescription. This is a bulk package and not intended for dispensing. 100 No. 3263 7833217

    NDC 0006-0042-68
    100 TABLETS
    HYDRODIURIL® 25 mg
    (HYDROCHLOROTHIAZIDE)
    Dist. by:
    MERCK & CO., INC.
    West Point, PA 19486, USA

    You would give _____ tablet(s) per day.

Critical Thinking Exercises

Use a separate sheet of paper for your answers.

A.D., age 56, is hypertensive. She has maturity-onset diabetes mellitus. Vital signs: BP 162/90 mm Hg, P 90 beats/min, R 24 breaths/min. A.D. was prescribed hydrochlorothiazide (HydroDIURIL) 50 mg daily.

1. A.D. is prescribed an oral antidiabetic (hypoglycemic) drug. Why should A.D.'s blood glucose level be closely monitored?

2. What type of diuretic is hydrochlorothiazide (HydroDIURIL)?

3. What are the similarities and differences in the actions of thiazide diuretics and loop diuretics?

4. What are the similarities and differences of thiazide diuretics and loop diuretics in their blood chemistry (i.e., electrolytes, uric acid, and blood glucose levels)?

5. If A.D.'s serum calcium level was 12.5 mg/dl, which diuretic should she avoid? Why?

6. What are four client teaching strategies that should be included in A.D.'s care?

   a.

   b.

   c.

   d.

Digoxin 0.25 mg daily was added to her drug regimen. Her serum potassium level is 3.7 mEq/L.

7. What is the average serum potassium range? Why should A.D.'s serum potassium level be closely monitored?

8. What are the signs and symptoms of digitalis toxicity?

9. What groups of diuretics can affect electrolyte balance?

10. When is it a benefit to use the combination of potassium-wasting and potassium-sparing diuretics?

43 Antihypertensives

Study Questions

Define the following:

1. Alpha-adrenergic blockers

2. Beta-adrenergic blockers

3. Calcium channel blockers

4. Angiotensin-converting enzyme (ACE) inhibitors

5. Angiotensin II receptor blockers (ARBs)

Complete the following:

6. The hormones atrial natriuretic peptide (ANP) and brain natriuretic peptide (BNP) are released by the _____ of the heart when the volume (decreases/overloads) within the heart chambers. *(Circle correct answer.)*

7. Four causes of essential hypertension are _____, _____, _____, and _____ .

8. Nonpharmacologic measures to decrease blood pressure include _____ , _____ , _____ , and _____ .

9. When hypertension cannot be controlled by nonpharmacologic means, antihypertensive drugs may be prescribed. Three of the sympatholytic groups are _____ , _____ , and _____ .

10. Three additional categories of antihypertensives in addition to the sympatholytics are _____ , _____ , and _____ .

11. The Joint National Committee on Prevention, Detection, Evaluation, and Treatment of High Blood Pressure (JNC-7) uses three classifications for defining elevated systolic blood pressure (SBP): _____ , _____ , and _____ .

12. The most common antihypertensive agent for treating stage I hypertension is the _____ .

13. Thiazide diuretics may be combined with other antihypertensive agents such as _____ and _____ .

14. Many antihypertensive drugs can cause fluid retention. To decrease body fluid, what drug group is often administered with antihypertensive drugs? _____

15. ACE inhibitors may be combined with the antihypertensive agent _____ .

16. A client with a blood pressure of 182/105 mm Hg has what stage of hypertension according to JNC-7? _____

17. Beta-adrenergic blockers reduce cardiac output by diminishing the sympathetic nervous system response. With continued use of beta blockers, vascular resistance is (increased/diminished) and blood pressure is (lowered/increased). *(Circle correct answers.)*

18. The cultural group that does not respond well to beta blockers or ACE inhibitors is _____ .

19. Atenolol and metoprolol are examples of (cardioselective/noncardioselective) antihypertensive drugs. *(Circle correct answer.)*

20. The generic names for beta blockers end with which four letters? _____

21. The alpha blockers are useful in treating hypertensive clients with lipid abnormalities. The effects they have on lipoproteins include _____ and _____ .

22. An example of a cardioselective alpha blocker is _____ .

23. Two direct-acting arteriolar vasodilators for treating acute hypertensive emergencies are _____ and _____ .

24. The newest group of antihypertensive drugs that are prescribed when clients cannot take ACE inhibitors is _____ .

25. A frequent side effect of ACE inhibitors is _____ .

Match the generic drug name with the category of antihypertensive.

Drug	Antihypertensive Category
____ 26. captopril	a. beta blocker
____ 27. verapamil	b. selective alpha blocker
____ 28. prazosin	c. angiotensin antagonist (ACE inhibitor)
____ 29. methyldopa	
____ 30. hydralazine	d. calcium blocker
____ 31. candesartan	e. centrally acting sympatholytic
	f. direct-acting vasodilator
	g. angiotensin II receptor antagonist (A-II blocker)

Give the rationale for the nursing interventions related to ACE inhibitors.

Nursing Intervention	Rationale
32. Monitor vital signs.	32.
33. Monitor WBC, BUN, serum creatinine, protein, potassium, and blood glucose levels.	33.
34. Inform client that dizziness and lightheadedness may occur during the first week.	34.
35. Instruct the client not to discontinue ACE inhibitor abruptly without notifying health care provider.	35.
36. Instruct the client to report bruising, petechiae, and/or bleeding.	36.
37. Instruct the client to take the drug 20 minutes to 1 hour before meals.	37.

NCLEX Review Questions

Select the best response.

38. The JNC-7 developed new guidelines for determining hypertension. The category for prehypertension is:
    a. less than 120 mm Hg/less than 80 mm Hg.
    b. 120-139 mm Hg/80-89 mm Hg.
    c. 140-159 mm Hg/90-99 mm Hg.
    d. greater than 160 mm Hg/greater than 100 mm Hg.

39. Another name for the cardioselective beta-adrenergic blocker is:
    a. alpha blocker agent.
    b. beta blocker agent.
    c. alpha-beta blocker agent.
    d. beta-angiotensin agent.

40. The nonselective alpha-adrenergic blockers are useful for:
    a. treating mild to moderate hypertension.
    b. treating severe hypertension caused by adrenal medulla tumor.
    c. preventing hyperlipidemia.
    d. administration with all drugs.

41. Direct-acting vasodilators used to treat hypertension act on:
    a. smooth muscles of the blood vessels.
    b. skeletal muscles.
    c. renal tubules.
    d. cardiac valves.

42. With use of direct-acting vasodilators, sodium and water are retained, and peripheral edema occurs. A drug category that is given to avoid fluid retention is:
    a. anticoagulants.
    b. antidysrhythmics.
    c. cardiac glycosides.
    d. diuretics.

43. Which of the following is NOT an action of A-II blockers (ARBs)?
    a. blocks angiotensin II
    b. increases sodium retention
    c. causes vasodilation
    d. decreases peripheral resistance

44. An angiotensin receptor blocker (ARB) can be combined with the thiazide diuretic HydroDIURIL. The purpose of combining these two drugs is to:
    a. decrease rapid blood pressure drop.
    b. promote potassium retention.
    c. enhance the antihypertensive effect by promoting sodium and water loss.
    d. increase sodium and water retention for controlling blood pressure.

45. Angiotensin II receptor blockers (ARBs or A-II blockers) may be prescribed for hypertensive clients instead of an ACE inhibitor. A common side effect of ACE inhibitors is:
    a. coughing.
    b. sneezing.
    c. dizziness.
    d. shortness of breath.

46. The use of ACE inhibitors is NOT effective for treating hypertension in the African-American population. This is because African-Americans:
    a. are susceptible to low-renin hypertension.
    b. respond mostly to loop and thiazide diuretics.
    c. are susceptible to high-renin hypertension.
    d. have increased sodium and water retention.

47. ACE inhibitors can be effective for treating hypertension in African-Americans if the ACE inhibitor is given with which other drug?
    a. beta blocker
    b. calcium blocker
    c. angiotensin II blocker
    d. diuretic

48. Herb-drug interactions may occur if the client is taking certain herb supplements. An herb history should be obtained. Use of ma huang or Ephedra with an antihypertensive drug may:

    a. increase the hypertensive state.

    b. decrease or counteract the effects of the antihypertensive drug.

    c. increase the hypotensive effects of the antihypertensive drug.

    d. not have any effect on the antihypertensive drug.

Situation: D.D., age 59, has essential hypertension. He is taking captopril 25 mg t.i.d. D.D. tells the health care provider that he feels fine, his blood pressure is within normal range, and he feels he does not need the drug. Questions 49 to 59 relate to this situation.

49. Captopril is from which group of antihypertensives?

    a. beta blocker

    b. calcium blocker

    c. direct-acting vasodilator

    d. angiotensin antagonist (ACE inhibitor)

50. The action of captopril is to:

    a. dilate the arteries.

    b. inhibit angiotensin II (a vasoconstrictor).

    c. increase sodium and water excretion.

    d. inhibit the alpha receptors.

51. The protein-binding power of captopril is:

    a. highly protein-bound.

    b. moderately to highly protein-bound.

    c. moderately protein-bound.

    d. low protein-bound.

52. If D.D. takes captopril with a highly protein-bound drug, what might occur?

    a. There is no drug displacement, because captopril is not highly protein-bound.

    b. There will be moderate drug displacement of captopril, which is moderately to highly protein-bound.

    c. Captopril and the highly protein-bound drug compete for protein sites.

    d. The concentration of captopril is increased.

53. What drug interaction could occur if D.D. takes captopril with nitrates, diuretics, or adrenergic blockers?

    a. hypertensive reaction

    b. hypotensive reaction

    c. no effect

    d. hypoglycemic reaction

54. Captopril may not be as effective with which of the following group(s) of people?

    a. children

    b. middle-age adults

    c. elderly

    d. Caucasian

55. If D.D. takes captopril with a potassium-sparing diuretic, what might occur?

    a. hypokalemia

    b. hyperkalemia

    c. hypocalcemia

    d. hypercalcemia

56. D.D. states that he wishes to stop taking the drug. How might the nurse respond?

    a. "Yes, you could stop taking captopril because your blood pressure has been normal."

    b. "Stop taking the drug for a month and see what happens."

    c. "Captopril is controlling your blood pressure and should not be stopped until you discuss this with the health care provider."

    d. "Stop taking captopril, exercise, and avoid salt."

57. D.D.'s antihypertensive drug was changed to nifedipine (Procardia) 10 mg t.i.d. What type of antihypertensive drug is nifedipine?

    a. beta blocker

    b. calcium blocker

    c. angiotensin antagonist

    d. centrally acting sympatholytic

58. The protein-binding power of nifedipine (Procardia) is:
    a. highly protein-bound.
    b. moderately to highly protein-bound.
    c. moderately protein-bound.
    d. low protein-bound.

59. Side effects that D.D. may encounter with the use of nifedipine include all of the following EXCEPT:
    a. dizziness.
    b. lightheadedness.
    c. headache.
    d. increased blood pressure.

Situation: J.R. is taking amlodipine (Norvasc) 10 mg daily. He is 77 years old. His blood pressure before Norvasc was 168/88 mm Hg and now is 136/76 mm Hg. Questions 60 to 63 pertain to this situation.

60. Amlodipine (Norvasc) is what type of drug?
    a. diuretic
    b. ACE inhibitor
    c. angiotensin II blocker
    d. calcium channel blocker

61. Norvasc promotes:
    a. vasoconstriction.
    b. vasodilation.
    c. peripheral vascular resistance.
    d. peripheral clotting.

62. Norvasc:
    a. is highly protein-bound.
    b. is moderately protein-bound.
    c. is low protein-bound.
    d. has a very short half-life.

63. J.R. complains of swelling in his ankles. The nurse should tell J.R. that:
    a. swelling is common with Norvasc. He should cut the tablet in half.
    b. he should not be taking that drug because of his age. Suggest another antihypertensive drug.
    c. swelling may occur with Norvasc. Call the health care provider to determine if the drug should be changed or another drug should be added.
    d. he should stop taking the drug for several days and check that the swelling has decreased.

64. Zebeta is classified as a/an:

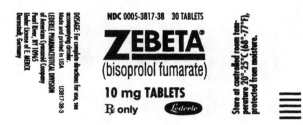

    a. diuretic.
    b. beta blocker.
    c. calcium blocker.
    d. ACE inhibitor.

65. Procardia is classified as a/an:

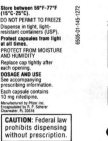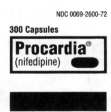

    a. diuretic.
    b. beta blocker.
    c. calcium blocker.
    d. ACE inhibitor.

66. Pindolol is classified as a/an:

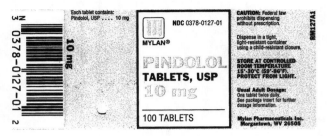

    a. diuretic.

    b. beta blocker.

    c. calcium blocker.

    d. ACE inhibitor.

67. The advantage(s) of beta-adrenergic blockers for their antihypertensive effect is/are the following: *Select all that apply.*

    a. increase serum electrolyte levels

    b. minimize hypoglycemic effect

    c. maintain renal blood flow

    d. help prevent bronchoconstriction

    e. can be abruptly discontinued without causing rebound symptoms

    f. prevent hypolipidemia

68. The angiotensin receptor blocker (ARB) has gained popularity for treating hypertension. Example(s) of ARB agents is/are: *Select all that apply.*

    a. irbesartan (Avapro).

    b. losartan potassium (Cozaar).

    c. valsartan (Diovan).

    d. lisinopril (Prinivil).

    e. metoprolol (Lopressor).

69. A new antihypertensive agent/group, the direct renin inhibitors, has been approved by the FDA for treatment of hypertension. Indicate the correct responses.

    a. It is effective for treating severe hypertension.

    b. It can be combined with another antihypertensive drug such as an ARB.

    c. It can cause hypokalemia when taken as a monotherapy drug.

    d. Aliskiren (Tekturna) is an example of a direct renin inhibitor.

    e. Telmisartan (Micardis) is an example of a direct renin inhibitor.

    f. Diazoxide (Hyperstat) is an example of a direct renin inhibitor.

Critical Thinking Exercises

Use a separate sheet of paper for your answers.

S.H., 82 years old, has essential hypertension. He is taking atenolol (Tenormin) 25 mg, daily, and hydrochlorothiazide 25 mg, daily. His vital signs are BP 138/88 mm Hg, P 74 beats/min, R 22 breaths/min. He lives by himself and has a care person who is with him for 4 hours in the morning and 4 hours in the evening. The care person assists S.H. with his medication and food.

1. What type of antihypertensive agent is atenolol (Tenormin)? Is the drug dosing for S.H. within normal range?

2. What is the pharmacologic action of atenolol (Tenormin)?

3. From what drug group is hydrochlorothiazide? Why would this drug be ordered for S.H.?

4. What type of electrolyte imbalance may occur with the use of hydrochlorothiazide? Why?

5. With his blood pressure within normal range, should the drug be discontinued or the drug dose be reduced?

6.   What important client teaching points should the nurse discuss with S.H.'s care person?

7.   What are the similarities and differences between atenolol and amlodipine?

8.   What are some of the side effects of atenolol?

9.   What laboratory tests should be monitored?

44 Anticoagulants, Antiplatelets, and Thrombolytics

Study Questions

Complete the following word search. Clues are given below. Circle your responses.

```
P  O  Q  W  U  D  J  R  S  A  A  B  C  P  S
F  A  J  V  I  E  D  R  H  B  E  P  N  M  O
I  G  N  S  D  T  Q  P  T  W  J  K  P  R  V
B  G  C  T  H  R  O  M  B  O  L  Y  T  I  C
R  R  J  W  I  S  C  H  E  M  I  A  Y  Z  E
I  E  A  T  M  C  E  G  E  U  T  F  L  V  A
N  G  O  A  W  C  O  P  Q  C  B  N  J  I  R
O  A  J  S  K  A  R  A  W  U  Z  Y  A  B  C
L  T  W  T  M  N  G  P  G  J  C  D  Q  I  M
Y  I  K  R  L  H  N  Y  V  U  E  O  T  U  Z
S  O  Y  O  J  A  D  H  M  N  L  M  W  H  J
I  N  R  K  Y  B  M  R  T  Q  W  A  Z  D  P
S  K  N  E  J  Q  R  T  S  W  Z  I  N  V  N
J  A  C  D  E  P  Q  R  S  V  C  E  K  T  M
```

a. clumping together of platelets to form a clot

b. inhibits blood clot formation

c. breakdown of fibrin for preventing clot formation

d. lack of blood supply to tissues

e. category of drugs used to destroy blood clot formation

f. antiplatelets are prescribed to prevent myocardial infarction and _____

Locate and circle the abbreviations for:

g. international normalized ratio

h. low molecular weight heparin

i. deep vein thrombosis

j. prothrombin time

Complete the following:

1. A thrombus can form in a/an
    _____ and _____ .

2. Anticoagulants are used to inhibit
    _____ .

3. Anticoagulants and thrombolytics (have/do
    not have) the same action. *(Circle correct
    answer.)*

4. The most frequent use of heparin is to
    prevent _____ _____ .

5. Heparin can be given (orally/subcutaneously/
    intravenously). *(Circle correct answers.)*

6. The new low molecular weight heparins
    (LMWHs) are derivatives of
    _____ . The advantage of the use
    of LMWHs is to _____ .

7. The international normalized ratio (INR) is a
    new laboratory test to monitor the therapeutic
    effect of (warfarin/heparin). *(Circle correct
    answer.)*

8. Heparin can (decrease/increase) the platelet
    count, causing thrombocytopenia. *(Circle
    correct answer.)*

9. A thrombus disintegrates when a
    thrombolytic drug is administered within
    _____ hours following an acute
    myocardial infarction.

10. The action of the thrombolytic drugs
    streptokinase and urokinase is the conversion
    of _____ to _____ .

11. The major complication with the use of
    thrombolytic drugs is _____ .

12. A synthetic anticoagulant that indirectly
    inhibits thrombin production but is closely
    related in structure to heparin and LMWH is
    _____ .

Match the drug with its drug group.

Drug	Drug Group
____ 13. warfarin	a. anticoagulant: LMWH
____ 14. aspirin	
____ 15. enovaparin (Lovenox)	b. direct thrombin inhibitor (parenteral)
____ 16. dalteparin sodium (Fragmin)	c. Coumarin
____ 17. protamine sulfate	d. antiplatelet
	e. anticoagulant antagonist
____ 18. clopidogrel (Plavix)	f. thrombolytic
____ 19. streptokinase	
____ 20. bivalirudin (Angiomax)	
____ 21. alteplase (tissue plasminogen activator [tPA])	

22. List four specific nursing interventions related
    to clients receiving anticoagulants:

    a.

    b.

    c.

    d.

NCLEX Review Questions

Select the best response.

23. Anticoagulants will:
    a. dissolve blood clots.
    b. be administered with thrombolytics to dissolve blood clots.
    c. prevent new clot formation.
    d. promote clot formation.

24. Clients receiving warfarin therapy have their INR maintained at:
    a. 1.3 to 2.0.
    b. 2.0 to 3.0.
    c. 3.0 to 4.5.
    d. greater than 5.0.

25. LMWHs are frequently prescribed to:
    a. prevent cerebrovascular accident, or stroke.
    b. enhance the action of warfarin.
    c. prevent deep vein thrombosis following knee or hip replacement surgery.
    d. prevent GI bleeding caused by a peptic ulcer.

26. Recently three new LMWHs were approved by the FDA. The one drug that is NOT an LMWH is:
    a. ardeparin (Normiflo).
    b. danaparoid (Orgaran).
    c. tinzaparin sodium (Innohep).
    d. clopidogrel (Plavix).

27. An example of an antiplatelet agent for angioplasty and acute coronary syndrome is:
    a. abciximab.
    b. protamine sulfate.
    c. warfarin.
    d. aminocaproic acid.

28. Clopidogrel (Plavix) is:
    a. more effective when prescribed singly as an antiplatelet drug.
    b. more effective when prescribed with aspirin after MI and stroke.
    c. an inexpensive antiplatelet drug for stroke.
    d. an antiplatelet drug that can be used instead of an anticoagulant drug.

Situation: R.B. was given heparin for early treatment of deep vein thrombophlebitis. Later, warfarin (Coumadin) was prescribed. Questions 29 to 36 relate to this situation.

29. Effects of heparin are monitored by which of the following laboratory test(s)?
    a. CBC, WBC
    b. PTT and APTT
    c. PT, INR
    d. BUN

30. Enoxaparin sodium is an anticoagulant used to prevent and treat deep vein thrombosis and pulmonary embolism. This drug is in which drug group?
    a. standard heparin
    b. LMWH
    c. oral anticoagulant
    d. thrombolytic

31. In the event of hemorrhage, which of the following medications is most likely to be administered intravenously?
    a. urea
    b. cimetidine
    c. phenytoin
    d. protamine sulfate

32. The protein-binding power of warfarin is:
    a. highly protein-bound.
    b. moderately to highly protein-bound.
    c. moderately protein-bound.
    d. low protein-bound.

33. If R.B. was taking a highly protein-bound drug with warfarin, what might occur?
    a. no drug displacement of warfarin or the highly protein-bound drug
    b. moderate drug displacement of warfarin, which is moderately protein-bound
    c. drug displacement of warfarin, which is also highly protein-bound
    d. drug displacement of the highly protein-bound drug but not displacement of warfarin

34. Which of the following medications is administered to decrease bleeding and increase clotting for bleeding resulting from excess free Coumadin?
    a. vitamin E
    b. vitamin K
    c. glucagon
    d. calcium gluconate

35. Of the following drugs/foods, which does NOT alter the action of heparin?
    a. aspirin
    b. oral hypoglycemics
    c. phenytoin
    d. Maalox

36. Your health teaching plan for R.B. would include all of the following EXCEPT:
    a. comply with ongoing laboratory test regimen.
    b. report bleeding.
    c. take aspirin for headache.
    d. use an electric razor.

Situation: E.Z., a 51-year-old client in the emergency department, is receiving streptokinase. Questions 37 to 39 refer to this situation.

37. Assessment for an allergic reaction to streptokinase includes all of the following EXCEPT:
    a. nausea.
    b. hives.
    c. dyspnea.
    d. bronchospasm.

38. Which drug would you have readily available as an antidote?
    a. aminocaproic acid (Amicar)
    b. Apsac
    c. alteplase (tPA)
    d. calcium gluconate

39. Nursing care for E.Z. would include all of the following EXCEPT:
    a. record vital signs and report changes.
    b. observe for signs and symptoms of bleeding.
    c. monitor liver enzymes.
    d. assess for reperfusion dysrhythmias.

40. Anticoagulants are recommended for use in the following arterial disorder(s): *Select all that apply.*
    a. coronary thrombosis
    b. valvular prosthetic devices
    c. pulmonary embolism
    d. cerebrovascular accidents (CVAs)
    e. hip replacement surgery

41. The use(s) of low molecular weight heparin (LMWH) include(s) the following: *Select all that apply.*
    a. Can be taken orally.
    b. Has a lower risk of bleeding than heparin.
    c. Can be administered by the client at home.
    d. Check the international normalized ratio (INR).
    e. Overdose of LMWH is rare.

42. Nursing interventions for clients taking warfarin include the following: *Select all that apply.*
    a. Use a firm toothbrush when cleaning teeth and gums.
    b. Suggest the client carries a medical ID card or wears ID jewelry indicating that he/she is taking warfarin.
    c. Inform the client that smoking does not influence warfarin dose.
    d. Instruct the client that the health care provider should be notified before taking OTC drugs.
    e. Inform the client that many herbal products interact with warfarin.
    f. Advise the client to report bleeding, such as petechiae, ecchymosis, purpura, tarry stools, bleeding gums, or expectoration of blood.

43. Order: heparin 4000 units, subQ, q6h

Available:

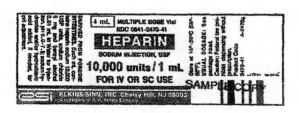

How many milliliters (ml) should the client receive? _____

Critical Thinking Exercises

Use a separate sheet of paper for your answers.

B.C., age 63, had a myocardial infarction (heart attack). While hospitalized, he received heparin 5000 units subcutaneously q6h for 5 days. Heparin is available as 5000 units/ml and 10,000 units/ml. On the fifth day, warfarin 5 mg daily was started. His INR is 2.7.

1. a. Which heparin vial would you select?

    b. How many ml of heparin should B.C. receive per dose?

2. Can heparin be given orally? Explain.

3. What laboratory test is used to monitor heparin doses? What is the normal range?

4. How many tablet(s) of warfarin (Coumadin) should the nurse administer to B.C. per day?

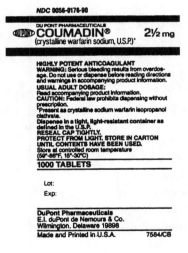

5. What is INR? For what drug is INR ordered? How does INR compare with prothrombin time (PT)?

6. What side effects might occur with the use of warfarin?

7. What are the protein-binding power and half-life of warfarin?

8. What client teaching is essential for B.C. when he is taking warfarin?

45 Antilipidemics and Peripheral Vasodilators

Study Questions

Complete the following:

1. "Friendly" lipoproteins are the
   _____.

2. The "bad" lipoproteins include
   _____ , _____ , and
   _____.

3. Clients should fast for _____ hours
   before a lipid profile.

4. Nonpharmacologic method for cholesterol
   reduction is that the total fat intake should be
   _____% and the cholesterol intake
   should be _____ mg or less.

5. The most common discomfort (side effect) of
   many antilipidemics is _____.

6. An antilipidemic medication may take
   several (days/weeks) to decrease the blood
   lipid levels. (Circle correct answer.)

7. The desired cholesterol level is
   _____.

8. Some clients report a decreased libido with
   the drug _____.

9. Peripheral vasodilators are more effective in
   disorders resulting from vasospasms than
   _____.

10. The hemorrheologic group such as
    pentoxifylline (Trental) increases
    _____ blood flow.

Match the drug with its drug group.

	Drug		Drug Group
____11.	colestipol hydrochloride	a.	statins
____12.	gemfibrozil (Lopid)	b.	bile-acid seques-trant
____13.	atorvastatin (Lipitor)	c.	fibrates
____14.	simvastatin (Zocor)	d.	antihyperlipid-emic
____15.	cholestyr-amine resin (Questran)		
____16.	ezetimibe (Zetia)		

Give the rationale for the nursing interventions related to antilipidemics.

Nursing Intervention	Rationale
17. Monitor the client's blood lipid levels.	17.
18. Monitor laboratory tests for liver function.	18.
19. Advise the client to take the antilipidemic with sufficient water or with meals.	19.
20. Instruct the client to have an annual eye examination.	20.
21. Instruct the client to maintain a low-fat diet.	21.
22. Inform the client that it may take several weeks for the blood lipid levels to decline.	22.

NCLEX Review Questions

Select the best response.

23. Elevated apolipoproteins can be an indicator of LDL and coronary heart disease (CHD). Which Apo is an indicator of low-density lipoprotein that could lead to CHD?
    a. Apo A-1
    b. Apo A-2
    c. Apo B
    d. Apo C

24. A severe side effect of a "statin" drug is:
    a. rhabdomyolysis.
    b. headache.
    c. diarrhea.
    d. convulsions.

25. Homocysteine is a protein in the blood that has been linked to cardiovascular disease and stroke. It may also promote:
    a. blood clotting.
    b. urine retention.
    c. increased blood flow.
    d. lowering of lipid levels.

26. An herb that has been taken for intermittent claudication, though it has not been approved by the FDA, is:
    a. St. John's wort.
    b. ginkgo biloba.
    c. ginger.
    d. ginseng.

Situation: A.B.'s lipid levels are as follows: cholesterol, 258 mg/dl; LDL, 160 mg/dl; HDL, 38 mg/dl. A.B.'s diet consisted of less than 30% total daily fat intake and less than 300 mg of daily cholesterol intake. After 2 months A.B.'s lipid levels were the following: cholesterol, 246 mg/dl; LDL, 150 mg/dl; HDL, 42 mg/dl.
What are the desired lipid levels for cholesterol, LDL, and HDL?

27. Cholesterol: _____

28. Low-density lipoprotein (LDL):
    _____

29. High-density lipoprotein (HDL):
    _____

30. Why did A.B.'s serum lipids not drop after 2 months of a low-fat and low-cholesterol diet?
    a. A.B. most likely did not adhere to the diet.
    b. Diet modification will usually lower cholesterol levels by only 10% to 30%.
    c. A.B. was too obese and lost only 10 pounds.
    d. A.B.'s exercise program should have been increased.

A.B. was prescribed simvastatin (Zocor) 10 mg, daily, to take in the evening.

31. A.B. asked if she could eat whatever she wanted because of the Zocor. Your response could be:
    a. "Yes, as long as you take Zocor."
    b. "Diet is not important if you take Zocor and exercise."
    c. "You should maintain a low-fat and low-cholesterol diet and exercise."
    d. "With Zocor, diet is not important but you should lose weight and exercise."

Situation: E.B. is 54 years old and is taking isoxsuprine hydrochloride (Vasodilan) for peripheral vascular disease. Questions 32 to 34 relate to this situation.

32. Vasodilan is also prescribed for treatment of all of the following conditions EXCEPT:
    a. transient ischemic attack.
    b. Raynaud's disease.
    c. Buerger's disease.
    d. Paget's disease.

33. The usual dose of Vasodilan is:
    a. 10-20 mg t.i.d.
    b. 20-30 mg t.i.d.
    c. 30-40 mg t.i.d.
    d. 40-50 mg t.i.d.

34. List four points you would include in E.B.'s health teaching plan:

    a.

    b.

    c.

    d.

35. Assessment of adequate blood flow to the extremities includes the following: *Select all that apply.*
    a. pallor
    b. coolness of extremities
    c. pain
    d. heat
    e. movement of all extremities

36. Antilipidemics other than the "statins" are prescribed for reducing cholesterol and LDL levels, which include: *Select all that apply.*
    a. bile-acid sequestrants.
    b. alpha-adrenergic antagonists.
    c. direct thrombin inhibitors.
    d. nicotinic acid.
    e. antiplatelets.
    f. cholesterol absorption inhibitors.

37. Rosuvastatin (Crestor) is a: *Select all that apply.*
    a. HMG-CoA reductase inhibitor.
    b. cholesterol absorption inhibitor.
    c. statin drug.
    d. combination of two antilipidemics.
    e. bile-acid sequestrant.

38. The client is receiving Crestor 5 mg, PO, daily. Available: Crestor 10 mg and 20 mg tablets.
    a. Which bottle would you select?
    b. How many tablets would you give?

Critical Thinking Exercises

Use a separate sheet of paper for your answers.

R.T.'s cholesterol level is 267 mg/dl. Her LDL level is 146 mg/dl and her HDL level is 44 mg/dl. She is 36 years old and weighs 210 pounds. R.T. was initially prescribed atorvastatin (Lipitor) 10 mg daily, and later it was increased to 20 mg daily.

1. R.T. wants to know what the desired cholesterol level is. How would you respond to her question?

2. What is atorvastatin? For what reason(s) would R.T. receive this drug? Is the drug dose within normal range?

3. What information do you need to know from R.T. concerning taking atorvastatin and pregnancy?

4. What is the protein-binding power of atorvastatin? What effect is likely to occur when taking a highly protein-binding drug such as warfarin with atorvastatin?

5. R.T. wants to know when she should take atorvastatin. How would you respond?

6. What laboratory tests should be monitored while R.T. is taking atorvastatin?

7. What client teaching is essential for R.T.'s drug therapy?

46 Drugs for Gastrointestinal Tract Disorders

Define the following:

1. Adsorbents

2. Cannabinoids

3. Chemoreceptor trigger zone (CTZ)

4. Emetics

5. Opiates

6. Osmotics

7. Purgatives

Matching

8. Match the following parts of the GI system to the figure:

____ pancreas
____ trachea
____ salivary glands
____ duodenum
____ esophagus
____ diaphragm
____ ileocecal valve (junction)
____ anus
____ liver

____ oral cavity
____ superior esophageal sphincter
____ stomach
____ esophagus
____ large intestine (colon)
____ gallbladder
____ rectum
____ small intestine

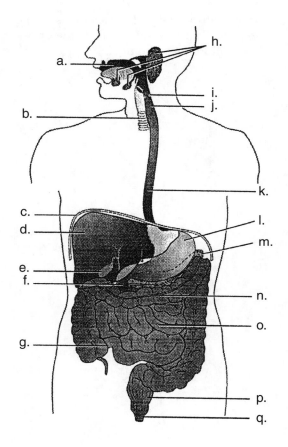

Complete the following:

9. The two main centers that cause vomiting when stimulated are _____ and _____ in the medulla.

10. The five groups of prescriptive antiemetics are _____ , _____ , _____ , _____ , and _____ .

11. Many antiemetics act as _____ to dopamine, histamine, and acetylcholine, which are associated with vomiting.

12. Which group of drugs should NOT be used until the cause of vomiting is identified? _____

13. Nonpharmacologic methods to decrease nausea and vomiting include:

    a.

    b.

    c.

    d.

    e.

14. Over-the-counter (OTC) antihistamines such as Dramamine and the prescribed scopolamine transdermal patch used for motion sickness are best taken _____ minutes before travel.

15. Antiemetic drugs (are/are not) recommended for use during pregnancy. *(Circle correct answer.)*

16. Drugs from the _____ group are most commonly used in the treatment of motion sickness.

17. The major ingredient of the cannabinoids is _____ .

18. Diphenidol (Vontrol) is recommended for nausea, vomiting, and vertigo resulting from _____ disease.

19. In addition to antiemetic effects, benzquinamide also (increases/decreases) cardiac output and blood pressure. *(Circle correct answer.)*

20. The mode of action of charcoal is _____ .

21. The four groups of antidiarrheals are _____ , _____ , _____ , and _____ .

22. A common side effect of opium preparations is _____ .

23. Use of opiates and opiate-related drugs may lead to drug _____ and _____ .

24. Laxatives promote a _____ stool; cathartics result in a _____ stool with cramping.

25. The four laxative/cathartic groups are _____ , _____ , _____ , and _____ .

26. Contact laxatives/cathartics increase peristalsis by _____ . This group is frequently prescribed before _____ and _____ .

27. Emollients act by promoting _____ in the intestine.

28. Saline cathartics are contraindicated for clients with _____ .

29. Bulk-forming laxatives (do/do not) cause laxative dependence. *(Circle correct answer.)*

30. Mineral oil absorbs essential _____ -soluble vitamins _____ , _____ , _____ , and _____ .

31. List four points to include in health teaching plans for clients experiencing constipation:

    a.

    b.

    c.

    d.

NCLEX Review Questions

Select the best response.

32. An expected action of opiates is to:
    a.   absorb toxic materials.
    b.   decrease intestinal motility.
    c.   gently stimulate peristalsis.
    d.   stimulate the chemoreceptor trigger zone.

33. Contraindications for the use of laxatives/cathartics include all of the following EXCEPT:
    a.   inflammatory disease of the GI tract.
    b.   undiagnosed severe pain.
    c.   cirrhosis.
    d.   bowel obstruction.

Situation: R.T., 50 years old, is receiving prochlorperazine (Compazine) for nausea and vomiting. Questions 34 to 37 refer to this situation.

34. The usual dose of Compazine varies with form and includes all of the following EXCEPT:
    a.   5-10 mg q3-4h IM PRN.
    b.   10 mg SR q12h PO.
    c.   5-25 mg supp PRN.
    d.   25 mg q3h PRN.

35. The nurse assesses R.T. for all of the following side effects of Compazine EXCEPT:
    a.   hypotension.
    b.   excessive saliva.
    c.   agitation.
    d.   urinary retention.

36. Specific nursing interventions for R.T. would include all of the following EXCEPT:
    a.   obtaining history of vomiting.
    b.   monitoring vital signs and bowel sounds.
    c.   encouraging fluids.
    d.   maintaining oral hygiene.

37. R.T.'s health teaching plan would include all of the following EXCEPT:
    a.   suggest nonpharmacologic methods.
    b.   stay busy to "keep your mind off" the nausea.
    c.   avoid driving or operating hazardous machinery.
    d.   avoid alcohol.

38. A client is taking dronabinol (Marinol) for nausea and vomiting caused by cancer chemotherapy. It is recommended that this drug be administered:
    a.   1-3 h before and for 24 h after chemotherapy.
    b.   12 h before and for 24 h after chemotherapy.
    c.   q3-4h PRN.
    d.   q6h PRN.

39. The usual adult dose of dronabinol is:
    a.   1-2 mg.
    b.   3-4 mg.
    c.   5-7 mg.
    d.   8-10 mg.

40. Antidiarrheals are contraindicated in clients with all of the following EXCEPT:
    a.   congestive heart failure.
    b.   narcotic dependence.
    c.   ulcerative colitis.
    d.   liver disease.

41. With severe diarrhea, it is important to monitor all of the following EXCEPT:
    a. electrolytes.
    b. vital signs.
    c. bowel sounds.
    d. WBC count.

42. Which of the following drugs is a somatostatin analogue frequently prescribed for metastatic cancer–related severe diarrhea?
    a. loperamide
    b. octreotide (Sandostatin)
    c. docusate potassium (Dialose)
    d. psyllium

43. Bulk-forming laxatives should be mixed in at least _____ ounces of fluid.
    a. 4
    b. 8
    c. 12
    d. 16

44. Use of opiate-related drugs for severe diarrhea may cause which of the following? *Select all that apply.*
    a. drowsiness
    b. constipation
    c. paralytic ileus
    d. urinary frequency
    e. abdominal cramping

45. The nurse recommends that a client with diarrhea avoid which of the following? *Select all that apply.*
    a. fried foods
    b. clear liquids
    c. bottled water
    d. raw vegetables
    e. milk products

46. The nurse should encourage a client with constipation to ingest which of the following? *Select all that apply.*
    a. cheese
    b. bran
    c. grains
    d. fruit
    e. water

Critical Thinking Exercises

Use a separate sheet of paper for your answers.

L.B., age 85, comes to your clinic complaining, "I can't move my bowels." L.B. lives independently in a studio apartment in housing for the elderly. Two months ago she fell and fractured her hip. She is currently taking digoxin, an antacid, and a narcotic PRN for pain.

1. You know that constipation is a major problem in the elderly. Identify at least six possible contributing factors to L.B.'s problem.

    a.

    b.

    c.

    d.

    e.

    f.

It is determined that L.B. does not have a fecal impaction and bisacodyl 10 mg PO is ordered.

2. Is this dose within the therapeutic range? At what time of day should this be taken?

3. What is the mode of action of bisacodyl?

4. What is the mode of action of bulk-forming laxatives?

5. What are the contraindications for use of bisacodyl?

6. Describe at least two drug-lab-food interactions. Relate these interactions to L.B.'s current drug regimen.

    a.

    b.

7. What specific instructions would you discuss
    with L.B. related to taking bisacodyl?

8. Describe at least six health teaching points to
    be included in L.B.'s care.

    a.

    b.

    c.

    d.

    e.

    f.

47 Antiulcer Drugs

Study Questions

Define the following:

1. Gastric mucosal barrier (GMB)

2. Gastroesophageal reflux disease (GERD)

3. Histamine$_2$-receptor antagonists

Complete the following:

4. Gastric secretion in the stomach attempts to maintain a pH of _____.

5. The gastric mucosal barrier is a defense against _____ substances.

6. Predisposing factors for peptic ulcers include the following:

   a.

   b.

   c.

   d.

7. The classic symptom of peptic ulcers is _____ pain.

8. The seven groups of antiulcer drugs are:

   a.

   b.

   c.

   d.

   e.

   f.

   g.

9. Antacids neutralize hydrochloric acid; they (do/do not) coat the ulcer. *(Circle correct answer.)*

10. Bromo-Seltzer and Alka-Seltzer (are/are not) recommended for treatment of peptic ulcers. *(Circle correct answer.)*

11. A combination of magnesium and aluminum salts neutralizes the gastric acid without causing _____ or _____.

12. Sucralfate (Carafate) is a mucosal _____ drug.

13. All proton pump inhibitors (can/cannot) be combined with antibiotics to treat *Helicobacter pylori*. *(Circle correct answer.)*

Match the descriptor in Column I with the drugs/ factor in Column II. Use each term only once.

Column I		Column II	
_____ 14.	risk factor for the development of PUD	a.	Pepto-Bismol
_____ 15.	neutralizes gastric acid	b.	magnesium hydroxide
_____ 16.	inhibition of gastric acid secretion	c.	*Helicobacter pylori*
		d.	sucralfate
_____ 17.	associated with recurrence of PUD	e.	cimetidine
		f.	omeprazole
_____ 18.	used as mucoprotective in conjunction with NSAIDs	g.	misoprostol
		h.	smoking
_____ 19.	binds free protein in base of ulcer	i.	antacids
		j.	metronidazole
_____ 20.	eradication rates require addition of this antimicrobial		
_____ 21.	causes antidiarrheal effect of some antacids		
_____ 22.	OTC agent used in combination to eradicate *H. pylori*		
_____ 23.	H_2 antagonist with multiple drug interactions		

Give the rationale for the nursing interventions related to antacids.

Nursing Intervention	Rationale
24. Assess renal function.	24.
25. Monitor urinary pH, calcium and phosphate levels, and electrolytes.	25.
26. Avoid administering antacids with other oral drugs.	26.
27. Shake suspension well before administering.	27.
28. Instruct the client to report pain, coughing, and vomiting of blood.	28.
29. Instruct the client not to take the drug with meals.	29.
30. Instruct the client to notify the health care provider if constipation or diarrhea occurs.	30.
31. Advise the client to check antacid labels for sodium content.	31.
32. Instruct the client in use of relaxation techniques.	32.

Complete the drug chart for omeprazole (Prilosec):

Proton Pump Inhibitor

Drug Name Omeprazole (Prilosec) **Pregnancy Category:**	**Dosage:**	**Assessment and Planning**	**Nursing Process**
Contraindications:	**Drug-Lab-Food Interactions:**		
Pharmacokinetics: *Absorption:* *Distribution:* **PB:** *Metabolism:* **t½:** *Excretion:*	**Pharmacodynamics:** *PO:* Onset: Peak: Duration:	**Interventions**	
Therapeutic Effects/Uses: **Mode of Action:**		**Evaluation**	
Side Effects:	**Adverse Reactions:**		
	Life-Threatening:		

NCLEX Review Questions

Select the best response.

33. Ideal dosing for antacids is:
    a. with meals and 1 hour after.
    b. 1 hour before meals.
    c. 1 and 3 hours after meals.
    d. with meals.

34. For best results, antacids should be taken with _____ ounces of water.
    a. 2-4
    b. 4-6
    c. 6-8
    d. at least 8

35. Popular drugs in the treatment of gastric and duodenal ulcers are:
    a. histamine blockers.
    b. antacids.
    c. pepsin inhibitors.
    d. tranquilizers.

36. The group of drugs used to prevent acid reflux in the esophagus is:
    a. antacids.
    b. pepsin inhibitors.
    c. prostaglandin analogues.
    d. histamine blockers.

Situation: D.Z. is being treated for peptic ulcers. She is taking Pro-Banthine. Questions 37 to 39 refer to this situation.

37. Propantheline bromide (Pro-Banthine) belongs to which drug group?
    a. tranquilizers
    b. anticholinergics
    c. suppressors of gastric acid
    d. antacids

38. For best results, the nurse knows that Pro-Banthine should be taken:
    a. with meals.
    b. before meals.
    c. 2 hours after meals.
    d. with two glasses of fluid.

39. D.Z. is also receiving an antacid. The best time to administer the antacid is:
    a. with belladonna.
    b. 2 hours before meals.
    c. 2 hours after meals.
    d. with meals.

Situation: J.M., a senior in college, complains of pain in the stomach after eating. He reports that pain is intensified at exam time. The health care provider recommends an antacid. Questions 40 and 41 relate to this situation.

40. Cimetidine may cause an increase in which of the following laboratory tests?
    a. platelets
    b. BUN
    c. WBCs
    d. blood sugar

41. The enhancement of these drug effects is due to cimetidine:
    a. inhibiting hepatic metabolism.
    b. inhibiting renal excretion.
    c. prolonging the half-life.
    d. displacing protein-binding sites.

42. A synthetic prostaglandin analogue used for the prevention and treatment of peptic ulcer is:
    a. Pepcid.
    b. Zantac.
    c. Indocin.
    d. Cytotec.

43. Which of the following drugs inhibits gastric acid secretions to a greater extent than histamine antagonists?

    a. Prilosec

    b. Pepcid

    c. Pro-Banthine

    d. Quarzan

44. Which of the following drugs are proton pump inhibitors?

    a. esomeprazole (Nexium)

    b. pantoprazole (Protonix)

    c. rabeprazole (AcipHex)

    d. all of the above

45. Which of the following are side effects of Pro-Banthine? *Select all that apply.*

    a. bradycardia

    b. dry mouth

    c. constipation

    d. urinary retention

    e. decreased gastric secretions

46. A client is taking cimetidine (Tagamet). Side effects include which of the following? *Select all that apply.*

    a. headache

    b. back pain

    c. nausea

    d. loss of libido

    e. gynecomastia

47. The nurse is aware of cimetidine's enhancement of which of the following drugs? *Select all that apply.*

    a. laxatives

    b. oral anticoagulants

    c. propranolol (Inderal)

    d. phenytoin (Dilantin)

    e. fluconazole (Diflucan)

Critical Thinking Exercises

Use a separate sheet of paper for your answers.

S.S., 63 years old, has a high-stress job as a county judge. He complains of abdominal distress after eating. He is currently taking aluminum hydroxide (Amphojel) 600 mg q4h while awake.

1. Is the dose within the therapeutic range? What are the nursing responsibilities, if any?

2. What is the mode of action of aluminum hydroxide? Compare its action with that of ranitidine and sucralfate.

3. Describe drug-drug and drug-lab interactions.

4. What is a common side effect of aluminum hydroxide?

5. What is the major contraindication for use of aluminum hydroxide? What are indications for cautious use?

6. What dietary recommendations would you make to S.S.?

7. Describe important health teaching to include with S.S.

48 Drugs for Disorders of the Eye and Ear

Study Questions

Complete the following word search. Clues are given in questions 1-15. Circle your responses.

```
Z  R  C  A  A  F  O  R  E  I  G  N  B  O  D  Y  L  B  D
Y  O  A  M  C  N  O  S  M  O  T  I  C  S  S  S  I  L  I
X  R  R  A  G  O  U  M  N  U  A  M  N  R  C  I  W  O  U
I  N  B  V  L  Q  N  R  D  K  N  S  A  I  L  N  S  O  R
N  A  O  N  A  P  H  J  I  C  U  E  G  U  V  C  N  D  E
H  A  N  O  U  T  M  Y  U  A  T  E  Y  F  A  R  E  S  T
I  E  I  I  C  T  G  W  Q  N  L  O  X  D  J  E  R  U  I
B  S  C  T  O  F  K  W  K  P  C  S  P  Z  G  A  D  G  C
I  A  Z  A  M  K  L  E  O  B  U  T  H  M  V  S  L  A  S
T  R  P  R  A  P  P  L  C  I  I  Y  I  B  E  E  I  R  Z
O  D  M  D  H  P  C  X  B  B  U  Z  Y  V  S  J  H  D  Q
R  Y  A  Y  O  Y  W  P  E  N  J  I  T  M  I  I  C  Y  P
S  H  R  H  C  M  G  E  S  A  E  R  C  E  D  T  A  S  E
S  N  Z  E  M  Y  D  R  I  A  T  I  C  S  R  A  I  C  S
A  A  T  D  C  E  R  A  L  U  C  O  A  R  T  N  I  S  T
```

1. Topical anesthetics are used during an eye exam and before removal of a _____ _____ from the eye.

2. Lubricants are used to moisten contact lenses and/or to replace _____ .

3. Miotics are used to lower _____ pressure.

4. Carbonic anhydrase inhibitors were developed as _____ . They are effective in treating _____ .

5. Osmotic drugs are used to (decrease/increase) the amount of aqueous humor. (*Circle correct answer.*)

6. Mannitol is contraindicated for clients with the condition of _____ or _____ .

7. Diabetic clients taking Glyrol require monitoring of _____ .

8. The drug group used to paralyze the muscles of accommodation is _____ .

9. BufOpto atropine is frequently used for refraction in _____ .

10. Instruct clients with glaucoma to avoid atropine-like drugs because they (decrease/increase) intraocular pressure. (*Circle correct answer.*)

11. Antiinfectives are used to treat infections of the eye, including inflammation of the membrane covering the eyeball and lining the eyelid known as _____ .

12. Drugs that interfere with production of carbonic acid, leading to decreased aqueous humor formation and decreased intraocular pressure, belong to the group _____ .

13. Beta-adrenergic blockers used to treat open-angle glaucoma may (increase/ decrease) the effect of systemic beta blockers. *(Circle correct answer.)*

14. The group of eye medications contraindicated in persons allergic to sulfonamides is _____ .

15. The volume of vitreous humor is reduced by the _____ group of drugs.

NCLEX Review Questions

Select the best response.

16. Your client has a medication ordered to dilate his eyes. Such a medication belongs to which group of drugs?
    a. mydriatics
    b. osmotics
    c. carbonic anhydrase inhibitors
    d. ceruminolytics

17. Your client is taking a carbonic anhydrase inhibitor. You will assess for which side effect associated with this group of drugs?
    a. nausea
    b. increased blood pressure
    c. renal calculi
    d. urinary retention

18. Which of the following drugs is most effective in treating glaucoma in African-American clients?
    a. latanoprost (Xalatan)
    b. bimatoprost (Lumigan)
    c. travoprost (Travatan)
    d. unoprostone (Rescula)

19. Your client is taking a prostaglandin analogue, and you assess for the most common adverse reaction, which is:
    a. light intolerance.
    b. ocular hyperemia.
    c. conjunctivitis.
    d. blurred vision.

20. Your client had her ears irrigated. To determine the results of this irrigation, visualization of which structure is required?
    a. semicircular canals
    b. tympanic membrane
    c. external acoustic meatus
    d. auricle

21. Preparations that are helpful for loosening wax from the ear canal belong to which group?
    a. carbonic anhydrase inhibitors
    b. osmotics
    c. prostaglandin analogues
    d. ceruminolytics

Situation: E.Q. is receiving Isopto-Eserine eye drops for treatment of glaucoma. Questions 22 to 24 refer to this situation.

22. You would assess E.Q. for possible side effects, including all of the following EXCEPT:
    a. headache.
    b. nausea.
    c. brow pain.
    d. decreased vision.

23. Nursing care for E.Q. would include all of the following EXCEPT:
    a. monitoring for postural hypotension.
    b. assessing for increased bronchial secretions.
    c. increasing fluid intake.
    d. maintaining oral hygiene.

24. Health teaching for this medication includes all of the following EXCEPT:
    a. ensure first dose is administered by health care provider.
    b. follow-up with tonometry readings.
    c. increase caloric intake.
    d. stress importance of regular medical supervision.

25. Solutions commonly used to irrigate the ear include the following: *Select all that apply.*
    a. Burow's solution.
    b. hydrogen peroxide 3%.
    c. hypotonic HCl solution 10%.
    d. acetic acid.

26. C.G., 7 years old, is receiving Bactrim (trimethoprim/sulfamethoxazole) for an inner-ear infection. Nursing care for C.G. includes the following: *Select all that apply.*
    a. obtaining culture and sensitivity
    b. assessing for hematuria and oliguria
    c. restricting fluids
    d. monitoring intake and output

27. When administering eardrops to a 7-year-old child, the nurse should do the following: *Select all that apply.*
    a. Pull down and back on the auricle.
    b. Pull up and back on the auricle.
    c. Tilt head to unaffected side.
    d. Instill medication at room temperature.

Critical Thinking Exercises

Use a separate sheet of paper for your answers.

D.Z. is 82 years old and comes to the office for her regular glaucoma follow-up. She denies any problems but admits to having blurred vision. She reports self-administration of pilocarpine, 2 gtt q4h.

1. Describe the mode of action of pilocarpine. Why is it used in the treatment of glaucoma?

2. Is the dose that D.Z. reports taking within the therapeutic range? What are the related nursing responsibilities, if any?

3. What is the most likely cause of D.Z.'s blurred vision?

4. Systemic absorption of pilocarpine is contraindicated in what conditions?

5. As part of your assessment, you ask D.Z. about any side effects of pilocarpine. What side effects would you include?

6. What client teaching would be appropriate for D.Z.?

7. What are the advantages and disadvantages of the Ocusert system? Do you think this would be appropriate for D.Z.? State your rationale.

49 Drugs for Dermatologic Disorders

Study Questions

Match the description with the correct term.

Term		Description
____ 1.	macule	a. round, palpable lesion, <1 cm in diameter
____ 2.	vesicle	
____ 3.	plaque	b. hard, rough, raised lesion; flat on top
____ 4.	papule	c. flat lesion with varying colors
		d. raised lesion filled with fluid and <1 cm in diameter

Label the structures of the skin as follows:

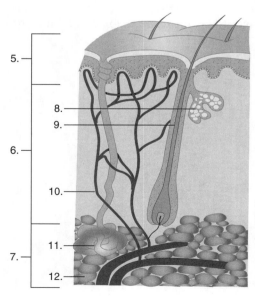

5. _____

6. _____

7. _____

8. _____

9. _____

10. _____

11. _____

12. _____

NCLEX Review Questions

Select the best response.

13. Your client has severe acne. Drugs frequently used to treat this condition are:
    a. antibiotics and glucocorticoids.
    b. antibiotics and coal tar products.
    c. podophyllum and anthralin.
    d. Sulfamylon and keratolytics.

14. Psoriasis affects what percent of the population in the United States?
    a. 1%-2%
    b. 3%-4%
    c. 5%-6%
    d. 10%

15. Psoriatic scales are loosened with which of the following medications?
    a. podophyllum
    b. antibiotics
    c. keratolytics
    d. benzoyl peroxide

16. Drugs commonly used to treat moderate to severe psoriasis include which of the following?
    a. antibiotics
    b. biologic agents
    c. keratolytics
    d. silver nitrate

17. Efalizumab (Raptiva), a humanized therapeutic antibody, is administered:
    a. orally.
    b. transdermally.
    c. subcutaneously.
    d. intramuscularly.

18. Contact dermatitis is commonly caused by:
    a. irritation.
    b. burns.
    c. inhalation.
    d. smoke.

19. A moderately severe sunburn is an example of what degree sunburn?
    a. first
    b. second
    c. third
    d. full thickness

Situation: J.T., 18 years old, is receiving treatment for acne vulgaris. Questions 20 to 23 refer to this situation.

20. The usual dose of tetracycline for this condition is:
    a. 250-500 mg b.i.d.
    b. 500-1000 mg b.i.d.
    c. 500 mg daily.
    d. 1 g daily.

21. A major side effect of tetracycline is:
    a. urinary retention.
    b. photosensitivity.
    c. hypersensitivity.
    d. hepatotoxicity.

22. Health teaching for J.T. about tetracycline includes all of the following about drug interactions EXCEPT:
    a. tetracycline increases the effects of oral anticoagulants.
    b. tetracycline decreases the effects of oral contraceptives.
    c. tetracycline increases the effects of oral contraceptives.
    d. antacids decrease absorption of tetracycline.

23. Areas for general health teaching with J.T. include all of the following EXCEPT:
    a. not using harsh skin cleansers.
    b. reporting adverse effects.
    c. eating a diet high in fiber.
    d. alerting health care provider if pregnant or possibly pregnant.

24. To control severe psoriasis, the anticancer drug _____ may be prescribed.
    a. benzoyl
    b. tretinoin
    c. etretinate
    d. methotrexate

25. The FDA-approved drug for the treatment of baldness is:
    a. tretinoin.
    b. methoxsalen.
    c. etretinate.
    d. minoxidil.

26. Contact dermatitis may be treated with the following drugs: *Select all that apply.*
    a.   Burow's solution
    b.   calamine
    c.   Percocet
    d.   Benadryl

27. Antipruritics used in the treatment of contact dermatitis include the following: *Select all that apply.*
    a.   Peri-Colace
    b.   fluconazole
    c.   Decadron
    d.   Aristocort

28. Drugs known to cause alopecia include the following: *Select all that apply.*
    a.   antineoplastic agents
    b.   sulfonamides
    c.   selected NSAIDs
    d.   oral contraceptives

Critical Thinking Exercises

Use a separate sheet of paper for your answers.

C.S., 2 years old, has a third-degree burn over her right chest and shoulder and second-degree burns on her hands caused when she hit the handle of a pot filled with boiling water. Mafenide acetate is ordered to be applied to chest, shoulder, and hands, $\frac{1}{16}$-inch layer, b.i.d.

1. What are the depths and characteristics of second- and third-degree burns?

2. Is the dose within the therapeutic range for C.S.?

3. Describe the mode of action of mafenide acetate. What other drug is used for the prevention and treatment of sepsis in second- and third-degree burns?

4. Identify important nursing assessments for C.S.

5. Explain at least three nursing interventions for C.S.

    a.

    b.

    c.

6. What possible side effects of mafenide acetate would you discuss with C.S.'s family?

7. What health teaching is important to include with C.S.'s family?

50 Endocrine Drugs: Pituitary, Thyroid, Parathyroid, and Adrenal Disorders

Study Questions

Using these definitions, locate and circle the term in the word search below.

a. Growth hormone hypersecretion after puberty
b. Anterior pituitary gland
c. Initials for adrenocorticotropic hormone
d. Initials for antidiuretic hormone
e. Severe hypothyroidism in children
f. Ductless glands that produce hormones
g. Growth hormone hypersecretion during childhood

h. Cortisol hormone secreted from the adrenal cortex
i. Pituitary gland
j. Aldosterone hormone secreted from the adrenal cortex
k. Severe hypothyroidism in adults
l. Posterior pituitary gland
m. Toxic hyperthyroidism because of hyperfunction of the thyroid gland
n. T_4 hormone secreted by the thyroid gland
o. T_3 hormone secreted by the thyroid gland

```
T  F  M  L  E  I  B  G  H  M  X  Y  I  B  P  N  L  D  E  T  S  A  T
B  T  R  I  I  O  D  O  T  H  Y  R  O  N  I  N  E  N  M  E  C  Q  H
S  H  Y  P  O  P  H  Y  S  I  S  B  E  A  C  L  S  S  L  G  D  O  Y
V  Y  R  U  I  M  T  S  D  L  A  N  G  J  E  L  I  F  L  I  P  M  R
H  R  T  A  C  T  H  I  K  N  I  G  R  B  T  T  A  F  O  T  Y  R  O
F  O  I  D  B  S  A  U  O  X  X  A  A  C  N  D  E  C  J  L  K  D  X
I  T  Z  H  G  F  U  I  O  H  J  L  L  A  M  O  I  P  L  I  B  A  I
R  O  O  B  E  X  S  R  S  U  T  B  G  I  D  T  E  T  O  N  E  B  N
J  X  I  B  N  S  Y  E  Y  A  M  I  N  P  R  A  V  J  H  Q  O  D  E
Y  I  P  M  E  H  T  O  B  J  G  I  D  O  O  L  K  M  O  L  A  S  N
A  C  R  E  T  I  N  I  S  M  S  W  C  M  V  D  I  U  Q  E  R  Y  M
W  O  G  N  A  T  M  J  K  T  Y  O  O  T  A  L  U  G  E  R  U  H  I
B  S  P  D  L  I  Y  R  E  G  L  U  C  O  C  O  R  T  I  C  O  I  D
P  I  Y  O  V  R  I  A  K  A  C  R  O  M  E  G  A  L  Y  E  M  N  F
A  S  O  C  Y  L  P  U  R  A  E  B  H  T  E  S  S  C  P  O  L  Q  C
L  K  K  R  E  I  E  E  R  S  O  N  A  L  T  E  L  N  E  F  S  O
R  E  J  I  U  G  N  E  U  R  O  H  Y  P  O  P  H  Y  S  I  S  V  L
J  H  I  N  N  I  C  E  Y  A  M  K  N  P  E  A  V  J  H  Q  O  D  E
S  T  C  E  M  Y  X  E  D  E  M  A  T  A  C  L  S  F  L  G  T  O  R
P  A  D  E  N  O  H  Y  P  O  P  H  Y  S  I  S  S  L  F  E  M  N  W
```

Complete the following:

1. The pituitary gland is divided into two major lobes, the _____ and _____.

2. The growth hormone of the anterior pituitary gland (adenohypophysis) acts on all body tissues, especially the _____ and _____.

3. A child with a growth hormone (GH) deficiency may develop _____, and another child with an oversecretion of GH may develop _____.

4. Prolonged GH therapy can antagonize insulin secretion, thus causing the condition _____.

5. The tropic hormone from the anterior pituitary gland that stimulates the release of glucocorticoids and mineralocorticoids is _____.

6. The thyroid-stimulating hormone (TSH) drug Thytropar is the diagnostic drug to differentiate between _____ and _____ hypothyroidism.

7. The drug used in the treatment of diabetes insipidus is _____.

8. List four nursing interventions associated with drugs for disorders of the pituitary gland:

   a.

   b.

   c.

   d.

9. The two thyroid hormones secreted by the thyroid gland are _____ and _____.

10. Thyroid crisis (storm) may proceed to _____ and _____.

11. A serious adverse effect of antithyroid drugs is _____.

12. The parathyroid gland regulates the _____ (electrolyte) levels in the blood.

13. Parathyroid hormone is useful in treating _____ and the synthetic calcitonin drug is used to treat _____.

14. Tetany symptoms as a result of severe hypocalcemia include _____, _____, and _____.

15. The glucocorticoid drugs are administered orally, parenterally, and topically. The _____ route is not recommended for administration of glucocorticoids.

16. Drugs for adrenocortical insufficiency contain both glucocorticoids and mineralocorticoids; however, for use as an antiinflammatory and immunosuppressive drug, the (glucocorticoids/mineralocorticoids) are generally prescribed. *(Circle correct answer.)*

17. The glucocorticoid used to treat a severe inflammatory response such as that caused by head trauma or an allergic reaction is _____.

18. When a glucocorticoid is to be discontinued, the drug dose should be (stopped immediately/tapered over several days). *(Circle correct answer.)*

   State rationale:

   _____

   _____

19. An increase in aldosterone (a mineralocorti-coid) leads to _____ and _____.

20. Fludrocortisone (Florinef) is an oral form of mineralocorticoid. It can cause a negative nitrogen balance; therefore it is recommended that a diet high in _____ be included.

Match the description from Column II with the applicable term in Column I.

Column I		Column II
____ 21. hyperglycemia	a.	adrenal hyposecretion
____ 22. buffalo hump		
____ 23. hypoglycemia	b.	adrenal hypersecretion
____ 24. seizures		
____ 25. fatigue		
____ 26. impaired clotting		
____ 27. cataract formation		
____ 28. hypotension		
____ 29. hypervolemia		
____ 30. peptic ulcer		

Give the rationale for the nursing interventions related to glucocorticoid drug administration.

Nursing Intervention	Rationale
31. Monitor vital signs.	31.
32. Monitor weight after taking a cortisone preparation for more than 10 days.	32.
33. Monitor laboratory values, especially electrolytes and blood glucose.	33.
34. Instruct the client to take the cortisone preparation at mealtime or with food.	34.
35. Advise the client to eat foods rich in potassium.	35.
36. Instruct the client not to abruptly discontinue the cortisone preparation. Drug dose is normally tapered.	36.
37. Report changes in muscle strength and signs of osteoporosis.	37.
38. Teach client to report signs and symptoms of drug overdose.	38.

NCLEX Review Questions

Select the best response.

Situation: E.A., 49 years old, is being treated for hypothyroidism. E.A. is taking levothyroxine (Synthroid) 100 mcg/day. Questions 39 to 44 refer to this situation.

39. The usual maintenance dose of Synthroid is:
    a. 25-50 mcg/day.
    b. 50-200 mcg/day.
    c. 200-300 mcg/day.
    d. 300-500 mcg/day.

40. Clients report feeling the effect of levothyroxine (Synthroid) within:
    a. 3-4 days.
    b. 4-7 days.
    c. 1-3 weeks.
    d. 3-5 weeks.

41. The nurse assesses E.A. for symptoms of hyperthyroidism. Which one of the following is NOT a symptom of hyperthyroidism?
    a. tachycardia
    b. tinnitus
    c. chest pain
    d. excess sweating

42. The nurse suggests that E.A. avoid foods that can inhibit thyroid secretion, including all of the following EXCEPT:
    a. strawberries.
    b. cabbage.
    c. radishes.
    d. string beans.

43. The best time of the day to take Synthroid is:
    a. before breakfast.
    b. with breakfast.
    c. after breakfast.
    d. with lunch.

44. E.A.'s health teaching plan would include all of the following EXCEPT:
    a. take medication at same time each day.
    b. wear Medic-Alert information device.
    c. increase food and fluid intake.
    d. avoid over-the-counter (OTC) drugs.

Situation: L.T., 56 years old, is taking prednisone for an exacerbation of arthritic knee pain. Questions 45 to 52 refer to this situation.

45. The usual dose of prednisone is:
    a. 0.5-6 mg/day.
    b. 5-60 mg/day.
    c. 60-100 mg/day.
    d. 100-125 mg/day.

46. While L.T. is taking this medication, close monitoring of which of the following is required?
    a. sodium
    b. potassium
    c. hemoglobin
    d. hematocrit

47. The best time to take this drug is:
    a. before meals.
    b. with meals.
    c. 1 hour after meals.
    d. at bedtime.

48. Which one of the following drugs does NOT alter the action of prednisone?
    a. NSAIDs, including aspirin
    b. potassium-wasting diuretics
    c. acetaminophen
    d. oral anticoagulants

49. Specific nursing interventions for L.T. include all of the following EXCEPT:
    a. monitor vital signs.
    b. monitor for signs and symptoms of hypokalemia.
    c. obtain complete medication history.
    d. follow physical therapy regimen.

50. Which one of the following would NOT be included in the health teaching plan for L.T.?
    a.   Take glucocorticoids only as ordered.
    b.   Wear Medic-Alert device or carry card.
    c.   Force fluids.
    d.   Do not abruptly stop medication.

51. When an herbal laxative such as cascara or senna and herbal diuretics such as celery seed or juniper are taken with a corticosteroid, what imbalance may occur?
    a.   hypervolemia
    b.   hyperkalemia
    c.   hypokalemia
    d.   hypernatremia

52. Ginseng taken with a corticosteroid may cause:
    a.   CNS depression.
    b.   CNS stimulation and insomnia.
    c.   serum potassium excess.
    d.   counteraction of the effects of the corticosteroid.

53. A drug that is used to diagnose adrenal gland dysfunction is:
    a.   metyrapone (Metopirone).
    b.   mitotane (Lysodren).
    c.   ketoconazole (Nizoral).
    d.   prednisolone (Delta-Cortef).

54. The nurse advises a client to avoid potassium loss by eating which of the following foods? *Select all that apply.*
    a.   nuts
    b.   meats
    c.   vegetables
    d.   dried fruits
    e.   milk products

55. Which of the following drugs are known to interact with Synthroid? *Select all that apply.*
    a.   digitalis
    b.   diuretics
    c.   anticoagulants
    d.   acetaminophen
    e.   oral antidiabetics

56. The nurse assesses a client for the side effects of prednisone including which of the following? *Select all that apply.*
    a.   edema
    b.   anorexia
    c.   hypertension
    d.   mood changes
    e.   increased blood sugar

Critical Thinking Exercises

Use a separate sheet of paper for your answers.

M.N., age 52, is taking prednisone 10 mg t.i.d. for an acute neurologic problem. She also has a cardiac problem and is taking digoxin 0.25 mg daily, and hydrochlorothiazide 25 mg daily. Her serum potassium level is 3.2 mEq/L.

1. Is M.N.'s prednisone dosage within normal range?

2. From which drug groups are digoxin and hydrochlorothiazide?

3. What electrolyte imbalance(s) may occur with the use of prednisone and hydrochloro-thiazide?

4. How could M.N.'s electrolyte imbalance be avoided?

5. What effect could hypokalemia have on digoxin? Explain.

6. With continuous use of prednisone, what systemic side effects may occur?

7. What are the similarities and differences among prednisone, prednisolone, and dexamethasone?

8. When discontinuing prednisone, why is it recommended that the doses be tapered?

9. What should the nurse include in the teaching plan for M.N.?

51 Antidiabetics

Study Questions

Define the following:

1. Diabetes mellitus

2. Insulin

3. Hypoglycemic reaction

4. Type 1 diabetes

5. Type 2 diabetes

6. Ketoacidosis

7. Lipodystrophy

8. Polydipsia

9. Polyphagia

10. Polyuria

Complete the following:

11. Diabetes mellitus is characterized by the three *P*s: _____, _____, and _____.

12. Select all of the following drugs that may cause hyperglycemia.
    a. prednisone
    b. epinephrine
    c. levothyroxine
    d. hydrochlorothiazide

13. The beta cells of the pancreas normally secrete _____ units of insulin per day.

14. The two groups of antidiabetic agents are _____ and _____.

15. Insulin injection sites are rotated to prevent _____.

16. The only type of insulin that may be administered IV is _____.

17. Insulin requirements may vary. Usually (less/more) insulin is needed with increased exercise and (less/more) insulin is needed with infections and high fever. *(Circle correct answers.)*

18. Combination insulins are commercially premixed; e.g., Humulin 70/30. Some clients who need insulin (would/would not) benefit from commercially combined insulins. *(Circle correct answer.)*

19. The insulin most closely related to human insulin is (pork insulin/beef insulin). *(Circle correct answer.)*

20. List six signs and symptoms of a hypoglycemic (insulin) reaction:

    a.

    b.

    c.

    d.

    e.

    f.

21. List six signs and symptoms of diabetic ketoacidosis (hyperglycemia):

    a.

    b.

    c.

    d.

    e.

    f.

22. In maturity-onset, or type 2, diabetes, the oral antidiabetic (hypoglycemic) drug group that stimulates beta cells to secrete more insulin is _____ . For juvenile-onset, or type 1, diabetes, oral hypoglycemics (are/are not) prescribed. *(Circle correct answer.)*

23. List four health teaching points to be included for clients taking insulin:

    a.

    b.

    c.

    d.

24. List four health teaching points to be included for clients taking oral antidiabetic (hypoglycemic) drugs:

    a.

    b.

    c.

    d.

Match the terms with their definitions.

Term		Definition
_____ 25. NPH insulin	a.	oral hypoglycemic drug group
_____ 26. lipoatrophy		
_____ 27. sulfonylureas	b.	hyperglycemic hormone that stimulates glycogenolysis
_____ 28. glucagon		
_____ 29. Lispro insulin	c.	intermediate-acting insulin
	d.	long-acting insulin
	e.	tissue atrophy
	f.	rapid-acting insulin

Give the rationale for the nursing interventions related to insulin administration.

Nursing Intervention	Rationale
30. Monitor blood glucose levels.	30.
31. Instruct the client to report signs and symptoms of "insulin shock" (hypoglycemic reaction).	31.
32. Inform the client to have orange juice or a sugar-containing drink available if a hypoglycemic reaction occurs.	32.
33. Instruct the client to check the blood sugar daily.	33.
34. Instruct the client to adhere to the prescribed diet.	34.
35. Instruct family members on how to administer glucagon by injection for a hypoglycemic reaction.	35.
36. Advise the client to obtain a medical alert card or tag.	36.

Complete the drug chart for glimepiride (Amaryl):

Second-Generation Sulfonylurea

Drug Name Glimepiride (Amaryl) **Pregnancy Category:**	**Dosage:**	Assessment and Planning	Nursing Process
Contraindications:	**Drug-Lab-Food Interactions:**		
Pharmacokinetics: *Absorption:* *Distribution:* **PB:** *Metabolism:* **t½:** *Excretion:*	**Pharmacodynamics:** *PO:* **Onset:** **Peak:** **Duration:**	Interventions	
Therapeutic Effects/Uses: **Mode of Action:**		Evaluation	
Side Effects:	**Adverse Reactions:** **Life-Threatening:**		

NCLEX Review Questions

Select the best response.

37. Site and depth of insulin injection affect absorption. Insulin absorption is greater when given in:
    a. ventrogluteal and abdominal areas.
    b. deltoid and abdominal areas.
    c. deltoid and rectus femoris areas.
    d. dorsogluteal and ventrogluteal areas.

38. Lipoatrophy is a complication that occurs when insulin is injected repeatedly in one site. The physiologic effect that occurs is:
    a. a depression under the skin surface.
    b. a raised lump or knot on the skin surface.
    c. rash at a raised area on the skin surface.
    d. bruising under the skin.

Situation: R.K., 47 years old, takes insulin daily at 0700: 6 units of U100 regular and 14 units of U100 NPH. R.K.'s daily insulin dosage is regulated by using the sliding-scale (insulin coverage) method. He uses a glucometer at 1100, 1600, and bedtime (2100) to check his blood sugar. Questions 39 to 46 refer to this situation.

39. Insulin must be stored:
    a. in the refrigerator.
    b. in a cool place.
    c. wrapped in aluminum.
    d. in the light.

40. Before use, the nurse/client must prepare the insulin by:
    a. shaking the bottle well.
    b. allowing air to escape from the bottle.
    c. rolling the bottle in the hands.
    d. adding diluent to the bottle.

41. The nurse is giving R.K. his 0700 insulin and prepares:
    a. two separate injections.
    b. one injection; draw up regular insulin first.
    c. one injection; draw up NPH insulin first.
    d. one injection; draw up both simultaneously and mix well.

42. In administering R.K.'s insulin, the following syringe is used:
    a. 2 ml syringe.
    b. 5 ml syringe.
    c. U40 insulin syringe.
    d. U100 insulin syringe.

43. R.K. needs to develop a "site rotation pattern" for insulin injections. The American Diabetes Association suggests all of the following EXCEPT:
    a. choose an injection site for a week.
    b. inject insulin each day at the injection site at 1½ inches apart.
    c. change the injection area of the body every day.
    d. with two daily injection times, use the right side in the morning and the left side in the evening.

44. The nurse reviews with R.K. that regular insulin peaks in _____ hours.
    a. ½ to 1
    b. 2 to 6
    c. 6 to 8
    d. 8 to 10

45. NPH insulin peaks in _____ hours.
    a. 1 to 2
    b. 2 to 6
    c. 6 to 12
    d. 12 to 15

46. At what times is R.K. most likely to have a hypoglycemic reaction?
    a. 1300 and 1900
    b. 1200 and 2000
    c. 1000 and 2200
    d. 0900 and 1500

47. Lantus is a long-acting insulin. Which one of the following statements regarding Lantus is NOT correct?
    a. It is given in the evening and has a 24-hour duration of action.
    b. Some clients complain of pain at the injection site.
    c. It is safe because hypoglycemia cannot occur.
    d. It is available in a 3 ml cartridge insulin pen.

48. Insulin resistance can be a problem for some clients taking insulin. There are various causes for insulin resistance such as:
    a. antibody development in clients taking animal insulin over time.
    b. clients taking increased units of Humulin insulin over time.
    c. clients who are allergic to dust, mold, cat dander, and other allergens.
    d. clients with diabetes who are malnourished.

49. A method to determine if the client has insulin resistance is:
    a. chemistry laboratory tests.
    b. urinalysis to check for glucose.
    c. skin test with different insulin preparations.
    d. history of other allergies.

50. The insulin pump, though expensive, has become popular in the management of insulin. This method of insulin delivery:
    a. is more effective for use by the type 2 diabetic client.
    b. is effective in lessening long-term diabetic complications.
    c. can be used with modified insulins (NPH) as well as regular insulin.
    d. can be used with the needle inserted at the same site for weeks.

Situation: A.B., a 55-year-old obese female, has type 2 diabetes mellitus. She is receiving the oral hypoglycemic (antidiabetic) drug acetohexamide (Dymelor) daily in the morning. Questions 51 to 57 refer to this situation.

51. The oral hypoglycemic action is to:
    a. increase the number of insulin cell receptors.
    b. increase the number of insulin-producing cells.
    c. replace receptor sites.
    d. replace insulin.

52. A.B. asks if Dymelor is oral insulin. The best response would be:
    a. "Yes, it is the same as injected insulin, except it is taken orally."
    b. "Yes, it is similar; however, hypoglycemic reactions (insulin shock) do not occur with Dymelor."
    c. "No, it is not the same as insulin, and Dymelor can be taken even when the blood sugar remains greater than 250 mg/dl."
    d. "No, it is not the same as insulin. Dymelor can be used only when there is some beta cell function."

53. Acetohexamide (Dymelor) is a/an
    _____ hypoglycemic drug.
    Its duration of action is _____
    than tolbutamide (Orinase).
    a.   short-acting; shorter
    b.   intermediate-acting; longer
    c.   intermediate-acting; shorter
    d.   long-acting; longer

54. Health teaching related to acetohexamide
    includes avoidance of alcohol because of:
    a.   poor nutritional state.
    b.   decreased mental alertness.
    c.   inability to drive.
    d.   increased half-life of acetohexamide.

55. The effects of second-generation
    sulfonylureas include all of the following
    EXCEPT that:
    a.   they have less hypoglycemic potency
         than first-generation sulfonylureas.
    b.   effective doses are less than with
         first-generation sulfonylureas.
    c.   they have less displacement from
         protein-binding sites by other highly
         protein-bound drugs.
    d.   they increase tissue response and
         decrease glucose production by the
         liver.

56. New antidiabetic drugs are the nonsulfonyl-
    ureas. These drugs are used to control serum
    glucose levels following a meal. They act by:
    a.   raising the serum glucose level
         following a meal.
    b.   increasing the absorption of glucose
         from the small intestine.
    c.   causing a hypoglycemic reaction.
    d.   decreasing hepatic production of
         glucose from stored glycogen.

57. Correct the incorrect responses in question 56.
    _____
    _____
    _____

58. An example of a nonsulfonylurea is acarbose
    (Precose), an alpha-glucosidase inhibitor that
    acts by:
    a.   increasing insulin production; thus it
         can cause a hypoglycemic reaction.
    b.   inhibiting digestive enzymes in the
         small intestine, which releases glucose
         from the complex carbohydrates in the
         diet (less sugar is available).
    c.   stimulating the beta cells to produce
         insulin.
    d.   increasing glucose metabolism.

59. The newest class of nonsulfonylureas is the
    thiazolidinedione group. This group of oral
    antidiabetics does not promote insulin release
    but:
    a.   promotes absorption of glucose from
         the large intestine.
    b.   increases the uptake of glucose in the
         liver and small intestine.
    c.   increases insulin sensitivity for
         improving blood glucose control.
    d.   decreases glucose utilization.

60. The first thiazolidinedione, troglitazone
    (Rezulin), was removed from the market in
    2000. The reason for this drug's withdrawal
    by the FDA is that it caused:
    a.   kidney failure.
    b.   severe liver dysfunction.
    c.   blood dyscrasia.
    d.   peptic ulcer disease.

61. Clients taking thiazolidinedione drugs such
    as pioglitazone (Actos) and rosiglitazone
    (Avandia) should have which laboratory
    test(s) monitored?
    a.   BUN
    b.   hemoglobin and hematocrit
    c.   cardiac enzymes
    d.   liver enzymes

62. Herb-drug interaction needs to be assessed by clients taking herbs and antidiabetic agents. Ginseng and garlic taken with insulin or oral antidiabetic drugs:

    a. can decrease the effect of insulin and antidiabetic drugs, thus causing a hyperglycemic effect.

    b. can lower the blood glucose level, thus causing a hypoglycemic effect.

    c. may decrease insulin requirements.

    d. can be taken with insulin without any effect but can cause a hypoglycemic reaction with oral antidiabetic drugs.

63. Recommended guidelines for use of oral antidiabetics include which of the following? *Select all that apply.*

    a. underweight client

    b. onset at age 40 or older

    c. normal renal and hepatic function

    d. fasting blood sugar less than 200 mg/dl

    e. diagnosis of diabetes mellitus for <10 years

64. Which of the following will cause a drug interaction with acetohexamide? *Select all that apply.*

    a. aspirin

    b. antacids

    c. sulfonamides

    d. anticoagulants

    e. anticonvulsants

65. Contraindications for the use of oral antidiabetic drugs include which of the following? *Select all that apply.*

    a. pregnancy

    b. breast-feeding

    c. severe infection

    d. type 2 diabetes

    e. renal dysfunction

Critical Thinking Exercises

Use a separate sheet of paper for your answers.

N.V., age 39, was diagnosed with diabetes mellitus 15 years ago. Symptoms of diabetes occurred 3 weeks after he had hepatitis. N.V. takes 42 units of NPH and 8 units of regular insulin daily.

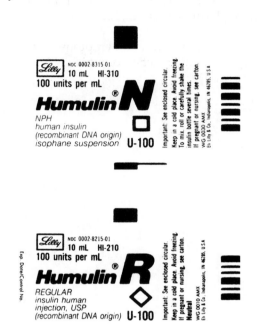

1. Why do you think N.V. is taking Humulin regular and Humulin NPH insulins rather than the same type of insulin from pork and beef?

2. Indicate on the insulin syringe the amount of regular and NPH insulin that is to be given.

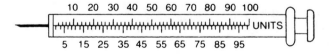

3. Could N.V. take a sulfonylurea or a nonsulfonylurea instead of insulin? Explain.

4. What instruction should you give N.V. concerning insulin injection sites?

5. N.V. weighs 72 kg. As a diabetic, is N.V. within the "average" insulin dosage?

6. When is it likely that N.V. might have a hypoglycemic (insulin) reaction?

7. What are the signs and symptoms of a hypoglycemic reaction of which N.V. should be aware?

8. What client teaching strategies should the nurse include for N.V.?

9. What effect can occur when mixing two insulins together, such as NPH and regular insulins, and Lente and regular insulins?

10. What teaching points should you give N.V. and significant others about reversing the onset of a hypoglycemic reaction?

52 Female Reproductive Cycle I: Pregnancy and Preterm Labor Drugs

Study Questions

Define the following:

1. Eclampsia

2. Gestational hypertension

3. HELLP

4. L/S (lecithin/sphingomyelin) ratio

5. Preeclampsia

6. Preterm labor

7. Progesterone

8. Surfactant

9. Teratogens

10. Tocolytic therapy

Complete the following:

11. Therapeutically prescribed drugs such as antibiotics (are/are not) ordered in lower doses during pregnancy. *(Circle correct answer.)*

12. Maternal physiologic changes during pregnancy that affect drug dosing include: _____ , a woman's reduced gastrointestinal motility and increased gastric pH, _____ , and _____ .

13. Highly protein-bound drugs (do/do not) readily cross the placenta. *(Circle correct answer.)*

14. The placenta (does/does not) act as a protective barrier to keep substances from going from the maternal circulation into the fetal circulation. *(Circle correct answer.)*

15. Drug excretion is (slower/faster) in the fetus than in the mother. *(Circle correct answer.)*

16. The mechanism by which drugs cross the placenta is similar to the way drugs infiltrate _____ tissue.

17. Important factors that determine the teratogenicity of any drug ingested during pregnancy include _____ , _____ , and _____ .

18. Surfactant is composed of the two phospholipids _____ and _____ .

19. The L/S ratio is a predictor of
_____ and _____.

20. a. Administration of the glucocorticoid
_____ (name), preferably
_____ hours (but less than
_____ days) before delivery
in the _____ week of
gestation or before, may promote fetal
lung maturity.

    b. The goal in administering
glucocorticoids during this time
is _____.

21. In addition to the delivery of an
uncompromised infant, the two primary
treatment goals in gestational hypertension
(PIH) are prevention of _____ and
_____.

22. The first and second most common
complaints of pregnancy associated with
client requests for medication are
_____ and _____.

23. The nonanemic pregnant woman is generally
instructed to increase iron intake from a
recommended _____
mg nonpregnant daily allowance to
_____ mg, while anemic clients
generally receive _____ mg
of elemental iron. These supplements
generally continue following delivery for
_____ weeks. Clients who exhibit
a validated iron deficiency anemia generally
respond to iron supplementation therapy
within _____ weeks as evidenced by
increased _____ (blood test) values.

24. Vitamin and mineral megadoses during
pregnancy (will/will not) improve health.
(Circle correct answer.)

25. Cultural variations exist in regard to the
use of prenatal vitamins. One country in
which some individuals are known to view
vitamins as a hot food to avoid in pregnancy
is _____.

26. List four nonpharmacologic measures to
decrease nausea and vomiting during early
pregnancy:

    a.

    b.

    c.

    d.

27. List four nonpharmacologic measures
preferred for the management of heartburn:

    a.

    b.

    c.

    d.

28. List four teaching goals for clients with
gestational hypertension:

    a.

    b.

    c.

    d.

Match the letter(s) of the substance in Column II with the associated adverse effect in Column I. Some substances may have more than one adverse effect.

Column I	Column II
____ 29. increased risk of spontaneous abortion	a. alcohol
	b. caffeine
____ 30. smaller head circumference without catch-up	c. cocaine
	d. heroin
	e. methadone
____ 31. hypertonicity, tremulousness in baby	f. barbiturates
	g. tobacco/nicotine
____ 32. abruptio placentae and premature delivery	h. tranquilizer
____ 33. degenerative placental lesions	
____ 34. decreased intervillous blood flow	
____ 35. inadequate maternal calorie and protein intake	
____ 36. ataxia, syncope, vertigo	
____ 37. rapidly crosses placenta and causes CNS depression in the fetus	

NCLEX Review Question

Select the best response.

38. During pregnancy, the amount of iron necessary is _____ that of the prepregnant state.
    a. the same as
    b. twice
    c. triple
    d. one-half

39. Side effects of iron include all of the following EXCEPT:
    a. nausea.
    b. constipation.
    c. epigastric pain.
    d. jaundice.

40. You advise the client that all of the following foods are rich in iron EXCEPT:
    a. lettuce.
    b. liver.
    c. spinach.
    d. cereal.

41. The pregnancy RDA for folic acid is:
    a. 100-400 mcg.
    b. 400-800 mcg.
    c. 800-1000 mcg.
    d. 1000-1200 mcg.

42. To enhance both drugs' effectiveness, iron and antacids should be administered:
    a. at the same time.
    b. 2 hours apart.
    c. with the antacid first.
    d. with the iron first.

43. The drug most commonly selected and ingested by clients during pregnancy is:

    a. ferrous sulfate.

    b. Tigan.

    c. Mylanta.

    d. acetaminophen.

Situation: W.C. is receiving a beta-sympathomimetic drug to stop her preterm labor. Questions 44 to 46 refer to this situation.

44. Nursing interventions for W.C., who is receiving a beta-sympathomimetic drug, include all of the following EXCEPT:

    a. monitoring maternal and fetal vital signs every 15 minutes when receiving IV dose.

    b. monitoring daily weight.

    c. being alert to hypoglycemia and hypokalemia in newborn delivered within 5 hours of discontinuing the drug.

    d. restricting all fluids.

45. The health care provider for W.C., who is receiving a beta-sympathomimetic drug, should be notified of any of the following findings EXCEPT:

    a. auscultated dysrhythmias.

    b. respirations greater than 30 breaths/min.

    c. systolic blood pressure greater than 100 mm Hg.

    d. fetal baseline heart rate greater than 180 beats/min.

46. Health teaching for W.C., who is receiving a beta-sympathomimetic drug, includes all of the following EXCEPT:

    a. palpitations are uncommon.

    b. notify health care provider of frequent contractions while taking the drug.

    c. consult health care provider before taking any other medications.

    d. take medications as directed.

47. A client receiving magnesium sulfate for preeclampsia requires all of the following nursing interventions EXCEPT:

    a. providing continuous fetal monitoring and documentation every 15 minutes.

    b. having airway suction equipment readily available.

    c. having antidote calcium gluconate at the bedside.

    d. monitoring vital signs every 4 hours.

48. While caring for a client receiving magnesium sulfate, you notify the health care provider of any of the following EXCEPT:

    a. absence of patellar reflexes.

    b. respirations greater than 15 breaths/min.

    c. absent bowel sounds.

    d. change in affect.

49. Magnesium toxicity is manifested by which of the following?

    a. rapid decrease in blood pressure and respiratory paralysis

    b. rapid increase in blood pressure and respiratory paralysis

    c. sudden fever and somnolence

    d. muscle pain and excessive weight gain

50. The client being treated during labor with magnesium sulfate asks how long she will need this drug. Your best response is that the drug will probably be discontinued:

    a. at the time of delivery.

    b. 1-4 hours after delivery.

    c. 24 hours after delivery.

    d. 48-72 hours after delivery.

51. Antacids may cause drug interactions with the following: *Select all that apply.*

    a. digitalis

    b. anticonvulsants

    c. tetracyclines

    d. iron

52. Use of aspirin late in pregnancy is related to the following:
    a. increased maternal blood loss at delivery
    b. low birth weight infant
    c. increased risk of anemia
    d. decreased hemostasis in newborn

53. Ms. Varnell is receiving magnesium sulfate IV for gestational hypertension. Expected side effects from this medication would include the following: *Select all that apply.*
    a. flushing
    b. lethargy
    c. tachycardia
    d. slurred speech
    e. hyperreflexia

Critical Thinking Exercises

Use a separate sheet of paper for your answers.

S.B. is a 38-year-old mother of 5- and 7-year-old children, is currently 28 weeks' pregnant, and has recently separated from her husband of 15 years. S.B. frantically calls the OB triage unit from the department store in the local mall where she works. She states that she has been unable to get through to her doctor's office because of busy signals and interruptions by her customers. She states that she is "terrified I might be going into labor." She stutters that she had a "baby born early" 5 years ago. She desperately says, "This just can't be happening again. I have no benefits yet in this job. My husband has been out of work due to his company downsizing; he has no benefits either. Plus he is keeping company with another lady in the meantime, which is why we are apart. Please, please tell me what to do now." She further conveys, "I'm having contractions about every eight minutes and I feel like there is some kind of pressure inside my lower belly. My children are in school and daycare and will be home three hours from now."

1. If you were the nurse in the OB triage unit who received this call from S.B., what data supplied in her brief telephone history support a diagnosis of PTL?

2. What additional data would you collect during evaluation at the triage unit to support the accuracy of the preliminary PTL diagnosis?

3. What risk factors are present that increase the likelihood of the PTL diagnosis for S.B.?

4. Considering that (1) you are talking with S.B. on the phone while she is at work, (2) your preliminary data analysis supports that S.B. is indeed at risk for PTL, and (3) S.B. has not been able to reach her personal health care provider, how would you counsel S.B.?

5. S.B.'s PTL contractions are not relieved following the conservative measures you suggested. Her doctor agrees that S.B. should be directed to the OB triage unit for further evaluation. The decision is made following interview, fetal monitoring, and cervical examination that S.B. is a suitable candidate for tocolytic therapy. Indicate four findings that, had they been present, would have contraindicated tocolytic therapy for S.B.:

    a.

    b.

    c.

    d.

6. You share with S.B. that the goal in tocolytic therapy is to (increase/decrease) *(Circle correct answer.)* the level of uterine contractions in order to stop preterm labor; this allows time for maturation of the lungs within the uterine environment.

7. The treatment plan for S.B. calls for the use of subQ terbutaline. Considering that the goal of tocolytic therapy is to depress or quiet the myometrial contractions, answer the following questions: (1) What information would you need to record on the fetal monitoring strip and/or document on the agency-specified flow sheet? (2) What information could you gain from the monitor strip in tracking the effectiveness of the tocolytic therapy? (3) What findings would you determine are important to convey specifically to the health care provider in addition to documenting them?

8. Criteria for determining that subQ tocolytic therapy is successful for S.B. are:

    Contractions decrease to _____ apart

    Cervical dilation and/or effacement _____.

9. Assume the decision is made for S.B. to continue taking oral terbutaline after discharge. The purpose of this oral therapy is to _____.

10. The high-risk unit nurse has worked with S.B. to address identified knowledge deficits, emphasizing the importance of medication compliance. S.B. states that she knows she must take her oral terbutaline on a schedule but questions, "If I go back to the store to work, it is hard to get free to go to the bathroom and to the break room for fluids; it is also difficult to get my purse, as we aren't allowed to keep purses at the counter where I work."

    a. Discuss some strategies for how S.B. could handle her medication needs while at work.

    b. If S.B. realizes that she missed taking a dose within the past hour and calls for advice, you correctly tell her to _____.

53 Female Reproductive Cycle II: Labor, Delivery, and Preterm Neonatal Drugs

Study Questions

Define the following:

1. Analgesia/sedation

2. Anesthesia

3. Bishop score

4. Cervical ripening

5. Dose ceiling effect

6. Ergot alkaloids

7. Kappa receptors

8. Labor augmentation

9. Labor induction

10. Mu receptors

11. Oxytocics

12. Oxytocin

13. Prostaglandin

14. Somatic pain

15. Stripping the membranes

16. Surfactant

17. Uterine inertia

18. Visceral pain

Complete the following:

19. Rales and moist breath sounds are expected, though they may be transient findings following the administration of _____ and _____.

20. Surfactant replacement therapy in the newborn with Survanta or Exosurf Pediatric is administered in one of two modes: _____ and _____.

21. When narcotic-agonists are administered during labor, birth should be anticipated to occur within _____ hours, or after _____ hours following administration, to prevent _____.

22. Argue in support of giving the medication at the time period selected.

_____

_____

23. The primary advantage of butorphanol tartrate (Stadol) and nalbuphine (Nubain) is their _____ effect. Discuss what this means specifically to labor.

24. The adverse effects of opioids depend on the responses activated by the _____ and _____ receptors.

25. Administer _____ by IM (Z track) only. Do not administer this drug subQ or IV.

26. When administering promethazine (Phenergan) by IV, administer at a rate not to exceed _____ mg/min.

27. The most common regional anesthestics used for women in labor are:

    a.

    b.

28. A primary concern for spinal anesthesia is _____.

29. List three treatment measures for postdural headaches:

    a.

    b.

    c.

30. Rescue doses of medication are given for continuous epidural infusions to _____.

31. Before labor induction a _____ score, an objective scoring system, is used to assess readiness for induction. List the five components of this scoring system.

    a.

    b.

    c.

    d.

    e.

32. List three mechanical methods used to induce labor.

    a.

    b.

    c.

33. Women receiving oxytocin need to be monitored for _____ and _____.

34. Discuss the possible complication(s) of administering methylergonovine maleate (Methergine) during labor and/or before the delivery of the placenta.

NCLEX Review Questions

Select the best response.

35. When pain medication is administered to the laboring client using the IV route, the medication should be given:
    a. at the beginning of the uterine contraction.
    b. in the middle of the uterine contraction.
    c. at the end of the uterine contraction.
    d. between uterine contractions.

36. If the client is abusing narcotics, a drug commonly used during labor is:
    a. Nembutal.
    b. Atarax.
    c. Stadol.
    d. Demerol.

37. Neonatal respiratory depression may require reversal by administration of:
    a. calcium gluconate.
    b. calcium carbonate.
    c. syrup of ipecac.
    d. naloxone (Narcan).

38. Before the administration of general anesthesia, the laboring woman is administered 30 ml of Bicitra. This medication is given to:
    a. prevent nausea and vomiting.
    b. decrease gastric acidity.
    c. maintain a patent airway.
    d. enhance anesthesia induction.

39. Before administration of an epidural, the woman in labor should:
    a. receive a bolus of crystalloids, 500-1000 ml IV.
    b. be monitored for mitral valve disease.
    c. verbally consent to the procedure.
    d. be typed and crossmatched for blood administration.

40. Ms. Surles is receiving an epidural and her blood pressure is beginning to drop. Your first action based upon your emergency protocol is to:
    a. expect an order to transfuse with 1 unit of PRCs.
    b. expect an order to administer 5-15 mg ephedrine IV.
    c. turn her on her left side.
    d. administer oxygen 2-4 L by nasal cannula.

41. The woman in labor is questioning you about labor being longer for women who receive an epidural. Your best response is:
    a. "This is not accurate as women who receive epidurals have the same length of labor as those receiving IV pain relief medications."
    b. "No, women with spinal anesthesia have a longer labor."
    c. "Yes, women do have a longer labor, approximately 15-30 minutes longer; they can feel movement and pressure but not pain."
    d. "Yes, women do have a longer labor, approximately 2-3 hours longer; they have no pain or pressure with epidurals."

42. Scores of _____ or greater on the Bishop score are associated with successful labor induction.
    a. 5
    b. 6
    c. 8
    d. 10

43. Women commonly receive ergot alkaloids during the:
    a. first stage of labor.
    b. second stage of labor.
    c. third stage of labor.
    d. fourth stage of labor.

44. Before administering methylergonovine (Methergine) it is important to obtain a baseline:
    a. fetal heart rate.
    b. maternal respiratory rate.
    c. maternal hourly urinary output.
    d. blood pressure.

45. With the administration of naloxone (Narcan) the woman in labor will experience:
    a. increased pain relief.
    b. increased pain.
    c. increased fetal heart rate decelerations.
    d. increased fetal variability.

Situation: S.R., a primipara, is 3 cm dilated and requesting medication for pain. Questions 46 to 48 refer to pain control in labor.

46. You are aware that many factors influence the choice of pain control. The MOST important factor is:
    a. intensity of contractions.
    b. amount of time likely until delivery.
    c. frequency of contractions.
    d. client requests.

47. You know that with the use of barbiturates in labor:
    a. delivery time is unpredictable.
    b. narcotic antagonists will not counteract respiratory depression.
    c. narcotics offer more complete relief.
    d. active labor is the most appropriate time for their use.

48. Client teaching for S.R. about an analgesic includes all of the following EXCEPT:
    a. expected effects on labor.
    b. expected effects on newborn.
    c. expected time delivery will occur.
    d. restrictions placed on her mobility.

49. Which of these statements about the client who receives continuous lumbar epidural block anesthesia in repeated doses is accurate?
    a. Before 8 cm dilation, there is a risk of arresting the first stage of labor.
    b. The method is suitable for vaginal delivery, but not for a cesarean delivery because the density of the block cannot be manipulated.
    c. Following injection, the client needs to be placed flat immediately to ensure dispersion of the local anesthetic toward the diaphragm.
    d. Each time the injection procedure occurs, documentation must be complete.

50. In relation to uterine contractions, spinal anesthesia should be administered:
    a. before.
    b. during.
    c. immediately after.
    d. 1-2 minutes after.

51. An example of a local anesthetic metabolized by pseudocholinesterase is:
    a. chloroprocaine (Nesacaine).
    b. mepivacaine (Carbocaine).
    c. lidocaine (Xylocaine).
    d. bupivacaine (Marcaine).

52. You assess a client receiving local anesthetic for side effects including all of the following EXCEPT:
    a. palpitations.
    b. "metallic taste" in mouth.
    c. nausea.
    d. hypertension.

Situation: Your client J.M. is having an IV oxytocin induction at 41+ weeks' gestation. Questions 53 to 56 refer to this situation.

53. You collect all of the following baseline data on J.M. EXCEPT:

    a. pulse rate and blood pressure.

    b. deep tendon reflexes.

    c. uterine activity.

    d. fetal heart rate.

54. You observe J.M. and her fetus for side effects and adverse reactions to oxytocin, including which of the following?

    a. tetanic uterine contractions

    b. fetal tachycardia

    c. generalized muscular weakness

    d. urinary retention

55. As a precaution, you have the antidote drug _____ readily available.

    a. prednisone

    b. Narcan

    c. calcium gluconate

    d. magnesium sulfate

56. In addition, you monitor J.M. for signs of uterine rupture, including any of the following EXCEPT:

    a. hypertension.

    b. sudden increased pain.

    c. hemorrhage.

    d. loss of fetal heart rate.

57. Systemic drug groups used during labor include which of the following? *Select all that apply.*

    a. NSAIDs

    b. narcotic agonists

    c. ataractics

    d. mixed narcotic agonists-antagonists

58. After receiving sedative-hypnotic drugs and antiemetic/antihistamines for analgesia during labor, the neonate is at risk for: *Select all that apply.*

    a. decreased FHR variability.

    b. hypotonia.

    c. urinary retention.

    d. CNS depression.

    e. hypothermia.

59. Ms. Wilson is complaining of labor pain. This pain, somatic, is pressure of the presenting part and stretching of the perineum and vagina. This pain is the pain of the: *Select all that apply.*

    a. first stage of labor.

    b. latent phase of labor.

    c. active phase of labor.

    d. transition phase of labor.

    e. second stage of labor.

    f. third stage of labor.

60. Anesthesia for cesarean deliveries may be: *Select all that apply.*

    a. general anesthesia.

    b. caudal block.

    c. spinal anesthesia.

    d. pudenal anesthesia.

    e. epidural anesthesia.

Critical Thinking Exercises

Use a separate sheet of paper for your answers.

Kendra, 28 years old, is the mother of a 2-year-old child; she is 38 weeks' pregnant and admitted to the OB unit in active labor. She states "I'm having contractions about every two-three minutes. It hurts." When questioned further she rates her pain as an 8 on a scale of 1-10, describing it as "intense cramping" in "my lower belly." "Can't you do something?" In review of her fetal heart rate strip you note contractions every 2-3 minutes, lasting 50-60 seconds and with an intensity of 55-65 mm Hg.

1. If you were the nurse in the OB unit who received this call from Kendra, what objective data supplied support the need for more effective pain management?

2. What additional subjective data support the need for more effective pain management?

3. Kendra has asked for an epidural. What risk factors are contraindications for an epidural?

4. Kendra asks the nurse if her labor will be longer with an epidural. The nurses' best response is _____.

5. Following Kendra's admission interview, fetal and uterine monitoring, and cervical exam, she requests pain medication: "Now; I can't wait until the epidural, please." Until Kendra receives the epidural the health care provider writes an order for nalbuphine (Nubain) IV 10 mg. When will the nalbuphine (Nubain) be administered in relationship to her uterine contractions? Discuss the rationale for this timing.

6. Kendra asks where the epidural is injected in her back. The nurses' best response is:

7. Before receiving the epidural, Kendra will receive a bolus _____ ml of _____ (type of IV fluids). You share with Kendra that the goal of this bolus of IV fluid is to prevent _____.

8. After receiving the epidural, Kendra blood pressure begins to drop. List two immediate nursing actions to address this problem.

   a.

   b.

9. Kendra's blood pressure is continuing to fall. You would anticipate the health care provider to order _____.

10. One hour after delivery, Kendra's uterus is boggy and she is saturating a pad within 35 minutes. What medication/dose would you anticipate the health care provider order to be added to Kendra's IV fluids?

54 Postpartum and Newborn Drugs

Define the following:

1. Episiotomy

2. Erythromycin ophthalmic ointment (Ilotycin Ophthalmic)

3. Hepatitis B

4. Hepatitis B immunoglobulin

5. Lactation

6. Phytonadione (vitamin K_1, Mephyton, AquaMEPHYTON)

7. Prolactin

8. Puerperium

9. Recombinant hepatitis B

10. Rh immune globulin D

11. Rh sensitization

12. Rubella syndrome

13. Titer

Complete the following:

14. Two drugs commonly used for the relief of perineal pain resulting from episiotomy/ laceration are _____ and _____.

15. Three common drugs for the relief of hemorrhoids are _____, _____, and _____.

16. High levels of _____ are necessary to initiate the onset of lactation.

17. Explain the purpose/action of a stool softener ordered for a postpartum client:

18. You have an order to administer bisacodyl USP at lunch so the client can swallow it with her milk. Select the best response and discuss your rationale.

    Administer as ordered.
    _____ (*Check if correct.*)

    Question the order.
    _____ (*Check if correct.*)

    Why?
    _____
    _____
    _____

19. A postpartum client with a repaired fourth-degree laceration has benzocaine topical spray. She asks if she can also use a heat lamp on her perineum for additional comfort.

    What would you tell her?
    _____

    Support your answer.
    _____

20. What is the correct procedure for application of an ointment (e.g., Anusol) to hemorrhoids in a postpartum client?
    _____
    _____

    What is the rationale for the method you described?
    _____

    What would possibly occur if you managed this client as if she were a nonmaternity client?
    _____

21. The lubricant laxative _____ should not be given with meals or immediately after.

22. Erythromycin ophthalmic ointment is prescribed as prophylactic treatment for gonococcal _____ and _____ caused by *Neisseria gonorrhoeae*, which, if left untreated, can cause _____ in the newborn.

23. REEDA is used to assess and document the status of perineal wounds, such as an episiotomy. The acronym REEDA means:
    R: _____
    E: _____
    E: _____
    D: _____
    A: _____

24. One form of administering iced witch hazel compresses is pouring witch hazel over ice and placing a packet of 4 × 4 absorbent pads into the solution before applying one at a time against the perineal tissue. Given that a newly delivered postpartum client has an alteration in skin integrity because of her episiotomy with risk for infection, how could the nurse instruct the mother to apply the compresses against her perineum and keep both skin and compress as clean as possible?

25. A postoperative cesarean birth mother states that she has not passed gas since delivery. While assessing this client, the nurse observes that the abdomen is distended. The nurse will assess for _____ (sound) by percussion. Also, as a part of the assessment, the nurse should evaluate for the presence of _____ sounds. To do this assessment correctly, the nurse places a stethoscope _____ (where). In addition, this client may be ordered to receive _____ (medication name) to help relieve her distention.

    Describe the process by which this medication must be ingested _____, followed by _____ ounces of water. If the client remains distended, is uncomfortable, and does not pass gas, what additional type of medication will likely be employed?
    _____

NCLEX Review Questions

Select the best response.

26. Relief of afterbirth pains may be a concern for the multiparous postpartum client. Factors associated with an increased risk of afterbirth pains include: *Select all that apply.*
    a. primigravida.
    b. breast-feeding.
    c. multiparity.
    d. preeclampsia.

27. Lactation suppression therapy includes: *Select all that apply.*
    a. ice packs.
    b. tight supportive bra.
    c. warm compresses.
    d. warm shower water directed to the breasts.
    e. lactation.

28. The best time(s) to administer the standard dose of Rh immune globulin D is (are):
    a. at 28 weeks' gestation.
    b. before amniocentesis and at 38 weeks' gestation.
    c. at 28 weeks' gestation and again within 72 hours after delivery.
    d. after chorionic villus sampling and at 38 weeks' gestation.

29. A microdose of Rh immune globulin D is indicated after:
    a. amniocentesis.
    b. abortion of <13 weeks.
    c. abortion of >16 weeks.
    d. chorionic villus sampling.

30. Rubella can be a devastating infection to the fetus depending on which of the following?
    a. gestational age at exposure
    b. genetic predisposition
    c. severity of maternal infection
    d. negative rubella titer

31. Which of the following is NOT a commonly reported side effect of the caine drugs used in local or topical agents ordered for postpartum clients?
    a. stinging
    b. burning
    c. itching
    d. petechiae

32. Which of the following is NOT a commonly reported side effect of the hydrocortisone local or topical drugs used in products ordered with occlusive dressings for postpartum clients?
    a. burning
    b. alopecia
    c. folliculitis
    d. swelling

33. The newborn is administered the following ophthalmic ointment immediately after birth:
    a. erythromycin.
    b. bacitracin.
    c. gentamicin.
    d. penicillin.

34. Client teaching regarding ophthalmic and parenteral drugs administered to the neonate immediately after birth includes:
    a. swelling of eyes usually disappears in the first 24-48 hours.
    b. all parenteral medications can be administered in one injection.
    c. the injection is not painful for the baby.
    d. if the mother has had hepatitis immunizations then the newborn will not receive the hepatitis B immunization.

35. Which of the following statements about vitamin K administration to the newborn is NOT correct?

    a. Vitamin K is administered in the vastus lateralis muscle.

    b. The newborn is unable to synthesize vitamin K because of limited intestinal flora.

    c. A filter needle is used to draw up and administer the medication.

    d. A 25-gauge 3/4-inch needle is used to administer the medication.

36. The newborn is to receive the vitamin K injection. Place an X on the muscle where the injection should be given.

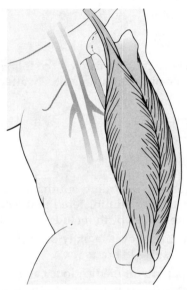

From Nichols F, Zwelling E: *Maternal-newborn nursing: theory and practice,* Philadelphia, 1997, Saunders.

Critical Thinking Exercises

Use a separate sheet of paper for your answers.

M.F., a newly delivered postpartum client, is transported from the labor/delivery suite to the postpartum unit where you are a staff nurse. Another nurse fills in and receives the transfer report about M.F.; you overhear a comment that M.F. is Rh-negative and rubella-negative.

1. What information from M.F.'s past and current history must you consider to address the question of whether she will be a candidate for Rh immune globulin D?

2. If M.F. is a candidate for Rh immune globulin D, what are two potential knowledge deficits M.F. might exhibit?

3. M.F. asks you what the Coombs test is and why her caregivers seem so interested in this test. You explain to M.F. that it is a test that screens for the presence of (antigen/antibodies) to the Rh (antigen/antibodies). The outcome is expressed as an (antigen/antibody) titer. You continue to explain that M.F. is referred to as sensitized or nonsensitized. You tell her that Rh immune globulin D candidates are (sensitized/nonsensitized) Rh-negative clients. The goal is, through the use of Rh immune globulin D, to _____ her from becoming _____ by suppressing the active (antigen/antibody) response by coating the (antigen/antibody). (*Circle correct answers.*)

Match items in Column II with those in Column I.

Column I
Test

_____ 4. direct
Coombs test

_____ 5. indirect
Coombs test

Column II
Test Subject

a. mother

b. baby

Result

_____ 6. negative indi-
rect Coombs

_____ 7. positive indi-
rect Coombs

Interpretation

a. Antigen-antibody
immunologic reac-
tion has occurred
(as shown by
reaction of rabbit
immune serum to
antibodies coat-
ing the RBCs;
an agglutination
reaction; some
quantity of anti-
bodies is present).

b. Antigen-antibody
immunologic
reaction has not
occurred (no anti-
bodies are present).

Substance

_____ 8. antigen

_____ 9. antibody

Descriptor

a. protein developed
by the body in
response to pres-
ence of a foreign
body; found in
plasma

b. invader; usually a
protein

Rh System

_____ 10. Rh-positive
individual

_____ 11. Rh-negative
individual

**Relationship to
the D Antigen***

a. red cells contain D
antigen

b. red cells lack D
antigen

Complete the following:

12. M.F. needs to understand that if the baby
she just delivered is Rh (positive/negative),
she could, based on factors from her history
and/or this pregnancy, labor, and delivery,
develop anti-D (antibodies/antigens) as an
outcome. Therefore her caregiver's goal is
to ascertain that the D (antibody/antigen) is
_____. Likewise, a laboratory report
of the baby's blood type and sensitization
status (based on detection of red blood cells
coated with antibody) is reviewed. If M.F.
and the baby both test (positive/negative)
for sensitization, general practice is for M.F.
to receive Rh immune globulin D within
_____ hours postpartum to prevent
isoimmunization, which could present difficulties for a fetus in a subsequent pregnancy.
(Circle correct answers.)

13. There are safety measures that the nurse
must observe when he or she administers Rh
immune globulin D to a client. Among these
is agreement of lot numbers on the vial with
crossmatch lab slips; match between the ID
band and the lab slip numbers; signed
consent; return of vial and lab slips; and
careful screening for known hypersensitivity
reactions to immune globulins. Discuss the
rationale for these safety measures.

14. M.F.'s history indicated she is rubella-negative.
You check her chart and find that she is listed
in one section of the chart as rubella-immune
and in another section of the chart as
rubella-susceptible. Describe appropriate
nursing actions to resolve the discrepancy.

15. Assume that M.F. is to receive both Rh
immune globulin D and rubella vaccine.
What would you explain to M.F. about the
interaction of the two drugs?

16. Based on her history, what would you convey
to M.F. as her postdischarge responsibility in
regard to the rubella vaccine she received?

55 Drugs for Women's Health and Reproductive Disorders

Study Questions

Define the following:

1. Estrogen replacement therapy (ERT)

2. Hormone replacement therapy (HRT)

3. Progestin

4. Oral contraceptives

Complete the following:

5. The two main types of oral contraceptives are:
   a. _____-_____
      combination products, the pill.
   b. _____-_____
      products, the mini pill.

6. List the serious side effects (ACHES) associated with oral contraceptives:
   A =
   C =
   H =
   E =
   S =

7. The newest combination product(s) designed to give low doses of both hormones with minimal side effects is/are the _____.

8. The mini pill acts primarily by _____.

9. The nurse can accurately explain to a client that the Depo-Provera injection acts by _____ and _____ to make the uterine wall mucosa less hospitable for _____.

10. G.P, a 17-year-old postpartum client, has decided to use long-acting injectable Depo-Provera as a birth control method because of the 3-month interval and the fact that she often "forgot" to take her oral contraceptives. The nurse gives the first injection on October 10 and advises the client that she will need to schedule subsequent injections for January 10, April 10, July 10, and again on October 10. The nurse circles these dates on the small purple wallet reminder card supplied with the product. The client responds, "Thanks! This is great and easy to remember." Comment on the way the nurse chose to handle follow-up injection planning and documentation and expected standards of practice.

11. Common symptoms associated with premenstrual syndrome (PMS) are:

    a.

    b.

    c.

    d.

    e.

    f.

12. List four points to be included in a client's health teaching plan for PMS:

    a.

    b.

    c.

    d.

13. The four most common physical changes associated with menopause are:

    a.

    b.

    c.

    d.

14. The most widely used treatment for the relief of menopause-associated changes is _____.

15. List four advantages and disadvantages of oral contraceptives:

Advantages	Disadvantages
a.	a.
b.	b.
c.	c.
d.	d.

16. List four major points to include in health teaching plans for oral contraceptives:

    a.

    b.

    c.

    d.

17. List four factors to be included in your health teaching with clients using HRT:

    a.

    b.

    c.

    d.

18. Progesterone-only methods of contraception result in regular menstrual cycles.
    a.   true
    b.   false

Match characteristics associated with the investigational drugs in Column II with the drugs in Column I. Some Column II characteristics may be used more than once.

Column I		Column II
_____ 19. misoprostol	a.	chemotherapeutic agent
_____ 20. methotrexate	b.	ulcer agent
	c.	destabilizes uterine lining
	d.	creates contractions that shed uterine lining in 24 hours
	e.	given 1 week after the first drug

NCLEX Review Questions

Select the best response.

21. Contraceptive methods that are available for poor pill-takers include:
    a. Depo-Provera injection.
    b. Ortho Evra patch.
    c. NuvaRing.
    d. Implanon.
    e. all of the above.

22. Which of the following modes of action is NOT correct for emergency contraception?
    a. delays ovulation
    b. interferes with hormones for implantation
    c. causes an abortion
    d. interferes with tubal transport of embryo

23. Which of the following statements about intrauterine devices is NOT correct?
    a. They are appropriate for all women.
    b. ParaGard's active ingredient is copper.
    c. Mirena's active ingredient is levonorgestrel.
    d. Mirena causes less menstrual bleeding and cramping.

24. The advantages of oral contraceptives include all of the following EXCEPT:
    a. relative safety.
    b. ease of use.
    c. low cost.
    d. high degree of effectiveness.

25. Which of the following does NOT contraindicate the use of oral contraceptives?
    a. breast cancer
    b. coronary artery disease
    c. pregnancy, confirmed or suspected
    d. emphysema

26. Considering concerns common to teenage girls in this society, which of these oral contraceptive-associated issues or side effects would be most likely to deter use?
    a. decreased tearing (dry eyes)
    b. risk of interaction with other drugs
    c. weight gain
    d. recommendation against smoking

27. Cautious use of oral contraceptives is recommended with all of the following EXCEPT:
    a. women who smoke.
    b. diabetes.
    c. grand multiparity.
    d. epilepsy.

28. The major risk associated with the use of leuprolide acetate for the treatment of endometriosis is:
    a. depression.
    b. decreased libido.
    c. cardiac dysrhythmias.
    d. potential loss of bone density.

29. Which of the following is correct regarding the administration of Lupron?
    a. Shake reconstituted product until clear; use 2 ml syringe.
    b. Reconstituted product is stable for 48 hours; use supplied syringe.
    c. Reconstituted solution is "milky"; use supplied syringe.
    d. Store product in refrigerator; use 2 ml syringe.

30. When teaching a client about the correct use of nafarelin acetate (Synarel nasal solution), include all EXCEPT which of the following?
    a. Precise guidelines must be followed.
    b. Medication is expensive; need to plan for 6 months' expenses to avoid interruptions in therapy.
    c. Clear nasal passage and administer spray in one nostril only.
    d. Avoid use of nasal decongestant sprays.

31. Which of the following is NOT a contraindication to HRT?

    a. impaired renal function

    b. history of thromboembolic disorder

    c. impaired liver function

    d. uncontrolled hypertension

Situation: N.M. has been taking Tri-Levlen for contraception. Questions 32 to 36 refer to this situation.

32. N.M. reports a variety of side effects. The side effect NOT due primarily to an excess in estrogen is:

    a. acne.

    b. nausea.

    c. fluid retention.

    d. breast tenderness.

33. As you listen to N.M.'s current drug history, you are alert to drugs that interact with oral contraceptives and are NOT concerned with her reported use of:

    a. phenytoin.

    b. caffeine.

    c. vitamins.

    d. theophyllines.

34. Which of the following laboratory values would NOT be expected to change for N.M.?

    a. thyroid and liver function

    b. blood glucose

    c. triglycerides

    d. BUN

35. N.M. calls and reports missing one pill. Your best response is to advise her to:

    a. skip this pill. Take her next pill at the normal time tomorrow.

    b. take the missed pill right away. Take tomorrow's pill at the usual time.

    c. discard current pill pack and start a new package of pills.

    d. do a pregnancy test; report the results.

36. The family planning nurse would be correct to tell N.M. to stop taking her oral contraceptive pills and notify her health care provider if she experiences:

    a. increased vaginal discharge.

    b. severe headaches.

    c. lighter/shorter periods.

    d. menstrual cramping.

Situation: M.B. is taking danazol (Danocrine) for the treatment of endometriosis. Questions 37 to 39 refer to this client situation.

37. Which of the following is NOT true about this drug?

    a. It is a pituitary gonadotropin-inhibiting agent.

    b. Menses cease during therapy.

    c. Ovulation occurs during therapy.

    d. It has no estrogenic action.

38. Which of the following is NOT a side effect of Danocrine?

    a. weight gain

    b. rash

    c. decrease in breast size

    d. hot flashes

39. M.B. asks, "What are the chances of conception during a cycle?" The most accurate response is:

    a. 4%.

    b. 6%.

    c. 8%.

    d. 10%.

Situation: E.H. is taking HRT for menopause. Questions 40 to 44 relate to this client situation.

40. This therapy is treatment for all of the following EXCEPT:

    a. gastrointestinal disturbances.

    b. vasomotor symptoms.

    c. prevention of osteoporosis.

    d. urogenital atrophy.

41. Use of progestin in HRT is to decrease:
    a. endometrial hyperplasia.
    b. risk of endometrial cancer.
    c. risk of breast cancer.
    d. risk of cervical cancer.

42. Which of the following is NOT an advantage of the Estraderm transdermal system?
    a. less expensive than tablets
    b. applied 2 times per week for 3 weeks using rotation of sites
    c. drug absorbed directly into bloodstream
    d. results in less nausea and vomiting

43. Which of the following statements are *TRUE* about combined birth control pills? *Select all that apply.*
    a. available in 24 day active pills
    b. available in 28 day active pills
    c. available as a chewable pill
    d. available without a prescription

44. Medications used to prevent and/or treat osteoporosis include the following: *Select all that apply.*
    a. estrogen.
    b. statins.
    c. bisphosphonates.
    d. SERMs.

45. Which of the following are true statements about HRT? *Select all that apply.*
    a. HRT may be used to prevent heart disease.
    b. HRT is indicated for the treatment of menopausal vasomotor symptoms.
    c. HRT should be used for the shortest period of time possible, at the lowest effective dose.
    d. Vaginal creams or rings may be used to treat urogenital atrophy.

Critical Thinking Exercises

Use a separate sheet of paper for your answers.

During her GYN intake interview with the nursing case manager at her company's new health care clinic, C.W., age 55, states, "I seem to be having more discomfort when I have intercourse. I don't lubricate when I want and need to; if Charlie hurries me, it is downright painful. This is probably my problem, but Charlie thinks that after a 35-year marriage, I just don't really want to have sex any more."

Sarah, the nurse, compiles a few more facts about C.W. for review and consideration. In addition to her dyspareunia, C.W. has urinary frequency and urgency, leukorrhea, itching, thinning vaginal epithelium with a glazed-looking appearance, and minimal elasticity upon speculum examination.

C.W. is Caucasian, thin overall, and reports no periods for nearly 2 years. She has no history of vaginal infections, and her hygiene is excellent.

1. The most likely physiologic explanation for C.W.'s current experiences during intercourse is _____. Given the fact that C.W. has had no periods for more than a year, Sarah knows that menopause (has/has not) occurred. (Circle correct answer.) Sarah asks C.W. if she has considered exploring the use of HRT. C.W. responds that she has thought about it, listens to every news report that addresses the issue, but is afraid to take hormones unless she can perceive more benefits than potential liabilities for her personally. How might Sarah advise C.W.?

2. While conducting an assessment of C.W. for other physical changes associated with menopause, what other physical characteristics might Sarah discuss with C.W.?

3. C.W.'s physical characteristics put her at particular risk for _____.

   Why is this risk an especially important consideration for C.W.?

4. In advising C.W., Sarah knows that the two major reasons women often choose NOT to use estrogen replacement therapy or do not continue it are _____ and _____. As a result, significant preventive health care benefits from the therapy _____.

5. Benefits of HRT that Sarah will want to discuss with C.W. include (in priority order):

   Give information to support the order in which you listed these.

6. As the discussion progresses, C.W. mentions that, "If the estrogen is so beneficial, it doesn't make sense why a person also has to take a medication with it that partially blocks these beneficial effects." Explain the reason the synthetic hormone progestin is added.

7. C.W. asks, "Do I need to swallow pills if I just want to get rid of these vaginal problems?" Sarah correctly responds:

8. Sarah reviews C.W.'s history for the presence of any factors that might contraindicate the use of estrogens. What factors should Sarah look for?

   If C.W. is perimenopausal with irregular periods, what additional contraindication should be ruled out?

9. If C.W. elects to start HRT and returns complaining of PMS-type complaints, what is the most likely cause? _____

   What should Sarah advise C.W. to do?

10. C.W. elects to try HRT. Several months go by and Sarah receives a call from C.W. stating that she is not having bleeding between her periods but is having bleeding during the last week of her cycle that lasts a few days but does not quite resemble her former periods. She also says that she is having an occasional hot flash during this period and that she thought these would completely disappear with the therapy. Sarah correctly advises C.W. that:

56 Drugs for Men's Health and Reproductive Disorders

Study Questions

Define the following:

1. Anabolic steroids

2. Androgens

3. Hirsutism

4. Spermatogenesis

5. Virilization

Complete the following:

6. The primary androgen _____ is synthesized in the testes and adrenal cortex.

7. The human sexual response cycle consists of five phases: desire, excitement, _____, _____, and _____.

8. The rate of testosterone production is controlled by a _____.

9. Synthetic androgens have (shorter/longer) half-lives. (*Circle correct answer.*)

10. Levels of testosterone in elderly men are _____ of the peak value.

11. The intermittent approach to androgen therapy allows for _____ between courses of therapy.

12. Clients who have elevated serum calcium levels and are prescribed androgen therapy need 3 to 4 liters per day of liquid intake to prevent kidney stones. Signs of hypercalcemia include the following: nausea and vomiting, lethargy, _____, _____, and _____.

13. The synthesis or actions of androgens may be blocked by _____.

14. When luteinizing hormone (LH) and follicle-stimulating hormone (FSH) levels are low, the drug _____ is injected intramuscularly. When reconstituted, the drug must be used _____.

15. Insufficient _____, _____, or _____ accounts for up to 5% of cases of delayed puberty.

16. The occurrence of testicular tumors peaks in early _____. Combinations of _____, _____, and _____ are used in their treatment.

17. The drug _____ is effective in stimulating libido in non-Parkinson's clients.

NCLEX Review Questions

Select the best response.

18. Sildenafil is contraindicated in men with which of the following severe conditions?
    a. renal disease
    b. cardiac disease
    c. hepatic disease
    d. CNS disorder

Situation: P.S. is a 17-year-old male receiving androgen therapy for hypogonadism. Questions 19 to 26 refer to this situation.

19. P.S. asks the nurse what androgen therapy does. The nurse's best response would be:
    a. "It ensures the ability to respond sexually."
    b. "It ensures adequate sperm production."
    c. "It promotes larger stature through protein deposition."
    d. "It stimulates the development of secondary sex characteristics."

20. P.S. observes that some of the football players at his school take hormones to help them bulk up. The nurse replies that:
    a. "This is safe as long as they use the proper dosage."
    b. "This can cause serious, often irreversible, health problems years later."
    c. "Most athletic organizations endorse this practice."
    d. "As long as they don't use other street drugs, this is probably safe."

21. P.S. asks how often and for how long he must have his testosterone enanthate injection. Therapy is expected to be given:
    a. daily for a month.
    b. biweekly for 4 months.
    c. biweekly for 4 years.
    d. weekly for a year.

22. In reviewing P.S.'s current medications, the nurse is aware that:
    a. androgens may decrease blood glucose levels in diabetics, so insulin dose may need adjustment.
    b. barbiturates potentiate androgens.
    c. there is no interaction with steroids.
    d. androgens decrease the effect of anticoagulants.

23. During one of his clinic visits, P.S. tells you that his great-aunt said that she took male hormones. He asks you why they would be given to a woman. An appropriate response would be:
    a. "Women are not treated with male hormones."
    b. "Women bodybuilders take androgens."
    c. "The doctor will explain this to you later."
    d. "Women with advanced breast cancer or severe menopausal symptoms may benefit from androgens."

24. Evidence that P.S. is receiving too much testosterone enanthate would include the following: *Select all that apply.*
    a. deepening of his voice
    b. continuous erection
    c. breast soreness
    d. urinary urgency

25. Before P.S. can begin his androgen therapy regimen, the following contraindications must be ruled out: *Select all that apply.*
    a. nephrosis
    b. hepatic insufficiency
    c. diabetes
    d. pituitary insufficiency

26. On one of his clinic visits, P.S. tells you that his grandfather is taking antiandrogens. He asks you why these drugs are used. Indications include the following: *Select all that apply.*
    a. cancer of the prostate
    b. male pattern baldness
    c. virilization syndrome in women
    d. precocious puberty in girls

Critical Thinking Exercises

Use a separate sheet of paper for your answers.

M.T., age 16, is the shortest male in his class. His parents bring him to the endocrine clinic because of their concern.

1. Why would the treatment team explore family feelings about this before initiating treatment?

2. What should the family be told about the effectiveness of androgen treatment for delayed growth?

3. How is an androgen selected for therapy?

4. Which body systems' functioning needs to be monitored during therapy?

5. How long can this therapy be expected to last?

57 Drugs for Infertility and Sexually Transmitted Diseases

Study Questions

Define the following:

1. Pelvic inflammatory disease

2. Basal body temperature

3. Ovulation

4. Infertility: primary, secondary

5. Sexually transmitted disease (STD)

6. Vertical transmission

Complete the following:

7. Sexually transmitted diseases, if not treated early, can result in _____, _____, and _____.

8. The infection of a fetus or neonate by the infected mother is _____ transmission.

9. The disease that is transmitted transplacentally is _____.

10. The modes of transmission of STDs are _____, _____, or by sexual contact with oral-fecal exposure.

11. Infants' eyes are treated with erythromycin 0.5% to prevent _____.

12. The only STDs for which a vaccine exists are _____ and _____.

13. A spirochete is the cause of the STD _____, and the drug of choice for its treatment is _____.

14. The most effective risk-reducing behavior for avoidance of STDs is _____ or sexual contact with _____.

15. Recurrent candidiasis may be indicative of _____ or _____.

16. There is no cure for genital herpes. The drugs used to treat a primary infection are _____, _____, or _____.

17. Infertility is diagnosed when the couple has engaged in frequent, unprotected coitus around the time of ovulation and not conceived in _____.

18. When infertile couples experience low levels of hormones, _____ is used to achieve physiologic levels.

19. No cause can be found for infertility in about _____% of cases of infertility.

20. When endometriosis causes infertility, it can be treated with _____ to _____.

21. Women with inadequate luteal phase progesterone output are treated with _____ intravaginally or intramuscularly.

22. Evaluation and intervention for infertility are both _____ and _____ draining for the couple.

23. Some women have been helped to conceive by taking guaifenesin (Robitussin) because it _____.

NCLEX Review Questions

Select the best response.

Situation: J.C., 19 years old, comes to the clinic complaining of dysuria and yellow-green discharge. Culture confirms *Neisseria gonorrhoeae*. Questions 24 and 25 refer to this situation.

24. Because she has presented with a sexually transmitted disease, which test should J.C. be counseled to consider?
    a. fasting blood sugar
    b. liver function
    c. HIV test
    d. fertility workup

25. All recent sexual partners need to be informed of J.C.'s gonorrhea, and until reculturing demonstrates cure, J.C. should:
    a. abstain or use condoms during sex.
    b. ask partners to take antibiotics.
    c. douche before intercourse.
    d. only engage in anal intercourse.

Situation: A.Z. has repeated gonorrhea and chlamydia as well as HPV, and is being followed up at the infectious disease clinic. Questions 26 to 32 refer to this situation.

26. In teaching A.Z. about the transmission of STDs, the nurse observes that the most risky form of sexual contact because of tissue trauma is:
    a. genital-genital.
    b. genital-anal.
    c. oral-genital.
    d. mouth-to-mouth.

27. A.Z. asks how long she must abstain from sex. The nurse responds:
    a. "Two months."
    b. "You may have sex using condoms."
    c. "Until the medication is finished."
    d. "Until your partner finishes his treatment."

28. A.Z. asks if gonorrhea and syphilis are the same. The nurse responds:
    a. "No, but if you have one, you should consider being tested for the other."
    b. "Yes, they are essentially the same."
    c. "No, syphilis cannot be cured."
    d. "No, gonorrhea has no serious effects."

29. A.Z. says she might be pregnant. What is the risk to her baby?
    a. If she is treated now and avoids sexual risk, there is no risk to her baby.
    b. Her baby will have an eye infection.
    c. Her baby will have a birth defect.
    d. She will need a cesarean delivery.

30. A.Z. wonders if her HPV will be cured. Which of the following is true?
    a. The lesion can be removed, but the HPV cannot be cured.
    b. Cryotherapy will cure her.
    c. Medications can eliminate recurrences.
    d. HPV cannot be cured, but it is not highly contagious.

31. The nurse tells A.Z. that HIV is spread in the following ways: *Select all that apply.*
    a. contact with contaminated blood
    b. sexual contact
    c. urine
    d. breast milk

32. The nurse tells A.Z. that she may want to be tested for HIV for the following reasons: *Select all that apply.*
    a. STDs indicate risky behavior.
    b. Repeated infections suggest immune compromise.
    c. Early detection is the best hope for cure.
    d. Treatment will prevent her from passing it on.

Situation: Jane and Joe have a fertility workup. Jane has been prescribed clomiphene citrate. Questions 33 to 35 relate to this situation.

33. The nurse explains to the clients that clomiphene citrate's action is to:
    a. stimulate ovulation.
    b. replace FSH.
    c. stimulate LH.
    d. normalize prolactin levels.

34. Jane and Joe ask you about the side effects of clomiphene citrate. Your best response is:
    a. decreased appetite.
    b. insomnia.
    c. breast discomfort.
    d. dehydration.

35. Contraindications for the use of clomiphene citrate include the following: *Select all that apply.*
    a. pregnancy.
    b. fibroids.
    c. depression.
    d. diabetes mellitus.

Critical Thinking Exercises

Use a separate sheet of paper for your answers.

Tess and Tom, both age 32, are being evaluated for infertility.

1. Why is Tess' history of several episodes of gonorrhea while she was in college significant?

2. Because of that history, it is suggested that Tess consider HIV testing. How are HIV and gonorrhea interrelated?

3. It is determined that Tom's sperm count is within the range of normal, but Tess is not ovulating regularly. A course of clomiphene citrate is recommended. What side effects can Tess expect? What adverse effects might require that the regimen be interrupted?

4. How does a woman's basal temperature change throughout her ovulatory cycle, and when should she engage in coitus? How might this affect the clients' relationship?

5. What stresses might a couple experience during infertility therapy? What damage might be inflicted on their relationship if pregnancy is not achieved?

58 Adult and Pediatric Emergency Drugs

Study Questions

Define the following:

1. Anaphylactic shock

2. Angina pectoris

3. Asystole

4. Extravasation

5. Hypoxemia

6. Torsades de pointes

Complete the following:

7. Adenosine is indicated in the treatment of _____.

8. Lidocaine may be commonly prescribed to treat ventricular dysrhythmias. List three signs and symptoms of lidocaine toxicity that must be recognized and reported to the primary health care provider:

   a.

   b.

   c.

9. Naloxone reverses the effects of _____ drugs. Name at least three drugs in this category that may be reversed by naloxone:

   a.

   b.

   c.

10. The nurse should remember that activated charcoal must not be given with _____ because the adsorptive properties of charcoal are decreased.

11. Clients should be taught to self-administer nitroglycerin translingual aerosol spray in the same manner as an albuterol inhaler.
    a. true
    b. false

12. Oxygen therapy should never be withheld from clients experiencing medical emergencies such as chest pain, trauma, or other causes of hypoxemia, even if they have a history of COPD.
    a. true
    b. false

13. Albuterol is a _____ (class of drug) used to treat clients experiencing _____ and _____.

NCLEX Review Questions

Select the best response.

14. Sublingual nitroglycerin may be prescribed for chest pain. What is the most important vital sign to assess BEFORE giving this drug?
    a. temperature
    b. blood pressure
    c. heart rate
    d. respiratory rate

15. Following administration of IV morphine to treat chest pain associated with acute myocardial infarction, the most important aspect of client monitoring is:
    a. measurement of central venous pressure.
    b. measurement of strict intake and output records.
    c. assessment of respiratory status.
    d. documentation of neurologic function.

16. An emergency drug indicated for the treatment of symptomatic bradycardia is:
    a. lidocaine.
    b. atropine.
    c. naloxone.
    d. epinephrine.

17. When monitoring a client with an isoproterenol (Isuprel) infusion, the nurse must be alert to the development of these dangerous adverse effects, which may require slowing or discontinuing drug administration:
    a. tachycardia and cardiac ectopy (PVCs and ventricular tachycardia).
    b. bradycardia and hypotension.
    c. bradycardia and hypertension.
    d. respiratory depression and cardiac ectopy.

18. Verapamil is classified as a:
    a. calcium channel blocker.
    b. beta blocker.
    c. cardiac glycoside.
    d. nitrate.

19. A dangerous adverse effect of IV procainamide administration is the development of:
    a. respiratory depression.
    b. hypertension.
    c. hypotension.
    d. urinary retention.

20. Amiodarone IV is used to treat:
    a. atrial dysrhythmias.
    b. ventricular dysrhythmias.
    c. a and b.
    d. none of the above.

21. The best indication for sodium bicarbonate is:
    a. metabolic alkalosis.
    b. metabolic acidosis.
    c. respiratory alkalosis.
    d. respiratory acidosis.

22. C.N. is admitted to the neurosurgical floor with a closed head injury. Mannitol is ordered to decrease intracranial pressure. Mannitol exerts its pharmacologic effects through:
    a. cerebral constriction.
    b. peripheral vasodilation.
    c. loop diuresis.
    d. osmotic diuresis.

23. Methylprednisolone (Solu-Medrol) is a controversial adjunctive therapy in the treatment of acute spinal cord injury. The nurse must be aware that the loading dose of this drug must be given within _____ hours of the injury.
    a. 2
    b. 4
    c. 6
    d. 8

24. Your client is receiving labetolol IV, a drug typically prescribed to treat which of the following?
    a. severe anxiety
    b. hypotension
    c. severe hypertension
    d. cardiac arrest

25. Dopamine should NOT be administered to clients with hypotension caused by:
    a. neurogenic shock.
    b. hypovolemic shock.
    c. septic shock.
    d. cardiogenic shock.

26. Dobutamine elevates BP through:
    a. vasoconstriction.
    b. vasodilation.
    c. increasing cardiac output.
    d. positive alpha effects.

27. J.S. has a diagnosis of septic shock. A norepinephrine drip is infusing through a central IV line. The bag of norepinephrine is almost empty. The nurse makes it a priority to prepare a new bag because:
    a. hypertensive crisis can result if the infusion is interrupted.
    b. profound hypotension can occur if the infusion is abruptly discontinued.
    c. the client is at high risk for bradycardia and heart block.
    d. the organisms responsible for septic shock will proliferate.

28. Dextrose 50% is most commonly prescribed:
    a. as a maintenance infusion to keep a vein open.
    b. to increase urine output.
    c. to treat hyperglycemia.
    d. to treat insulin shock.

29. The proper method of administering adenosine is:
    a. slow IV push.
    b. diluted in 50 ml of normal saline and infused via an electronic pump over 30 minutes.
    c. rapid IV push as a bolus.
    d. via a nebulizer.

30. Following administration of a total IV lidocaine dose of 3 mg/kg to an adult:
    a. a continuous infusion of lidocaine must be initiated to maintain a therapeutic serum level.
    b. a therapeutic serum level will be achieved and maintained.
    c. it is recognized that a lidocaine overdose has occurred.
    d. additional bolus doses must be administered to achieve a therapeutic serum level.

31. Vasopressin:
    a. is a vasoconstrictor.
    b. is an adjunct to epinephrine in the treatment of cardiac arrest.
    c. can induce myocardial ischemia in clients with coronary artery disease.
    d. all of the above.

32. To administer epinephrine 0.3 mg for IM injection, the nurse should select a:
    a. 1:10,000 solution of epinephrine.
    b. 1:100 solution of epinephrine.
    c. 1:1000 solution of epinephrine.
    d. 1:1 solution of epinephrine.

33. To administer epinephrine 1 mg for IV injection, the nurse should select a:
    a. 1:10,000 solution of epinephrine.
    b. 1:100 solution of epinephrine.
    c. 1:1000 solution of epinephrine.
    d. 1:1 solution of epinephrine.

34. The lowest adult dose of atropine for heart block or symptomatic bradycardia is 0.5 mg IV because at lower doses:
    a. vagal activity is completely blocked.
    b. paradoxical bradycardia can occur.
    c. miosis occurs.
    d. the client is at high risk for tachycardia.

35. Flumazenil is used to reverse the effects of which of the following?
    a. narcotics
    b. antipsychotics
    c. benzodiazepines
    d. paralytic agents

36. Magnesium sulfate is indicated for which of the following?
    a. treatment of torsades de pointes
    b. treatment of hypomagnesemia
    c. a and b
    d. none of the above

37. Furosemide exerts its effects on pulmonary edema through which two mechanisms?
    a. venodilation and diuresis
    b. bronchodilation and antiinflammatory actions
    c. vasoconstriction and diuresis
    d. bronchodilation and diuresis

38. Which of the following statements regarding epinephrine is/are true? *Select all that apply.*
    a. Epinephrine is a catecholamine.
    b. Indications for epinephrine include asystole and ventricular fibrillation.
    c. The action of epinephrine is enhanced if it is infused through alkaline solutions such as sodium bicarbonate.
    d. Metabolic acidosis decreases the effectiveness of epinephrine.

39. Nursing considerations when caring for a client with a nitroprusside infusion should include the following: *Select all that apply.*
    a. The solution must be protected from light.
    b. Thiocyanate levels should be monitored.
    c. A blue or brown color to the solution is typical.
    d. Continuous BP measurement is required.

40. Which of the following are commonly associated with atropine administration? *Select all that apply.*
    a. dry mouth
    b. urinary retention
    c. mydriasis
    d. miosis

Critical Thinking Exercises

Use a separate sheet of paper for your answers.

Case Study #1

T.M., an acutely ill 64-year-old male, is brought to the emergency department by his family to be treated for "the flu." His initial vital signs are as follows: BP 70/40 mm Hg, heart rate 140 beats/min, respiratory rate 32 breaths/min, and temperature 40.2° C PO. After examination and diagnostic studies, T.M. is diagnosed with pneumonia and septic shock.

A triple-lumen subclavian line is inserted for administration of fluids and IV medications and for measurement of central venous pressure (CVP). His initial CVP reading is 3 cm of H_2O. A 2000 ml normal saline fluid bolus is infused rapidly, which elevates his CVP to 9 cm of H_2O. His BP increases to 86/60 mm Hg, and his heart rate decreases to 110 beats/min. A dopamine infusion is initiated at 5 mcg/kg/min and titrated to 8 mcg/kg/min to achieve a systolic BP of >100 mm Hg. He is medicated with acetaminophen for fever. T.M. will be admitted to the ICU for placement of a pulmonary artery catheter and further aggressive management.

The following questions relate to the case study:

1. Why were IV fluids given to raise BP before initiating dopamine?

2. What are the beneficial pharmacologic effects of dopamine at the dose range in the case study?

3. How should dopamine be administered for precise dosing?

4. What are pertinent nursing considerations/assessments when monitoring a client receiving a dopamine infusion?

5. What actions should be taken if a dopamine infusion should infiltrate and produce tissue extravasation?

6.   T.M. had a heart rate of 140 beats/min on arrival in this case study. Is verapamil or adenosine indicated in this case to treat the client's tachycardia?

Case Study #2

C.S., a 56-year-old male, is admitted to coronary care step-down after a 3-day critical care unit stay for an inferior wall myocardial infarction. After dinner, C.S. summons nursing assistance for complaints of severe substernal chest pain with radiation into his left arm. He has an IV of D_5W infusing at KVO. He is receiving O_2 at 4 L by nasal cannula. C.S. has a PRN order for nitroglycerin (NTG) 0.4 mg SL for chest pain.

1.   Should the NTG 0.4 mg SL be administered based on the case study?

2.   What nursing assessment data should be collected before administering the NTG?

C.S. continues to complain of severe chest pain after three NTG tablets, 5 minutes apart. The health care provider is notified. Morphine sulfate, 2 mg IV push, is ordered, which may be repeated at 5-minute intervals until chest pain is relieved or until 10 mg has been administered.

3.   If respiratory depression occurs as a result of the morphine, what drug should be available to reverse the effects?

C.S. is transferred back to the critical care unit. IV NTG is ordered to be started at 10 mcg/kg/min and titrated to relieve chest pain while keeping systolic BP >100 mm Hg.

4.   What are pertinent nursing considerations when administering IV nitroglycerin?

5.   What actions should the nurse take if systolic BP falls to 96 mm Hg?

6.   What if the client's BP dropped precipitously to 75 mm Hg?

C.S.'s chest pain is relieved with the NTG infusion. He remains comfortable over the next 3 hours until his cardiac monitor alarms for a low heart rate of 38 beats/min. C.S. is found to be diaphoretic with a BP of 60 mm Hg by palpation. The nurse turns off the NTG infusion.

7.   What is the drug of choice for symptomatic bradycardia? What are the minimum and maximum adult doses?

8.   How does this drug exert its effects?

Answer Key

CHAPTER 1—
Drug Action: Pharmaceutic, Pharmacokinetic, and Pharmacodynamic Phases

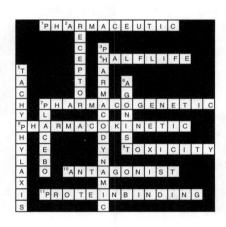

12. e
13. d
14. b
15. a
16. f
17. c
18. c
19. b
20. b
21. d
22. b

23. a
24. c
25. b
26. d
27. b
28. c
29. b
30. b
31. a
32. a
33. d
34. b
35. c
36. a
37. d
38. b
39. c
40. a
41. d
42. b, e
43. a, b, d

Critical Thinking Exercises

1. bleeding under skin

2. protein-binding; with two highly protein-bound drugs, the drugs compete for sites, causing more free drug. With more warfarin release, bleeding could occur; increased half-life may contribute to drug accumulation, especially with long protein-binding and half-life.

3. inform health care provider; request appropriate laboratory tests

4. inform client of your actions; tell client drug doses may be adjusted/changed

5. no; digoxin level is elevated; because of two highly protein-bound drugs: digoxin and warfarin. Digoxin is displaced from site; thus serum value increases.

6. may cause drug accumulation and drug toxicity because of a decrease in urine output

7. check vital signs, monitor urine output, report findings, and others

CHAPTER 2—
Nursing Process and Client Teaching

Questions 1-4: refer to text.

5. a
6. a
7. b
8. a
9. c
10. a
11. d
12. c
13. c
14. a
15. d
16. variable; related to potential for injury, knowledge deficit, and/or altered thought process
17. client-centered, clearly stated expected change, acceptable to both client and nurse, realistic and measurable, realistic deadline, shared with other health care providers
18. variable
19. general, skill, diet, side effects
20. include return demonstration, provide written instructions, use of colorful charts, provide time for questions, review community resources
21. forgetfulness, knowledge deficit, side effects, low self-esteem, depression, lack of trust in the health care system, language barriers, cost of medications, anxiety, and lack of motivation
22. b
23. a
24. c
25. c
26. c
27. d
28. b
29. d
30. a
31. d
32. a, b, c, e
33. a, b, d, e

CHAPTER 3—
Principles of Drug Administration

Questions 1-6: refer to text.

7. anticipate developmental needs, be creative
8. right client, right drug, right dose, right time, right route, right assessment, right evaluation, right documentation, client's right to education, and right to refuse; variable nursing implications
9. variable: age, body weight, toxicity, route, time of administration, emotional factors, pre-existing disease states, drug-drug interactions, etc.

10.

Route	Needle Size	Angle of Insertion	Sites
ID	26-27 gauge	10°-15°	area where inflammatory reaction can be observed
subQ	23, 25-27 gauge	45°-90°	abdomen, upper hips, upper back, lateral upper arms, lateral thighs
IM	18-23 gauge	90°	most common: ventrogluteal, dorsogluteal, deltoid, vastus lateralis
IV	20-21 gauge		most common: median cubital vein, basilic vein, cephalic vein, radial vein

```
S  I  L  A  R  E  T  A  L  S  U  T  S  A  V
O  M  D  V  Z  T  W  G  G  K  N  E  Y  I  E
B  U  D  L  E  A  M  F  L  O  H  S  C  P  N
J  I  R  D  O  N  O  T  U  D  X  Q  M  U  T
D  O  R  S  O  G  L  U  T  E  A  L  G  H  R
E  F  B  D  I  O  T  L  E  D  W  A  N  B  O
S  B  E  I  M  C  R  L  A  F  Z  I  Y  K  G
D  C  O  P  A  J  T  I  L  Q  O  T  R  N  L
R  E  F  U  S  A  L  R  E  A  S  O  N  A  U
D  E  N  E  P  O  E  M  I  T  E  T  A  D  T
S  L  A  I  T  I  N  I  F  Y  M  W  H  J  E
B  N  T  U  O  X  R  N  T  R  L  D  A  P  A
T  D  E  M  N  T  R  W  I  G  Q  M  H  U  L
```

11. ventrogluteal	36. b	13. ng
12. vastus lateralis	37. b	14. m
13. deltoid	38. a	15. gr
14. gluteal	39. b, c, d, e	16. fl oz
15. dorsogluteal	40. a, b, c	17. fl dr
16. a		18. qt
17. a		19. pt
18. b	**CHAPTER 4—**	20. minum
19. a	***Medications and***	
20. b	***Calculations***	21. c
21. a		22. T
22. b		23. t
23. c	***Section 4A***	24. gtt
24. b	1. metric; gram; liter; meter	25. a. 1000 mg; b. 1000 ml; c. 1000 mcg
25. a	2. right	26. 3000 milligrams
26. b	3. left	27. 1500 milliliters
27. a	4. gram; fluid ounce; fluid dram; and minim (also quart, pint)	28. 100 milligrams
28. c	5. in the home setting	29. 2.5 liters
29. b	6. cup; glass; spoonful (tablespoon, teaspoon)	30. 0.25 liter
30. a	7. g	31. 0.5 gram
31. b	8. mg	32. 4 pints
32. c	9. L, l	33. 32 fluid ounces
33. d	10. ml	34. 48 fluid ounces
34. d	11. kg	35. 2 pints
35. d	12. mcg	36. 16 fluid drams

37. 1 medium-sized glass = 8 ounces; 1 coffee cup = 6 ounces; 1 ounce = 2 tablespoons; 1 tablespoon = 3 teaspoons; 1 drop = 1 minim

38. convert grams to milligrams; drug label is in milligrams; 500 mg

39. 1000 mg; 15 gr

40. 0.5 g; 7½ gr

41. 100 mg; 1½ gr

42. 60 or 64 mg

43. ⅟₁₅₀ gr

44. 1 liter; 1 quart

45. 8 fl oz; 1 medium-sized glass

46. 1 ounce; 2 tablespoons; 6 teaspoons

47. 1 teaspoon

48. 15 (16) minim; 15 (16) drops

49. 1½ ounces; 9 teaspoons

50. 150 ml; 10 tablespoons

Section 4B

1. drug label

2. 1 g

3. 15 gr

4. ½ or $\overline{ss}$

5. 250 mg

6. 5 gr

7. ⅟₂₀₀ gr

8. 75 ml; 5 T

9. ½ ounce; 1 T; 3 t

10. 12 t

11. 2 ml

12. 2 t

13. Principen

14. ampicillin

15. 250 mg per 5 ml

16. oral suspension

17. milligrams. Convert to the unit on the drug label.

18. a. Yes. Convert grams to milligrams. Move the decimal point three spaces to the right.
    $0.2 \text{ g} = 0.200 \text{ mg}$

    b. BF: $\dfrac{D}{H} \times V = \dfrac{200 \text{ mg}}{100 \text{ mg}} \times 1 \text{ cap} =$
    2 capsules

    RP: H   : V   :: D   : X
    100 mg   : 1 cap :: 200 mg : X cap

    $100X = 200$
    $X = 2$ capsules

    FE: $\dfrac{H}{V} = \dfrac{D}{X} = \dfrac{100 \text{ mg}}{1 \text{ cap}} = \dfrac{200 \text{ mg}}{X \text{ cap}} =$

    $100X = 200$
    $X = 2$ capsules

    DA: cap $= \dfrac{1 \text{ cap} \times \overset{10}{\cancel{1000 \text{ mg}}} \times 0.2 \, \cancel{g}}{\underset{1}{\cancel{100 \text{ mg}}} \times 1 \, \cancel{g} \times 1}$
    $= 2$ capsules

19. a. No. Conversion is NOT needed. The units in the drug order and on the drug label are the same.

    b. BF: $\dfrac{D}{H} \times V = \dfrac{25 \text{ mg}}{12.5 \text{ mg}} \times 5 \text{ ml} =$

    $12.5\overline{)125.0}$ $\overset{10}{}$ = 10 ml

    RP: H   : V   :: D   : X
    12.5 mg : 5 ml :: 25 mg   : X ml

    $12.5X = 125$
    $X = \dfrac{125}{12.5} = 10$ ml

    DA: ml $= \dfrac{5 \text{ ml} \times \overset{2}{\cancel{25 \text{ mg}}}}{\underset{1}{\cancel{12.5 \text{ mg}}} \times 1}$
    $= 10$ ml

20. a. Yes; conversion is needed. Convert grams to milligrams. Move the decimal point three spaces to the right.
    $0.25 \text{ g} = 0.250 \text{ mg}$

    b. BF: $\dfrac{D}{H} \times V = \dfrac{\overset{2}{\cancel{250 \text{ mg}}}}{\underset{4}{\cancel{125 \text{ mg}}}} \times 5 \text{ ml}$
    $= 10$ ml

    RP: H   : V   :: D   : X
    125 mg   : 5 ml :: 250 mg   : X ml

    $125X = 1250$
    $X = 10$ ml

    FE: $\dfrac{H}{V} = \dfrac{D}{X} = \dfrac{125 \text{ mg}}{5 \text{ ml}} = \dfrac{250 \text{ mg}}{X} =$

    $125X = 1250$
    $X = 10$ ml

    DA: ml $= \dfrac{5 \text{ ml} \times \overset{8}{\cancel{1000 \text{ mg}}} \times 0.25 \, \cancel{g}}{\underset{1}{\cancel{125 \text{ mg}}} \times 1 \, \cancel{g} \times 1}$
    $= 10$ ml

21. a. No; conversion is NOT needed. The units in the drug order and on the drug label are the same.

    b. BF: $\dfrac{D}{H} \times V = \dfrac{100 \text{ mg}}{50 \text{ mg}} \times 1 \text{ ml} =$
    $\dfrac{100}{50} = 2$ ml

    RP: H   : V   :: D   : X
    50 mg   : 1 ml :: 100 mg   : X ml

    $50X = 100$
    $X = 2$ ml

    DA: ml $= \dfrac{1 \text{ ml} \times \overset{2}{\cancel{100 \text{ mg}}}}{\underset{1}{\cancel{50 \text{ mg}}} \times 1}$
    $= 2$ ml

22. a. Yes. Convert milligrams to grams. The drug label is in grams.
    $500 \text{ mg} = .500 \text{ g} \ (0.5 \text{ g})$

    According to the drug label, the drug solution after reconstitution is $3 \text{ ml} = 1 \text{ g}$.

b. BF: $\dfrac{D}{H} \times V = \dfrac{0.5\text{ g}}{1\text{ g}} \times 3\text{ ml} =$

$\dfrac{1.5}{1} = 1.5$ ml

RP: H : V :: D : X
  1 g : 3 ml :: 0.5 g : X ml
       1X = 1.5 ml

DA: ml $= \dfrac{3\text{ ml} \times 1\text{ g} \times \overset{1}{\cancel{500\text{ mg}}}}{1\text{ g} \times \underset{2}{\cancel{1000\text{ mg}}} \times 1}$

  = 1.5 ml

23.

DA: tab $= \dfrac{1\text{ tab}}{\underset{1}{\cancel{25\text{ mg}}}} \times \dfrac{\overset{2}{\cancel{50}}\text{ mg}}{1} = 2$ tablets

  a. If the 100 mg drug label is selected, then the client should receive ½ tablet.

  b. Select the 25 mg drug label; give 2 tablets.

24.

DA: tab $= \dfrac{1\text{ tab}}{\underset{1}{\cancel{50\text{ mg}}}} \times \dfrac{\overset{20}{\cancel{1000\text{ mg}}}}{1\text{ g}} \times \dfrac{0.1\text{ g}}{1}$

  = 2 tablets

  Give 2 tablets (50 mg tablets) daily.

25. grain
26. gram
27. drops
28. liter
29. microgram
30. milliequivalent
31. milliliter
32. milligram
33. kilogram
34. fluid ounce
35. one-half
36. tablespoon
37. teaspoon
38. suppository
39. telephone order

40. intramuscular
41. intravenous
42. keep vein open
43. sublingual
44. subcutaneous
45. by mouth, orally
46. before meals
47. after meals
48. with
49. without
50. nothing by mouth
51. whenever necessary
52. every 8 hours
53. twice a day
54. three times a day
55. q.i.d. is four times a day, usually during the day (8 AM, 12 PM, 4 PM, 8 PM). q6h is every 6 hours (four times in 24 hours) such as 6 AM, 12 PM, 6 PM, 12 AM.
56. 1 mg (milligram) equals 1000 mcg (microgram).

Section 4C

1. 2 tablets of Cogentin 0.5 mg

BF: $\dfrac{D}{H} \times V = \dfrac{1\text{ mg}}{0.5\text{ mg}} \times 1\text{ tab} =$

$0.5\overline{)1.0\,}^{\,2.0} = 2$ tablets

RP: H : V :: D : X
  0.5 mg : 1 tab :: 1 mg : X tab

$0.5X = 1 = \dfrac{1}{0.5}$

  X = 2 tablets

FE: $\dfrac{H}{V} = \dfrac{D}{X} = \dfrac{0.5\text{ mg}}{1\text{ tab}} = \dfrac{1\text{ mg}}{X\text{ tab}} =$

$0.5X = 1$
  X = 2 tablets

DA: tab $= \dfrac{1\text{ tab} \times 1\text{ mg}}{0.5\text{ mg} \times 1}$

  = 2 tablets

2. 2 tablets of codeine 30 mg

  If codeine 15 mg bottle is used, give 4 tablets.

  To give codeine 60 mg, it would be more desirable to give fewer tablets using codeine 30 mg bottle.

3. 1½ tablets of propranolol 10 mg. It would be difficult to obtain ¾ of a tablet from propranolol 20 mg.

BF: $\dfrac{D}{H} \times V = \dfrac{15\text{ mg}}{10\text{ mg}} \times 1\text{ tab} = 1\frac{1}{2}$ tab

RP: H : V :: D : X
  10 mg : 1 tab :: 15 mg : X tab
       10X = 15

  $X = \dfrac{15}{10} = 1\frac{1}{2}$ tab

DA: tab $= \dfrac{1\text{ tab} \times \overset{3}{\cancel{15\text{ mg}}}}{\underset{2}{\cancel{10\text{ mg}}} \times 1} = 1\frac{1}{2}$ tab

4. ½ tablet of V-Cillin K 500 mg

BF: $\dfrac{D}{H} \times V = \dfrac{\overset{1}{\cancel{250}}\text{ mg}}{\underset{2}{\cancel{500}}\text{ mg}} \times 1\text{ tab} = \frac{1}{2}$ tab

RP: H : V :: D : X
  500 mg : 1 tab :: 250 mg : X tab
        500X = 250

  $X = \dfrac{250}{500} = \frac{1}{2}$ tab

DA: tab $= \dfrac{1\text{ tab} \times \overset{1}{\cancel{250\text{ mg}}}}{\underset{2}{\cancel{500\text{ mg}}} \times 1} = \frac{1}{2}$ tab

5.   3 tablets of cimetidine 200 mg

6.   ½ tablet of verapamil 120 mg

Verapamil 120 mg tablet

BF: $\dfrac{D}{H} \times V = \dfrac{\overset{1}{\cancel{60\,mg}}}{\underset{2}{\cancel{120\,mg}}} \times 1\ tab = \frac{1}{2}\ tab$

Verapamil 80 mg tablet

RP: H   : V   :: D   : X

   80 mg : 1 tab   :: 60 mg : X tablet

      80X = 60

        X = $\dfrac{60}{80} = \frac{3}{4}$ tablet

(Difficult to divide a tablet into ¾).

DA: tab = $\dfrac{1\ tab \times \overset{1}{\cancel{60\ mg}}}{\underset{2}{\cancel{120\ mg}} \times 1} = \frac{1}{2}$ tablet

7.   2 tablets of Artane sequels (sustained release [SR] capsule)
The drug order is for SR capsule/tablet.

8.   3 tablets of Desyrel 50 mg tablet
      1½ tablets of Desyrel 100 mg

9.   Select Coumadin 5 mg container. 1½ tablets of Coumadin 5 mg.

BF: $\dfrac{D}{H} \times V = \dfrac{7.5\ mg}{5\ mg} \times 1\ tab =$

$5\overline{)7.5}^{\,1.5} = 1\frac{1}{2}$ tablet

RP: H   : V   :: D   : X

   5 mg   : 1 tab :: 7.5 mg   : X tab

       5X = 7.5

         X = $\dfrac{7.5}{5} = 1\frac{1}{2}$ tablet

FE: $\dfrac{H}{V} = \dfrac{D}{X} = \dfrac{5\ mg}{1\ tab} = \dfrac{7.5\ mg}{X\ tab} =$

        5X = 7.5

          X = 1½ tablets

DA: tab = $\dfrac{1\ tab \times 7.5\ \cancel{mg}}{5\ \cancel{mg} \times 1} = \dfrac{7.5}{5}$

     = 1½ tablet

10.   d. The serum lithium level of 1.8 mEq/L is NOT within the normal range. The drug should be withheld and the health care provider notified.

11.   Select Nitrostat 0.3 mg. Conversion table indicates gr ⅟₂₀₀ is equal to 0.3 mg. Also, the drug label indicates 0.3 mg (gr ⅟₂₀₀).

12.   a. 4 tablets per dose

     b. 8 tablets per day

13.   Two bottles of Zithromax 15 ml bottle. The 22.5 ml bottle would not be sufficient for 5 days of Zithromax therapy.
    First day: 10 ml/day; days 2-5 days: 5 ml/day (total 30 ml)

14.   Label reads trihexyphenidyl 2 mg = 1 teaspoon or 5 ml. 2½ ml of Artane 2 mg/5 ml

BF: $\dfrac{D}{H} \times V = \dfrac{1\ mg}{2\ mg} \times 5\ ml =$

      $\dfrac{5}{2} = 2\frac{1}{2}$ ml

RP: H   : V   :: D   : X

   2 mg   : 5 ml   :: 1 mg   : X ml

       2X = 5

        X = 2½ ml

DA: ml = $\dfrac{5\ ml \times 1\ \cancel{mg}}{2\ \cancel{mg} \times 1} = 2\frac{1}{2}$ ml

15.   First day: 2 tablets of Vibra-Tabs; days 2-7: 1 tablet per day

---

16.   2 tablets of Lanoxin (digoxin) 0.125 mg
    The two tablets are equivalent to the digoxin dose; the 0.25 mg tablets are not available.

BF: $\dfrac{D}{H} \times V = \dfrac{0.25\ mg}{0.125\ mg} \times 1\ tab =$

$0.125\overline{)0.250}^{\,2} = 2$ tablets

RP: H   : V   :: D   : X

  0.125 mg : 1 tab   :: 0.25 mg   : X tab

      0.125X = 0.25

         X = 2 tablets

DA: tab = $\dfrac{1\ tab \times \overset{2}{\cancel{0.25\ mg}}}{\underset{1}{\cancel{0.125\ mg}} \times 1}$

     = 2 tab

17.   8 ml of Augmentin

BF: $\dfrac{D}{H} \times V = \dfrac{400\ mg}{250\ mg} \times 5\ ml =$

$\dfrac{2000}{250} = 8$ ml

RP: H   : V   :: D   : X

  250 mg : 5 ml   :: 400 mg   : X ml

      250X = 2000

        X = 8 ml

FE: $\dfrac{H}{V} = \dfrac{D}{X} = \dfrac{250\ mg}{5\ ml} = \dfrac{400\ mg}{X} =$

       250X = 2000

         X = 8 ml

DA: ml = $\dfrac{5\ ml \times \overset{8}{\cancel{400\ mg}}}{\underset{5}{\cancel{250\ mg}} \times 1} = \dfrac{40}{5} = 8$ ml

18.   10 ml of cefadroxil (Duricef) 500 mg/5 ml
    Convert grams to milligrams by moving the decimal point three spaces to the right.
    1 g = 1.000 mg

BF: $\dfrac{D}{H} \times V = \dfrac{1000\ mg}{500\ mg} \times 5\ ml =$

$\dfrac{5000}{500} = 10$ ml

RP: H   : V   :: D   : X

  500 mg   : 5 ml :: 1000 mg : X ml

      500 X = 5000

         X = 10 ml

$$DA: ml = \dfrac{5\ ml \times \overset{2}{\cancel{1000\ mg}} \times 1g}{\underset{1}{\cancel{500\ mg}} \times 1\ g \times 1}$$

$$= 10\ ml$$

19. Select 5 mg tablets. Give 2 tablets.

20. Select 25-250 mg strength. Give ½ tablet.

21. 6 ml of Ceclor per dose

$$BF: \dfrac{D}{H} \times V = \dfrac{150\ \cancel{mg}}{125\ \cancel{mg}} \times 5\ ml = 6$$

$$FE: \dfrac{H}{V} = \dfrac{D}{X} = \dfrac{125\ mg}{5\ ml} = \dfrac{150\ mg}{X} =$$

$$125X = 750$$

$$X = 6\ ml$$

$$DA: ml = \dfrac{5\ mg \times \overset{6}{\cancel{150\ mg}}}{\underset{5}{\cancel{125\ mg}} \times 1} = \dfrac{30}{5}$$

$$= 6\ ml$$

22. Convert 0.5 g to mg:
0.500 g = 500 mg

$$RP: H \quad : V \quad :: D \quad : X$$
$$250\ mg : 5\ ml :: 500\ mg : X$$
$$250X = 2500$$
$$X = 10\ ml$$

Section 4D

1. intradermal, subcutaneous, and intramuscular; also intravenous

2. subcutaneous and intravenous. Only regular insulin can be administered intravenously.

3. self-sealing rubber tops; reusable if properly stored

4. date to discard; dosage equivalence of solution; nurse's initials

5. solutions less than 1 ml and heparin dosages. Also pediatric dosages. Is NOT used for insulin administration.

6. units

7. a

8. c

9. b

10. b

11. c

12. d

13. Select the 5000 units vial. The drug order is for 3000 units of heparin. If 10,000 units is selected, give 0.3 ml.

$$BF: \dfrac{D}{H} \times V = \dfrac{3000\ units}{5000\ units} \times 0.6\ ml =$$

$$\dfrac{3}{5} = 5\overline{)3.0}\ \ 0.6 = 0.6\ ml$$

$$RP: H \qquad : V \quad :: D \qquad : X$$
$$5000\ units : 1\ ml :: 3000\ units : X\ ml$$

$$5000X = 3000$$
$$X = 0.6\ ml$$

$$FE: \dfrac{H}{V} = \dfrac{D}{X} = \dfrac{5000\ units}{1\ ml} = \dfrac{3000\ units}{X\ ml} =$$

$$5000X = 3000$$
$$X = 0.6\ ml$$

$$DA: ml = \dfrac{1\ ml \times \overset{3}{\cancel{3000\ units}}}{\underset{5}{\cancel{5000\ units}} \times 1}$$

$$= 0.6\ ml$$

14. Convert grains to milligrams. The dose on the cartridge is in milligrams. gr $\overline{ss}$ = gr ½ = 30 mg (see Table 2-4).

$$BF: \dfrac{D}{H} \times V = \dfrac{\overset{1}{\cancel{30}}\ mg}{\underset{2}{\cancel{60}}\ mg} \times 1\ ml =$$

0.5 ml or ½ ml

$$RP: H \qquad : V \qquad :: D \qquad : X$$
$$60\ mg \quad : 1\ ml \quad :: 30\ mg \quad : X\ ml$$

$$60X = 30 = \dfrac{30}{60} =$$
$$X = 0.5\ ml\ or\ ½\ ml$$

$$DA: ml = \dfrac{1\ ml \times \cancel{60\ mg} \times ½\ \cancel{gr}}{\cancel{60\ mg} \times 1\ \cancel{gr} \times 1}$$

$$= ½\ or\ 0.5\ ml$$

15. Convert grains to milligrams. The dose on the drug label is in milligrams. gr ⅙ = 10 mg (see Table 2-4 or 3-1).

$$BF: \dfrac{D}{H} \times V = \dfrac{10\ mg}{15\ mg} \times 1\ ml =$$

$$3\overline{)2.0}\ \overset{.667}{} = 0.66\ or\ 0.7\ ml$$

$$RP: H \qquad : V \qquad :: D \qquad : X$$
$$15\ mg \quad : 1\ ml \quad :: 10\ mg \quad : X\ ml$$
$$15X = 10$$
$$X = ⅔\ or\ .66\ ml$$
$$= 0.7\ ml$$

$$DA: ml = \dfrac{1\ ml \times \overset{4}{\cancel{60\ mg}} \times 1/6\ \cancel{gr}}{\underset{1}{\cancel{15\ mg}} \times 1\ \cancel{gr} \times 1}$$

$$= \dfrac{4/6}{1} = 0.66\ or\ 0.7\ ml$$

16. Withdraw 36 units of Humulin L insulin.

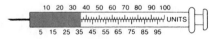

17. First withdraw 8 units of Humulin R (regular) insulin and then 44 units of Humulin N (NPH) insulin. TOTAL: 52 units of insulin.

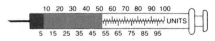

18. Digoxin 0.25 mg = 1 ml

$$BF: \dfrac{D}{H} \times V = \dfrac{0.25\ mg}{0.5\ mg} \times 2\ ml =$$

$$\dfrac{\overset{1}{\cancel{0.5}}}{\underset{1}{\cancel{0.5}}} = 1\ ml$$

$$RP: H \qquad : V \qquad :: D \qquad : X$$
$$0.5\ mg : 2\ ml :: 0.25\ mg : X\ ml$$
$$0.5X = 0.5$$
$$X = 1\ ml$$

$$\text{DA: ml} = \frac{2 \text{ ml} \times \overset{2}{\cancel{1000 \text{ mcg}}}}{\underset{1}{\cancel{500 \text{ mcg}}} \times 1 \text{ } \cancel{\text{mg}}}$$

$$\frac{\times 0.25 \text{ } \cancel{\text{mg}}}{\times 1} = 1 \text{ ml}$$

19. Select cyanocobalamin 1000 mcg. The drug order is for 400 mcg and the 100 mcg cartridge would not contain enough medication.

$$\text{BF: } \frac{D}{H} \times V = \frac{400 \text{ mcg}}{1000 \text{ mcg}} \times 1 \text{ ml} =$$
0.4 ml

RP: H   : V   :: D   : X
   1000 mcg : 1 ml   :: 400 mcg   : X ml

   1000X = 400

   X = 0.4 ml

$$\text{DA: ml} = \frac{1 \text{ ml} \times \overset{2}{\cancel{400 \text{ mcg}}}}{\underset{5}{\cancel{1000 \text{ mcg}}} \times 1}$$

$$= \frac{2}{5} = 0.4 \text{ ml}$$

20. Clindamycin 300 mg = 2 ml

$$\text{BF: } \frac{D}{H} \times V = \frac{\overset{1}{\cancel{300 \text{ mg}}}}{\underset{3}{\cancel{900 \text{ mg}}}} \times 6 \text{ ml} = \frac{6}{3} = 2 \text{ ml}$$

RP: H   : V   :: D   : X
   900 mg : 6 ml :: 300 mg   : X ml

   900X = 1800

   X = 2 ml

$$\text{DA: ml} = \frac{6 \text{ ml} \times \overset{1}{\cancel{300 \text{ mg}}}}{\underset{3}{\cancel{900 \text{ mg}}} \times 1}$$

$$= \frac{6}{3} = 2 \text{ ml}$$

21. Discard 0.4 ml of meperidine 100 mg.
     Administer 0.6 ml of meperidine 100 mg and 1.25 ml of atropine sulfate.
     Total volume: 1.85 ml.

Meperidine

$$\text{BF: } \frac{D}{H} \times V = \frac{\cancel{60} \text{ mg}}{\cancel{100} \text{ mg}} \times 1 \text{ ml} = 0.6 \text{ ml}$$

Atropine

RP: H   : V   :: D   : X
   0.4 mg : 1 ml   :: 0.5 mg : X ml

   $$0.4X = 0.5 = \frac{0.5}{0.4} = 1.25 \text{ ml}$$

22. Narcan 0.8 mg = 2 ml

$$\text{BF: } \frac{D}{H} \times V = \frac{0.8 \text{ mg}}{0.4 \text{ mg}} \times 1 \text{ ml}$$
= 2 ml

RP: H   : V   :: D   : X
   0.4 mg : 1 ml   :: 0.8 mg : X ml

   0.4X = 0.8

   X = 2 ml

$$\text{FE: } \frac{H}{V} = \frac{D}{X} = \frac{0.4 \text{ mg}}{1 \text{ ml}} = \frac{0.8 \text{ mg}}{X \text{ ml}} =$$

   0.4X = 0.8

   X = 2 ml

$$\text{DA: ml} = \frac{1 \text{ ml} \times \overset{5}{\cancel{1000 \text{ mcg}}}}{\underset{2}{\cancel{400 \text{ mcg}}} \times 1 \text{ } \cancel{\text{mg}}}$$

$$= \frac{\times 0.8 \text{ } \cancel{\text{mg}}}{\times 1} = \frac{4}{2} = 2 \text{ ml}$$

23. Hydroxyzine (Vistaril) 35 mg = 0.7 ml

24. Convert milligrams to grams, indicated on the drug label. Move the decimal point three spaces to the left.
     500 mg = 0.500 g or 0.5 g
     Drug label states to add 5.7 ml of sterile water to yield 6 ml of drug solution (oxacillin 1 g = 6 ml).

$$\text{BF: } \frac{D}{H} \times V = \frac{0.5 \text{ g}}{1 \text{ g}} \times 6 \text{ ml} =$$

$$\frac{3}{1} = 3 \text{ ml}$$

RP: H   : V   :: D   : X
   1 g   : 6 ml   :: 0.5 g   : X ml

   (1)X = 3

   X = 3 ml

$$\text{DA: ml} = \frac{6 \text{ ml} \times 1 \text{ } \cancel{\text{g}} \times \overset{1}{\cancel{500 \text{ mg}}}}{1 \text{ } \cancel{\text{g}} \times \underset{2}{\cancel{1000 \text{ mg}}} \times 1}$$

= 3 ml

25. Drug label states to add 2.7 ml of diluent to yield

a total of 3 ml of drug solution or 1.5 ml = 250 mg of oxacillin (oxacillin 500 mg = 3 ml).

$$\text{BF: } \frac{D}{H} \times V = \frac{300 \text{ mg}}{500 \text{ mg}} \times 3 \text{ ml} =$$

$$\frac{900}{500} = 1.8 \text{ ml}$$

RP: H   : V   :: D   : X
   500 mg : 3 ml   :: 300 mg : X ml

   500X = 900

   $$X = \frac{900}{500} = 1.8 \text{ ml}$$

$$\text{DA: ml} = \frac{3 \text{ ml} \times \overset{3}{\cancel{300 \text{ mg}}}}{\underset{5}{\cancel{500 \text{ mg}}} \times 1} = \frac{9}{5} = 1.8 \text{ ml}$$

26. Drug label states to add 1.8 ml of diluent to yield a total of 2 ml of drug solution or 1 ml = 250 mg of nafcillin. (nafcillin [Nafcil] 500 mg = 2 ml)
     Since the drug label states that 250 mg = 1 ml after the drug has been reconstituted, calculation of this problem is not necessary. Nafcillin 250 mg = 1 ml
     However, if you wish to work the problem:

$$\text{BF: } \frac{D}{H} \times V = \frac{250 \text{ mg}}{500 \text{ mg}} \times 2 \text{ ml} =$$

$$\frac{1}{1} = 1 \text{ ml}$$

RP: H   : V   :: D   : X
   500 mg : 2 ml   :: 250 mg : X ml

   (1) X = 1 ml

$$\text{DA: ml} = \frac{2 \text{ ml} \times \overset{1}{\cancel{250 \text{ mg}}}}{\underset{2}{\cancel{500 \text{ mg}}} \times 1}$$

= 1 ml

27. Trimethobenzamide (Tigan) 100 mg = 1 ml

28. 0.8 ml of Thorazine

$$\text{BF: } \frac{D}{H} \times V = \frac{20 \text{ mg}}{20 \text{ mg}} \times 1 \text{ ml} = \frac{4}{5} = 0.8 \text{ ml}$$

$$DA: ml = \frac{1\ ml\ \times \overset{4}{\cancel{20\ mg}}}{\underset{5}{\cancel{25\ mg}} \times 1} = \frac{4}{5}$$
$$= 0.8\ ml\ of\ Thorazine$$

29. Add 2 ml of diluent to yield 2.6 ml of drug solution. Change 400 mg to grams.
$(\underset{\frown}{400}\ mg = 0.4\ g)$

$$BF: \frac{D}{H} \times V = \frac{0.4\ g}{1\ g} \times 2.6\ ml = 1\ ml$$

$$DA: ml = \frac{2.6\ ml\ \times\ 1\ \cancel{g}\ \times\ \overset{2}{\cancel{400\ mg}}}{1\ \cancel{g}\ \times\ \underset{5}{\cancel{1000\ mg}}\ \times\ 1}$$
$$= \frac{5.2}{5} = 1\ ml$$

30. a. 750 mg of cefonicid is equivalent to 0.75 g.

    b. Drug label indicates that 2.5 ml of diluent should be added to the drug powder, which yields 3.1 ml of drug solution.

    c. $BF: \frac{D}{H} \times V = \frac{0.75\ g}{1\ g} \times 3.1\ ml =$
    2.32 ml or 2.3 ml

31. a. To change to grams, move decimal point, 750 mg, three spaces to the left = 0.75 g.

    RP: H : V :: D : X
    1 g : 2.4 ml :: 0.75 g : X ml
    X = 1.8 ml

$$DA: ml = \frac{2.4\ ml\ \times\ 1\ \cancel{g}\ \times\ \overset{3}{\cancel{7.50\ mg}}}{1\ \cancel{g}\ \times\ \underset{4}{\cancel{1000}\ mg}\ \times\ 1}$$
$$= \frac{7.2}{4} = 1.8\ ml\ per\ dose$$

    b. The remaining 0.6 ml of drug solution in the vial can be saved for 24 hours or 96 hours if refrigerated.

32. $BF: \frac{D}{H} \times V = \frac{1\ g}{1.5\ g} \times 2.6\ ml$
    $= 1.73\ or\ 1.7\ ml$

$$DA: ml = \frac{2.6\ ml\ \times\ 1\ g}{1.5\ g\ \times\ 1} = \frac{2.6}{1.5}$$
$$= 1.73\ or\ 1.7\ ml$$

Section 4E

1. drop factor, amount of fluid to be administered, and time period

2. macrodrip set: 10-20 gtt/ml; microdrip set: 60 gtt/ml

3. microdrip set

4. keep vein open; 250 ml IV bag

5. before administration

6. D_5W

7. NSS or 0.9% NaCl

8. D_5/½ NSS or 5% D/0.45% NaCl

9. D_5/LR or 5% D/LR

10. small; short

11. calibrated cylinder with tubing; intermittent IV drug administration

12. volumetric

13. uniform serum concentration of drug for avoiding drug "peaks and valleys"

Continuous Intravenous Administration

14. 27 to 28 gtt/min
    Method 2:

    a. 1000 ml ÷ 6 hours = 167 ml/hr

    b. $\dfrac{167\ ml\ \times\ \overset{1}{\cancel{10}}\ gtt/ml}{\underset{5}{\cancel{660}}\ minutes/hr} = \dfrac{167}{6} =$
    27-28 gtt/min

---

15. Inject KCl and MVI into the bag before administering IV fluids. Regulate IV flow rate to 31-32 gtt/minute.
    Drug calculation:
    Order: KCl 10 mEq in 1 liter of IV fluids
    Available: KCl 20 mEq/ 10 ml

    $BF: \dfrac{D}{H} \times V = \dfrac{10\ mEq}{20\ mEq} \times 10\ ml =$
    $\dfrac{10}{2} = 5\ ml$

    RP: H : V :: D : X
    20 mE : 10 ml :: 10 mEq : X ml
    X = 5 ml

    $FE: \dfrac{H}{V} = \dfrac{D}{X} = \dfrac{20\ mEq}{10\ ml} = \dfrac{10\ mEq}{X\ ml} =$
    20X = 100
    X = 5 ml

    $DA: ml = \dfrac{10\ ml\ \times\ \overset{1}{\cancel{10\ mEq}}}{\underset{2}{\cancel{20\ mEq}}\ \times\ 1}$
    $= 5\ ml$

    IV flow rate:

    Method 3: $\dfrac{1000\ ml\ \times\ \overset{1}{\cancel{15}}\ gtt/ml}{8\ hours\ \times\ \underset{4}{\cancel{60}}\ minutes} = \dfrac{1000}{32}$
    $= 31\text{-}32\ gtt/min$

16. Use the microdrip set. Regulate IV flow rate at 83 gtt/minute.

    a. 1000 ml ÷ 12 hours = 83 ml/hr

    b. $\dfrac{83\ ml\ \times\ \overset{1}{\cancel{60}}\ gtt/ml}{\underset{1}{\cancel{60}}\ min/hr} =$
    83 gtt/min

17. a. 1000 ml

    b. 2500 ml

    c. 100 ml/hr (actual amount is 104 ml/hr)

    d. macrodrip set, 10 gtt/ml

    e. 16-17 gtt/minute

    IV flow rate:

    $\dfrac{100\ ml\ \times\ \overset{1}{\cancel{10}}\ gtt/ml}{\underset{6}{\cancel{60}}\ minutes/hr} = \dfrac{100}{6} =$
    16-17 gtt/min

18. a. 500 ml of IV fluid is left.

b. Recalculated to run at 27-28 gtt/minute.

IV flow rate recalculated:

a. 500 ml ÷ 3 hr left = 167 ml/hr

b. $\dfrac{167\,ml \times \overset{1}{\cancel{10}}\,gtt/ml}{\underset{6}{\cancel{660}}\,minutes/hr} =$

$\dfrac{167}{6} = 27\text{-}28\,gtt/min$

Intermittent Intravenous Administration

19. Drug calculation:

BF: $\dfrac{D}{H} \times V = \dfrac{200}{300} \times 2\,ml = \dfrac{400}{300} = 1.3\,ml$

DA: $ml = \dfrac{2\,ml \times \overset{2}{\cancel{200}}\,mg}{\underset{3}{\cancel{300}}\,mg \times 1} = \dfrac{4}{3}$

$= 1.3\,ml$

IV flow calculation:

$\dfrac{\text{Amount of solution} \times gtt/ml}{\text{Minutes to administer}} = gtt/minute$

$\dfrac{50\,ml \times \overset{3}{\cancel{60}}\,gtt/ml}{\underset{1}{\cancel{20}}\,minutes} = 150\,gtt/min$

Answer: a. 1.3 ml of cimetidine; b. 150 gtt/minute

20. a. Add 10 ml of sterile water to cefamandole.

b. Total drug solution equals 1 g = 10 ml

Drug calculation: Convert milligrams to grams (gram is on the drug label). Move the decimal point three spaces to the left.

500 mg = .500 g = 0.5 g

RP: H   : V   :: D   : X

1 g   : 10 ml g :: 0.5 g   : X ml

(1) X = 5 ml

DA: $ml = \dfrac{10\,ml \times 1\,\cancel{g} \times \overset{1}{\cancel{500}}\,\cancel{mg}}{1\,\cancel{g} \times \underset{2}{\cancel{1000}}\,\cancel{mg} \times 1}$

$= 5\,ml$

IV flow calculation:

$\dfrac{55\,ml \times \overset{2}{\cancel{60}}\,gtt/ml}{\underset{1}{\cancel{30}}\,minutes} = 110\,gtt/minute$

5 ml drug ÷ 50 ml diluent = 55 ml

Answer: 5 ml of cefamandole, 110 gtt/minute

21. a. Add 6.6 ml of diluent to nafcillin.

b. Total drug solution equals 2 g = 8 ml

Drug calculation: Convert milligrams to grams (gram is on the drug label). Move the decimal point three spaces to the left.

1000 mg = 1.000 g = 1 g

BF: $\dfrac{D}{H} \times V = \dfrac{1\,g}{2\,g} \times 8\,ml = \dfrac{8}{2} = 4\,ml$

DA: $ml = \dfrac{8\,ml \times 1\,\cancel{g} \times \overset{1}{\cancel{1000}}\,\cancel{mg}}{2\,\cancel{g} \times \cancel{1000}\,\cancel{mg} \times 1}$

$= 4\,ml$

IV flow calculation:

$\dfrac{100\,ml \times 15\,gtt/ml}{40\,minutes} = \dfrac{1500}{40}$

$= 37\text{-}38\,gtt/minute$

Answer: 4 ml of nafcillin, 37-38 gtt/minute

22. Drug calculation: Convert milligrams to grams. Move the decimal point three spaces to the left.

250 mg = .250 g = 0.25 g

RP: H   : V   :: D   : X

1 g   : 3 ml :: 0.25 g   : X ml

(1) X = 0.75 ml

DA: $ml = \dfrac{3\,ml \times 1\,\cancel{g} \times \overset{1}{\cancel{250}}\,\cancel{mg}}{1\,\cancel{g} \times \underset{4}{\cancel{1000}}\,\cancel{mg} \times 1}$

$= \dfrac{3}{4} = 0.75\,ml$

IV flow calculation:

$\dfrac{100\,ml \times 15\,gtt/ml}{45\,minutes} = \dfrac{1500}{45} =$

33-34 gtt/min

Answer: 0.75 ml of kanamycin, 33-34 gtt/minute

23. a. Add 4 ml of sterile water to ticarcillin (Ticar).

b. Total drug solution equals 1 g = 4 ml

Drug calculation: Convert milligrams to grams. Move the decimal point three spaces to the left.

750 mg = .750 g = 0.75 g

BF: $\dfrac{D}{H} \times V = \dfrac{0.75\,g}{1\,g} \times 4\,ml =$

3 ml

FE: $\dfrac{H}{V} = \dfrac{D}{X} = \dfrac{1\,g}{4\,ml} = \dfrac{0.75\,g}{X\,ml} =$

1X = 3

X = 3 ml

IV flow calculation:

$\dfrac{75\,ml \times \overset{2}{\cancel{60}}\,gtt/ml}{\underset{1}{\cancel{30}}\,minutes} = 150\,gtt/minute$

Answer: 3 ml of ticarcillin, 150 gtt/minute

Volumetric IV Regulator

24. Drug calculation:

RP: H   : V   :: D   : X

160/800 mg : 10 ml   :: 80/400 mg : X ml

160/800X = 10 X 80/400

160/800X = 800/4000 = $\dfrac{\overset{5}{\cancel{800/4000}}}{\underset{1}{\cancel{160/800}}}$

= 5 ml

Volumetric pump regulator:

Amount of solution + $\dfrac{\text{minutes to administer}}{60\,minutes/hr} =$

125 ml + $\dfrac{90\,minutes}{60\,minutes} =$

125 ml + 5 ml (drug) + $\dfrac{90\,min}{60\,min}$

(invert the divisor and multiply)

$$130 \text{ ml} \times \frac{\overset{2}{\cancel{60 \text{ min}}}}{\underset{3}{\cancel{90 \text{ min}}}} = \frac{260}{3} = 87 \text{ ml/hr}$$

Answer: 5 ml of Septra; 87 ml/hr

25. Drug calculation: 75 mg of Vibramycin = 7.5 ml

$$\text{BF: } \frac{D}{H} \times V = \frac{75 \text{ mg}}{100 \text{ mg}} \times 10 \text{ ml} =$$

$$\frac{750}{100} = 7.5 \text{ ml}$$

$$\text{DA: ml} = \frac{10 \text{ ml} \times \overset{3}{\cancel{75 \text{ mg}}}}{\underset{4}{\cancel{100 \text{ mg}}} \times 1} = \frac{30}{4}$$

$$= 7.5 \text{ ml}$$

Volumetric pump regulator:

$$107.5 \text{ ml} + \frac{60 \text{ min}}{60 \text{ min}} =$$

$$107.5 \text{ ml} \times \frac{\overset{1}{\cancel{60 \text{ min}}}}{\underset{1}{\cancel{60 \text{ min}}}} = 107.5 \text{ ml/hr or } 108 \text{ ml/hr}$$

26. Drug calculation: Change 400 mg to grams (400 mg = 0.4 g)

$$\text{BF: } \frac{D}{H} \times V = \frac{0.4 \text{ g}}{1 \text{ g}} \times 4 \text{ ml} = 1.6 \text{ ml}$$

$$\text{DA: ml} = \frac{4 \text{ ml} \times 1 \text{ g} \times \overset{4}{\cancel{400 \text{ mg}}}}{1 \cancel{\text{ g}} \times \underset{10}{\cancel{1000 \text{ mg}}} \times 1}$$

$$= \frac{16}{10} = 1.6 \text{ ml}$$

400 mg of amikacin = 1.6 ml

Volumetric pump regulator:

$$125 \text{ ml} + \frac{\overset{1}{\cancel{60 \text{ minutes (1 hr)}}}}{\underset{1}{60 \text{ minutes}}} =$$

125 ml/hr (60 minutes)

27.

$$\text{BF: } \frac{D}{H} \times V = \frac{75 \text{ mg}}{100 \text{ mg}} \times 5 \text{ ml} = \frac{375}{100} =$$

3.75 ml

RP: H   : V   :: D   : X

100 mg : 5 ml :: 75 mg : X ml

$$100X = 375$$

$$X = 3.75 \text{ ml}$$

75 mg of minocycline = 3.75 ml

Volumetric pump regulator:

$$500 \text{ ml} \div \frac{120 \text{ minutes}}{60 \text{ minutes}} = 500 \times \frac{\overset{1}{\cancel{60}}}{\underset{2}{\cancel{120}}} =$$

$$\frac{500}{2} = 250 \text{ ml/hr}$$

28. Selection of the amount of diluent is 3.4 ml = 4.0 ml
Change 500 mg to 0.5 g or 2 g to 2000 mg

$$\text{BF: } \frac{D}{H} \times V = \frac{0.5 \text{ g}}{2 \text{ g}} \times 4 \text{ ml} =$$

1 mlm twice a day

$$\text{DA: ml} = \frac{4 \text{ ml} \times 1 \text{ g} \times \overset{1}{\cancel{500 \text{ mg}}}}{2 \cancel{\text{ g}} \times \underset{2}{\cancel{1000 \text{ mg}}} \times 1}$$

$$= \frac{4}{4} = 1 \text{ ml}$$

$$\frac{50 \text{ ml} \times \overset{2}{\cancel{60}} \text{ gtt}}{\underset{1}{\cancel{30}} \text{ minutes}} = 100 \text{ gtt/min}$$

29. Drug calculation:

$$\text{BF: } \frac{D}{H} \times V = \frac{1.5}{3} \times 10 = \frac{15}{3}$$

$$= 5 \text{ ml}$$

$$\text{DA: ml} = \frac{10 \text{ ml} \times \cancel{1.5} \text{ g}}{\underset{2}{\cancel{3}} \text{ g} \times 1} = \frac{10}{2}$$

$$= 5 \text{ ml}$$

Conversion factor is not needed.

IV flow calculation:

$$\frac{105 \text{ ml} \times \overset{2}{\cancel{60}} \text{ gtt/ml}}{\underset{1}{\cancel{310}} \text{ minutes}} = 210 \text{ gtt/min}$$

30. Drug calculation:

RP: H   : V   :: D   : X

1 g : 10 ml :: 0.5 g : X ml

$$X = 5 \text{ ml}$$

$$\text{ml} = \frac{10 \text{ ml} \times 1 \text{ g} \times \overset{1}{\cancel{500}} \text{ mg}}{1 \text{ g} \times \underset{2}{\cancel{1000}} \text{ mg} \times 1}$$

$$= 5 \text{ ml}$$

Volumetric pump regulator:

$$105 \text{ ml with drug solution} + \frac{45 \text{ minutes}}{60 \text{ minutes}}$$

= (invert the divisor)
(Drug will be infused entirely in 45 minutes)

$$\frac{105 \text{ ml} \times \overset{4}{\cancel{60}} \text{ min}}{\underset{3}{\cancel{45}} \text{ minutes}} = \frac{420}{3} = 140 \text{ ml/hr}$$

Section 4F

Orals

1. 2.5 ml of V-Cillin K 400,000 units/5 ml per dose.

Drug order is in units; use units that are on the drug label.

Dose is within safe parameters.

25,000 units × 21 kg = 525,000 units

90,000 units × 21 kg = 1,890,000 units

$$\text{BF: } \frac{D}{H} \times V = \frac{200,000 \text{ units}}{400,000 \text{ units}} \times 5 \text{ ml} =$$

$$\frac{10}{4} = 2.5 \text{ ml}$$

RP: H   : V   :: D   : X

400,000 units : 5 ml :: 200,000 units : X ml

$$400,000X = 500$$

$$X = 2.5 \text{ ml}$$

$$\text{DA: ml} = \frac{5 \text{ ml} \times \overset{1}{\cancel{200,000 \text{ units}}}}{\underset{2}{\cancel{400,000 \text{ units}}} \times 1}$$

$$= \frac{5}{2} = 2.5 \text{ ml}$$

2. Child's weight: 75 pounds = 34.1 kg
10 mg × 34.1 kg = 341 mg/day
15 mg × 34.1 kg = 511.5 mg/day

Child to receive 400 mg/day. Dose is within safe parameters.

Child should receive 4 ml of Ceftin per dose.

3. No; drug order per day is NOT within safe parameters.

    50 mg × 5 kg = 250 mg per day

    Order: 75 mg × 4 doses (q6h) = 300 mg per day

    Notify the health care provider.

4. 7.8 ml or 8 ml of acetaminophen 160 mg/5 ml

BF: $\dfrac{D}{H} \times V = \dfrac{250\,mg}{160\,mg} \times 5\,ml =$

$\dfrac{1250}{60} = 7.8\ or\ 8\ ml$

RP: H : V :: D : X

160 mg : 5 ml :: 250 mg : X ml

160X = 1250

X = 8 ml

FE : $\dfrac{H}{V} = \dfrac{D}{X} = \dfrac{160\,mg}{5\,ml} = \dfrac{250\,mg}{X\,ml} =$

160X = 1250

X = 7.8 or 8 ml

DA: ml = $\dfrac{5\,ml \quad \times 250\ \cancel{mg}}{160\ \cancel{mg} \times 1} = \dfrac{1250}{160}$

$= 7.8\ or\ 8\ ml$

5. 4 ml of cloxacillin (Tegopen) 125 mg/5 ml per dose

    Dose is within safe parameters.

    50 mg × 8 kg = 400 mg per day

    100 mg × 8 kg = 800 mg per day

    100 mg × 4 doses (q6h) = 400 mg per day

BF: $\dfrac{D}{H} \times V = \dfrac{100\,mg}{125\,mg} \times 5\,ml =$

$\dfrac{500}{125} = 4\ ml$

RP: H : V :: D : X

125 mg : 5 ml :: 100 mg : X ml

25X = 500

X = $\dfrac{500}{125}$ = 4 ml

DA: ml = $\dfrac{5\,ml \quad \times \overset{4}{\cancel{100\ mg}}}{\underset{5}{\cancel{125\,mg}} \times 1} = \dfrac{20}{5}$

$= 4\ ml$

6. 4 ml of erythromycin 200 mg/5 ml, q6h

    Dose is NOT within the drug parameters. The child is receiving less than the recommended dosage.

    160 mg × 4 (q6h) = 640 mg per day. Check with the health care provider.

    30 mg × 25 kg = 750 mg per day

    50 mg × 25 kg = 1250 mg per day

7. 3 ml of cefaclor (Ceclor) 125 mg/5 ml per dose

    Convert 22 pounds to kg (22 ÷ 2.2 = 10 kg)

    20 mg × 10 kg = 200 mg per day

    40 mg × 10 kg = 400 mg per day

    Order 75 mg × 3 (q8h) = 225 mg per day

    Drug dose is within safe parameters.

    Ceclor 125 mg/5 ml

BF: $\dfrac{D}{H} \times V = \dfrac{75\,mg}{125\,mg} \times 5\,ml =$

$\dfrac{375}{125} = 3\ ml$

DA: ml = $\dfrac{5\,ml \quad \times \overset{3}{\cancel{75}}\ mg}{\underset{5}{\cancel{125}}\ mg \times 1} = \dfrac{15}{5} = 3\ ml$

8. Child weighs 11.8 kg or 12 kg

    Yes; it is within the dose parameters:

    11.8 kg × 40 mg = 472 mg/day

    Child to receive 150 mg × 3 doses = 450 mg/day

6 ml of Augmentin per dose

BF: $\dfrac{D}{H} \times V = \dfrac{150\,mg}{125\,mg} \times 5\,ml = 6\ ml/dose$

FE : $\dfrac{H}{V} = \dfrac{D}{X} = \dfrac{125\,mg}{5\,ml} = \dfrac{150\,mg}{X\,ml} =$

125X = 750

X = 6 ml/dose

DA: ml = $\dfrac{5\,ml \quad \times \overset{6}{\cancel{150}}\ mg}{\cancel{125}\ mg \times 1} = \dfrac{30}{5} = 6\ ml/dose$

9. Child's body surface area (BSA) is 0.98 m^2.

    Safe dosage range: 60 mg × 0.98 m^2 = 58.8 or 59 mg

    250 × 0.98 m^2 = 245 mg (59 mg to 245 mg of Cytoxan)

10. Child's body surface area (BSA) is 0.87 m^2.

    250 mg × 0.87 m^2 = 218 mg per day AND

    218 ÷ 3 divided doses = 72.6 or 73 mg per dose

BF: $\dfrac{D}{H} \times V = \dfrac{73\,mg}{30\,mg} \times 5\,ml = \dfrac{365}{30} =$

12.1 or 12 ml

RP: H : V :: D : X

30 mg : 5 ml :: 73 mg : X ml

30X = 365

X = 12.1 or 12 ml

DA: ml = $\dfrac{5\,ml \quad \times 73\ \cancel{mg}}{30\ \cancel{mg} \times 1} = \dfrac{365}{30} = 12\ ml$

12 ml of Dilantin 30 mg/5 ml three times a day

Injectables

11. Child weighs 12 kg (26 ÷ 2.2 = 11.8 or 12 kg).

    Drug parameters: 25 mg × 12 kg = 300 mg per day

    50 mg × 12 kg = 600 mg per day

Drug order is 100 mg × 4 doses (q6h) = 400 mg per day

Child's drug dose is within safe parameters.

Drug label states to add 1.2 ml of diluent to equal ampicillin (Polycillin-N) 125 mg = 1.2 ml

BF: $\frac{D}{H} \times V = \frac{100\,mg}{125\,mg} \times 1.2\,ml = \frac{120}{125}$

$125\overline{)120}^{.96} = 0.96$ or 1 ml

RP: H   : V   :: D   : X

125 mg : 1.2 ml :: 100 mg   : X ml

125 X = 120

X = 0.96 or 1 ml

DA: ml = $\frac{1.2\,ml \times \overset{4}{\cancel{100\,mg}}}{\underset{5}{\cancel{125\,mg}} \times 1} = \frac{4.8}{5}$

= 0.96 ml or 1 ml

12.   Child weighs 18 kg (40 ÷ 2.2 = 18.18 or 18 kg).

Drug parameters:
3 mg × 18 kg = 54 mg
5 mg × 18 kg = 90 mg per day

Drug order is 25 mg. Drug dose is less than the drug parameters. Check with the health care provider. Drug dose order may be changed. Because the drug dose is NOT greater than the drug parameters, drug dose would be considered safe.

Pentobarbital (Nembutal) 25 mg = 0.5 ml.

13.   Child weighs 10 kg.
Drug parameters:
15 mg × 10 kg = 150 mg in 2 divided doses.
Drug order is 50 mg × 2 doses (q12h) = 100 mg

Drug dose is safe.
Drug label: Kantrex 75 mg/2 ml

BF: $\frac{D}{H} \times V = \frac{50\,mg}{75\,mg} \times 2\,ml =$

$\frac{100}{75} = 1.3\,ml$

FE: $\frac{H}{V} = \frac{D}{X} = \frac{75\,mg}{2\,ml} = \frac{50\,mg}{X\,ml} =$

75X = 100

X = 1.3 ml

RP: H   : V   :: D   : X

75 mg : 2 ml :: 50 mg   : X ml

75X = 100

X = 1.3 ml

Kanamycin (Kantrex) 50 mg = 1.3 ml

DA: ml = $\frac{2\,ml \times \overset{2}{\cancel{50}}\,mg}{\underset{3}{\cancel{75}}\,mg \times 1} = \frac{4}{3}$

= 1.3 ml/dose

14.   Drug dose is safe
5 mg × 9 kg = 45 mg q8h

7.5 mg × 9 kg = 67.5 mg q12h

BF: $\frac{D}{H} \times V = \frac{50\,mg}{100\,mg} \times 2\,ml =$

$\frac{100}{100} = 1\,ml$

DA: ml = $\frac{2\,ml \times \overset{1}{\cancel{50\,mg}}}{\underset{2}{\cancel{100\,mg}} \times 1}$

= 1 ml

15.   48 pounds ÷ 2.2 = 21.8 kg or 22 kg

Drug dose is safe (550-1100 mg).

Add 2 ml of diluent to yield 2 ml of drug solution (250 mg = 2 ml)

Cefazolin sodium 125 mg = 1 ml

16.   3 mg × 22 kg = 66 mg/day

5 mg × 22 kg = 110 mg/day

Child to receive 25 mg × 3 doses = 75 mg/day.
Drug dose is safe.

BF: $\frac{D}{H} \times V = \frac{25\,mg}{80\,mg} \times 2\,ml =$

$\frac{50}{80} = 0.63\,ml$ or 0.6 ml per dose

RP: H   : V   :: D   : X

80 mg : 2 ml :: 25 mg   : X ml

80X = 50

X = 0.6 ml per dose

DA: ml = $\frac{2\,ml \times 25\,mg}{80\,mg \times 1} = \frac{50}{80}$

= 0.63 ml or 0.6 mg per dose

CHAPTER 5—
The Drug Approval Process

Questions 1-4: refer to text.

5.   c

6.   c

7.   a

8.   b

9.   c

10.   VIPPS—Verified Internet Pharmacy Practice Site

11.   iron, flavored acetaminophen, chocolate-covered laxatives, and flavored liquid medicines

12.   a. provision of drug education and research into prevention and treatment of drug dependence

b. strengthen enforcement authority

c. establish treatment and rehabilitation facilities

d. designate categories for controlled substances according to abuse liability

13. Code of Ethics; variable
14. d
15. b
16. c
17. a
18. d
19. d
20. a
21. b
22. c
23. c
24. a
25. d
26. b
27. b
28. a
29. a
30. a, b
31. a, c
32. c
33. a
34. a, b, c
35. a, b, d

CHAPTER 6—
Transcultural and Genetic Considerations

Questions 1-6: refer to text.

7. d
8. a
9. d
10. a
11. a
12. b
13. d
14. a, b, c
15. b, c, d

Critical Thinking Exercises

1. Although direct eye contact is the norm in American health care systems, many cultural groups do not give direct eye contact. This family may look down or away from the health care provider as a result of the perception that the provider is superior or has increased knowledge. Most likely, persons who are not comfortable in this situation will not likely feel knowledgeable enough to question the health care provider and may actually nod affirmatively, which can be interpreted as agreement or understanding.

2. Obviously, these parents failed to understand the dosage of a teaspoon. This child received three times the dosage (3 teaspoons = 1 tablespoon).

3. Yes, it is dangerous because it could contribute to diarrhea, nausea, and vomiting. Further, this dose may cause liver impairment or hearing problems.

4. Overdosage may have been prevented if the parents were given a teaspoon measuring device along with the prescription. Further, the nurse may have observed the parent actually pouring and administering the correct amount.

5. As the parents are present-oriented, they may be inclined to discontinue the antibiotic when the child's symptoms disappear.

6. Ideally, a Chinese interpreter with a congruent dialect trained in the health care field would help to teach and clarify correct drug administration.

7. Prescriptions may need to be altered for chewable tablets, long-extended, or once-a-day formulas to simplify instruction. Detailed calendars and phrase charts may need to be developed using symbols such as the moon or the sun to illustrate correct timing of administration. This family may need a follow-up phone call or visit to ensure that the dosing requirements are correct and the drug is taken until completion.

CHAPTER 7—
Drug Interactions and Over-the-Counter Drugs

Questions 1-5: refer to text.

6. c
7. d

8. a

9. b

10. e

11. a

12. b, e

13. a, d

14. f

15. f

16. variable: symptoms may be masked; delay in professional diagnosis and treatment; OTC products may interact with other meds; need to consult health care provider before starting OTC products

17. c

18. a

19. b

20. d

21. c

22. a

23. d

24. c

25. b

26. a

27. b

28. b

29. b

30. a, c, d

31. a, b, d

32. a, c, e

CHAPTER 8—
Drugs of Abuse

Questions 1-8: refer to text.

9. anxiety, fine tremors, increased blood pressure, increased heart rate

10. b

11. d

12. d

13. a

14. a

15. c

16. a

17. a

18. a, b, e

19. a, b, c

CHAPTER 9—
Herbal Therapy with Nursing Implications

```
O  M  D  V  Z  T  W  A  E  T
F  R  E  S  H  H  E  R  B  C
J  I  R  D  O  S  L  I  O  A
D  S  B  I  D  Y  C  U  T  R
E  J  B  D  I  R  T  L  E  T
T  I  N  C  T  U  R  E  A  X
D  A  O  P  A  P  T  R  E  E
D  R  P  F  U  S  A  L  R  E  A
D  E  N  Y  P  S  E  U  I  W
S  X  A  K  T  I  L  I  F  Y
```

1. d

2. a

3. e

4. b

5. e

6. g

7. f

8. syrup

9. tea

10. tincture

11. extract

12. oil

13. fresh herb

14. d

15. g

16. h

17. j

18. a

19. f

20. b

21. c

22. e

23. i

24. c

25. a

26. b

27. b

28. b

29. a

30. c

31. d

32. c

33. b

34. c

35. a

36. b

37. b, d

38. a, b, e

Critical Thinking Exercises

1. Suggest that J.C. discuss his questions and potential benefits and risks of taking specific herbal preparations with his health care provider before taking any preparations.

2. Echinacea is recommended to boost the immune system on a short-term basis, less than 8 weeks. Need to discuss individual concerns with health care provider first. Caution is required when taking herbs with antidepressant and sedative-hypnotic effects together.
    What other meds, herbs, and conditions does person have?

3. FDA-proposed controls on dietary supplements containing Ephedra (ma huang) not to exceed 25 mg of ephedrine/day for <7 days and contraindicated in persons with diabetes mellitus, glaucoma, and hypertension. Use of this herb has diminished with reports of adverse events such as palpitations and stroke.

CHAPTER 10—
Pediatric Pharmacology

Questions 1-2: refer to text.

3. difficult to get pediatric sample; parents reluctant to take risks; potentially invasive nature of studies; smaller market share for meds

4. d

5. a. weight of child
    b. body surface area

6. a. minimum restraint; comforting
    b. simple explanation, firm approach, enlist imagination
    c. allow some choice
    d. involvement in administration process and information
    e. contract regarding plan of care, privacy

7. have child assist in placing EMLA on skin

and covering it with transparent dressing

8. so child does not fear "leakage" from the area

9. honesty, attention to vocabulary, forceful restraint not used, praise child after successful administration of med, never threaten or shame child into taking a med, teaching, developmental differences, etc.

10. b

11. a

12. c

13. a

14. a, b, d, e

15. b, c, d

Critical Thinking Exercises

1. Enlist parental support in medication administration.
    Use an oral syringe to administer oral medications in the buccal mucosa.
    Mix medication in a small amount of formula or age-appropriate food.
    Provide the least restrictive amount of restraint in order to not agitate the child.
    Squirt the medication into a bottle nipple as the child is sucking on it to allow the child to take the medicine.
    Use coke or cherry syrup to flavor medications.

2. Solicit the child's allergy history prior to the application of the topical anesthetic.

Ensure that the anesthetic is in place for the recommended amount of time prior to any painful procedures.

Use a transparent, nonocclusive dressing to ensure that the medication stays where applied.

Provide age-appropriate distraction to ensure the topical medication stays intact for the appropriate amount of time.

Make sure the cream forms a "pillow" over the potential IV site to ensure maximum effectiveness.

Provide age-appropriate explanations of the anesthetic and the invasive procedure.

3. Observe standard precautions.

Provide safe, atraumatic restraint for the child, enlisting the support of the parent or guardian.

Provide age-appropriate explanations of the procedure.

Select a needle and syringe appropriate for the client's size, muscle mass, site, and medication volume.

Select an angle appropriate for the client's size, injection site, and muscle mass.

Insert the needle into the skin.

Aspirate to ensure the needle is not in a blood vessel (may be controversial and is not done with many subcutaneous medications).

Inject the medication and count to five to ensure instillation of the medication.

Remove the needle and provide pressure with gauze if there is leakage.

Read medication insert or formulary to determine if massaging of the site is recommended.

Provide age-appropriate counseling and comfort following the procedure.

4. Pharmacokinetics and pharmacodynamics related to routes may differ based on the following criteria:

PO: specific medication characteristics, gastric acidity, amount of food in the stomach, age of the child, speed of peristalsis, type of medication (e.g., enteric-coated, time-release), type of medication (e.g., elixir, tablet, capsule), presence of antacids, first-pass effect

Injection/IV: hydration status, vascularity of the tissue/peripheral perfusion, type of medication, specific medication characteristics, presence of edema, amount of blood flow, use of muscle mass or extremity

Rectal: presence of stool in rectum, hydration status

Topical: porous nature of skin, skin surface area

5. Pharmacokinetics and pharmacodynamics related to age may differ based on the following criteria: acidity of stomach, body water content, nutrition and hydration status, organ and physiologic maturity, route of administration, level of mobility, compliance with medication regimen, gastric mobility and emptying, protein-binding capacity, metabolic rate

CHAPTER 11— *Geriatric Pharmacology*

1. drug metabolism that occurs in the liver and contributes to the clearance of drugs

2. taking drugs according to the prescribed drug regimen

3. not taking the prescribed drugs as indicated

4. taking many (multiple) drugs together

5. b

6. b

7. b

8. b

9. a

10. variable

11. a	21. d	2. warm bath before sleep, avoid caffeine products (coffee, cola, chocolates) before bedtime, soft music, routine bedtime patterns, seek health care provider help
12. c	22. c	
13. a, b	23. b	
14. d	24. a	
15. b	25. b	
16. c	26. a, c, e	
17. d	27. c, d, e	3. keep written record of each drug taken, keep drugs in daily or weekly pill box container, other suggestions
18. c		
19. b	*Critical Thinking Exercises*	
20. b	1. BUN, creatinine, creatinine clearance, serum protein, urinalysis	4. see the nursing process

CHAPTER 12—
Medication Administration in Community Settings

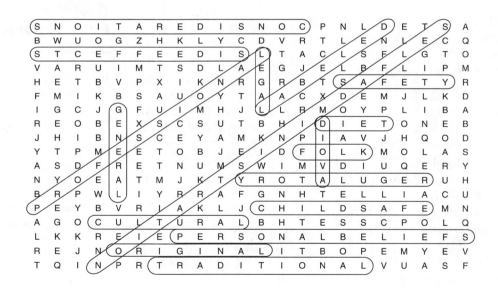

1. professional, legal, regulatory

2. avoid

3. general, diet, self-administration, side effects, cultural considerations

4. safety

5. original labeled, child safe

6. personal beliefs

7. traditional, folk

8. health care provider, pharmacist

9. report to health care provider

10. unused

11. self-administers

12. licensed

13. a

14. b

15. c

16. a, b, c, d, e, f, g, h

17. a, b, d

18. a, c, d

Critical Thinking Exercises

Meds given only with parent's written permission; prescription drugs require written authorization of health care provider; individual pharmacy labeled bottle for specific student; administration documented: name, med, dosage, time, and person giving; meds stored in locked, clean cabinet

CHAPTER 13—
The Role of the Nurse in Drug Research

Questions 1-4: refer to text.

5. d

6. a

7. g

8. b

9. c

10. f

11. e

12. i

13. j

14. h

15. k

16. client/family advocate; liaison between health care provider and research nurse

17. variable

18. variable

19. c

20. b

21. d

22. c

23. b

24. b

25. d

26. c

27. a, c, d

28. b, c, d, e, f

CHAPTER 14—
Vitamin and Mineral Replacement

Questions 1-4: refer to text.

5. a

6. b

7. b

8. a

9. a

10. a

11. a

12. a

13. b

14. b

15. a

16. d

17. c

18. e

19. a

20. b

21. administer with food to increase absorption; store in light-resistant container

22. variable: not to leave iron tablets within child's reach; telephone poison control center for overdoses; not to overdose; avoid megadoses of iron during first trimester; take iron with food if gastrointestinal upset occurs

23. d

24. c

25. d

26. b

27. a

28. c

29. d

30. a

31. c

32. a

33. b

34. c

35. b

36. d

37. d

38. d

39. a

40. c

41. b, c

42. a, b, c

43. a, c, d

Critical Thinking Exercises

1. Advise P.J. to eat three balanced and appropriately spaced meals each day. (Refer to the MyPyramid in Chapter 14 in the text.) Also advise P.J. to drink adequate fluids,

especially water, to maintain hydration.

2. With a balanced, nutritious diet, P.J. will get adequate vitamins and minerals from food.

CHAPTER 15—
Fluid and Electrolyte Replacement

1. serum calcium excess

2. serum potassium excess

3. serum sodium excess

4. serum calcium deficit (loss)

5. serum potassium deficit (loss)

6. serum sodium deficit (loss)

7. concentration of body fluids

8. effects of fluid on cellular volume

9. c

10. a

11. d

12. e

13. potassium: 3.5-5.3 mEq/L

14. sodium: 135-145 mEq/L

15. calcium: 9-11 mg/dl; 4.5-5.5 mEq/L

16. magnesium: 1.5-2.5 mEq/L

17. b

18. a

19. d

20. d

21. c

22. a

23. Potassium is extremely irritating to the gastric mucosa. It may cause bleeding or gastric ulcer if taken undiluted.

24. Potassium should never be given as a bolus or IV push. Inverting the IV bag with potassium ensures that the potassium is diluted. If the bag is NOT inverted several times, potassium can accumulate at the neck of the IV bag; thus a large portion of the potassium is given directly into the vein; cardiac dysrhythmias or arrest could result.

25. Potassium can cause tissue necrosis if it infiltrates into the fatty (subcutaneous) tissues.

26. 80% to 90% of potassium is excreted in the urine.

    With renal insufficiency, potassium can accumulate, causing hyperkalemia. Urine output should be at least 25 ml/hr and 600 ml/24 hr.

27. Serum potassium level should be 3.5 to 5.3 mEq/L. Hypokalemia occurs if the serum potassium level is <3.5 mEq/L; hyperkalemia occurs if it is >5.3 mEq/L.

28. If hypokalemia occurs, the T wave is flat or inverted and the ST segment is depressed. With hyperkalemia, the T wave is narrow and peaked and the QRS complex is spread.

29. Foods rich in potassium include citrus fruit juices, fruits, vegetables, nuts, and meats. Serum potassium level should be monitored while the client is taking potassium-wasting diuretics and cortisone. If serum level is low, potassium supplements should be taken.

30. Signs of hypokalemia include nausea, vomiting, cardiac dysrhythmias, abdominal distention, and soft and flabby muscles. Signs of hyperkalemia include nausea, abdominal cramps, oliguria, tachycardia and later bradycardia, weakness, and numbness or tingling in the extremities.

31. Hypokalemia enhances the action of digitalis preparation. Signs of digitalis toxicity include nausea, vomiting, anorexia, bradycardia (pulse < 60 beats/min), cardiac dysrhythmias, and visual disturbances. Serum potassium level should be checked while the client is receiving digoxin and a potassium-wasting diuretic or cortisone.

32. b

33. a

34. b

35. c

36. d

37. c

38. b

39. b

40. a

41. c

42. b

43. b

44. c

45. a

46. c

47. a

48. b

49. b

50. c

51. d

52. d

53. c

54. a

55. c

56. b

57. b

58. d

59. b

60. b, c, d

61. a, d

62. a, c

Critical Thinking Exercises

1. Crystalloids do not interfere with type and crossmatch of the blood. They will raise the blood pressure rapidly; however, the blood pressure will remain elevated longer with colloids than with crystalloids.

2. Whole blood is useful when replacing a large volume of blood. If a client has cardiac problems, packed red blood cells are recommended (less fluid volume, thus less fluid overload).

3. A.F. is showing signs of shock caused by loss of fluid volume and red blood cells to carry oxygen. The use of IV fluids should raise the blood pressure.

4. When client has shock-like symptoms, blood circulation is decreased, especially to the kidneys. Renal shutdown may occur if the decrease is severe. Less body fluids are circulated through the kidneys, and less urine output occurs.

5. Body fluid volume has increased.

6. Sodium should be part of the daily intravenous order. Giving only dextrose in water over 24 hours or more may cause fluid imbalance, such as intracellular fluid volume excess (water intoxication).

7. Dextrose in water and lactated Ringer's solution is isotonic. Dextrose in ½ normal saline solution is hypertonic.

8. If the client receives only hypertonic solutions, dehydration could result. Fluid is pulled from the cells to the vascular space and then excreted.

9. A.F.'s serum potassium level is low. A healthy client with a normal potassium level should receive 40 mEq of potassium daily. A.F. should receive a higher dosage of potassium since he has a potassium deficit. It would take 100-200 mEq of potassium intravenously to raise the serum potassium level by 1 mEq/L.

10. Nursing assessment: the type of intravenous fluids A.F. is receiving; checking vital signs; determining if blood loss is still occurring; and so forth.

CHAPTER 16—
Nutritional Support

Questions 1-4: refer to text.

5. a. gastrostomy

    b. jejunostomy

    c. nasoduodenal/ nasojejunal

    d. nasogastric

6. improving blood flow to major organs; enhancing wound healing; decreasing infection; decreasing hospital stay; improving organ function

7. a

8. b

9. d

10. b

11. b

12. a

13. c

14. c

15. b

16. d

17. c

18. a, b, c

19. a, c, d

20. d, b, e, c, a

Critical Thinking Exercises

1. The advantage of continuous and cyclic methods of enteral feeding for a severely ill client is that large amounts of highly concentrated (increased osmolality) solution are entered slowly into the GI tract; thus it is more tolerable for absorption.

Disadvantages of bolus administration and some intermittent methods are that the enteral feeding is highly concentrated and, when rapidly administered, diarrhea could occur. With continuous enteral feedings, the client is never free from the feeding, and other reasons.

2. T.A. would not receive adequate nutrition with IV solutions of crystalloids.

3. T.A. is to receive enteral feedings by the intermittent method. The enteral feedings may be given by drip or pump infusion for 30 to 60 minutes every 3 to 6 hours.

4. Share the family's concerns with the health care provider. Make appropriate referrals.

5. Elevate the head of the bed or place the client in the Fowler's position. Do not administer feedings while the client is lying flat. Check for residual feeding before administering a feeding.

6. Dilute the enteral feedings for several days until diarrhea stops. Dilute the medication. Check for GI bacteria.

7.

$$\frac{D \text{ (desired \%)}}{H \text{ (on hand vol.)}} \times \overset{V \text{ (desired}}{\text{total vol.)}} =$$

$$\frac{70}{100} \times 300 \text{ ml} = \frac{21000}{100} =$$

210 ml of Ensure Plus

Total amount − Amount of EF = amount of water

300 ml − 210 ml = 90 ml

Mix 210 ml of Ensure Plus and 90 ml of water for a total of 300 ml of solution.

CHAPTER 17—
Adrenergics and Adrenergic Blockers

Questions 1-5: refer to text.

6. smooth

7. adrenergic

8. sitting up

9. do

10. sympatholytics

11. Regitine

12. Minipress

13. beta blockers

14. hypertension

15. asthma, hypotension

16. The two drugs could counteract each other (as antagonists), thus negating a therapeutic action.

17. d

18. c, a

19. a

20. a

21. b

22. d

23. c

24. d

25. b

26. variable: monitor vital signs; report drug side effects such as tachycardia, palpitations, tremors, dizziness, and increased blood pressure; check urinary output and assess for bladder distention; offer food when giving adrenergic drugs orally, etc.

27. variable: monitor vital signs; report complaints of dizziness and nasal congestion; assess lungs for congestion and for edema in legs and feet; insulin or oral hypoglycemic agent may need adjustment, etc.

28. b

29. a

30. d

31. b

32. d

33. d

34. c

35. b

36. c

37. b

38. c

39. b

40. d

41. a, b, c

42. a, b, e

Critical Thinking Exercises

1. $beta_1$ and $beta_2$

2. Daily doses are safe. The client is receiving less than most suggested drug doses; however, the client's pulse rate and blood pressure are not elevated.

3. Yes. By blocking $beta_2$ receptors, the bronchial tubes constrict.

4. Propranolol decreases heart rate; therefore, K.S.'s pulse rate should be closely monitored, especially since his pulse rate is low-average.

5. Client teaching: check pulse rate; rise slowly to a standing position to avoid orthostatic hypotension, which causes dizziness and lightheadedness; decreased

libido may occur; mood changes may occur.

6. It would be unlikely that K.S. would develop rebound tachycardia or hypertension. He is on a low-average daily dose, his pulse rate is in the lower range, and his blood pressure is not elevated.

7. Propranolol could decrease the blood sugar level. Insulin dosage would have to be adjusted.

8. metoprolol, atenolol, acebutolol

CHAPTER 18—
Cholinergics and Anticholinergics

Questions 1-8: refer to text.

9. opposite

10. skeletal

11. cholinesterase

12. atropine

13. stimulate bladder and gastrointestinal tone, constrict pupils, increase neuromuscular transmission, decrease heart rate and blood pressure, and increase salivation

14. variable: monitor vital signs, observe for side effects, auscultate breath and bowel sounds, monitor intake and output, administer 1 hour before or 2 hours after meals, recognize effects on laboratory values

15. variable: monitor vital signs, observe for side effects, assess intake and output, report urinary retention, check for constipation, suggest hard candy for dry mouth, avoid alcohol

16. b
17. a
18. b
19. b
20. a
21. b
22. c
23. a
24. c
25. c
26. c
27. a
28. d
29. c
30. b
31. a
32. c
33. d
34. b
35. c
36. c
37. b
38. b, c, e, f
39. b, c, d, e

Critical Thinking Exercises

1. Anticholinergic. It has similar action and effects as atropine.

2. The dose (60 mg/day) is within therapeutic range (10-20 mg, t.i.d./q.i.d.).

3. contraindicated for clients having narrow-angle glaucoma, severe ulcerative colitis, paralytic ileus

4. similar to anticholinergics; urinary retention, increase in heart rate, dry mouth, constipation

5. The dose (6 mg/day) is within therapeutic range (6-10 mg/day).

6. 15 ml of trihexyphenidyl

$$\frac{D}{H} \times V = \frac{6}{2} \text{ mg} \times 5 \text{ ml} =$$

$$\frac{30}{2} = 15 \text{ ml}$$

7. Both drugs are anticholinergics. Trihexyphenidyl is used primarily for the early phase of parkinsonism for suppressing tremors and decreasing muscular rigidity. Dicyclomine is used to decrease gastrointestinal spasms.

CHAPTER 19—
Central Nervous System Stimulants

Questions 1-5: refer to text.

6. psychologic

7. normal waking

8. attention deficit hyperactivity disorder (ADHD)

9. are not

10. decongestants and

caffeine/barbiturates and antihypertensives

11. stimulation; toxicity or dysfunction

12. xanthine

13. 500

14. do

15. narcolepsy, ADHD, obesity, and reversal of respiratory distress

16. variable: monitor heart rate and blood pressure and report significant changes, assess for side effects, administer 6-8 hours before sleep, taper the dose when discontinuing the drug, avoid administering CNS stimulants to nursing mothers

17. Take drugs before meals; avoid alcohol and caffeine-containing foods; report weight loss; avoid hazardous equipment in the presence of tremors, nervousness, or tachycardia; and seek counseling

18. b

19. d

20. d

21. b

22. a

23. d

24. b

25. a

26. c

27. d

28. b

29. d

30. a

31. a, c

32. a, e

Critical Thinking Exercises

1. before meals to increase absorption

2. schedule children before lunch; have adequate space for number of children

3. fewer side effects

4. height, weight, and growth

5. CBC, differential WBC, and platelets

6. sugarless gum to relieve dry mouth; consult health care provider before taking OTC drugs that may contain caffeine. High caffeine plasma levels could be fatal. Need for three nutritional meals in presence of anorexia.

7. opportunity to discuss feelings and ask questions; need for appropriate counseling (not drugs alone!); long-term use may lead to drug abuse; diet; side effects and what to report to health care provider

CHAPTER 20—
Central Nervous System Depressants

Questions 1-5: refer to text.

6. sedative-hypnotics, general and local anes-

thetics, analgesics, narcotic analgesics, anticonvulsants, antipsychotics, and antidepressants

7. rapid eye movement (REM); and non–rapid eye movement (NREM)

8. sedation

9. arise at a specific hour; no naps; avoid caffeine drinks and large quantities of fluids 6 hours before bedtime; avoid heavy meals or exercise before bedtime; take a warm bath and/or listen to soft music at bedtime; avoid loud noises; drink warm milk

10. may

11. ultra-short

12. central nervous, pain, consciousness

13. ether

14. surgical; analgesia, excitement or delirium, medullary paralysis

15. spinal

16. respiratory distress or failure

17. saddle block

18. are

19. short

20. zolpidem tartrate (Ambien)

21. flumazenil (Romazicon)

22. esters and amides

23. variable: instruct the client about nonpharmacologic measures to induce/promote sleep; avoid alco-

hol, antidepressants, antipsychotic and narcotic drugs; not to drive or operate machinery; to report adverse effects, etc.

24. d
25. f
26. e
27. a
28. b
29. c
30. d
31. d
32. d
33. a
34. a
35. b
36. d
37. d
38. b
39. a, b, c
40. a, b, d, e
41. a, e

Critical Thinking Exercises

1. take a detailed history of insomnia; vital signs; assess renal function

2. promotes natural sleep; no hangover or undesirable effect

3. drug dependence; drug tolerance

4. yes; short-acting and decreased side effects

5. 15-30 minutes and 3-6 hours

6. prepare for bed and then take med (short-acting); incorporate nonpharmacologic measures to promote sleep; not for long-term use; dose should be tapered to avoid withdrawal symptoms

CHAPTER 21—
Anticonvulsants

Questions 1-5: refer to text.

6. one
7. electroencephalogram
8. idiopathic
9. generalized; partial
10. preventing; do not
11. are not
12. hydantoins, long-acting barbiturates, succinimides, oxazolidinones, benzodiazepines, carbamazepine, and valproate
13. phenytoin
14. OTC
15. intramuscular
16. variable: monitor serum drug levels, maintain protective environment, monitor nutrition, assess contraception in women
17. resources, current information, support groups, sharing information, sharing knowledge of community resources
18. d
19. a
20. d

21. c
22. b
23. a
24. a
25. b
26. b
27. d
28. c
29. c
30. variable: not to drive or operate hazardous machinery when drug therapy is started; report nystagmus, slurred speech, rash; advise health care provider if pregnant or contemplating pregnancy; wear medic-alert ID; not to abruptly stop drug, etc.
31. a
32. d
33. c
34. d
35. a
36. b
37. a, b, c
38. a, b, d
39. b, c, d, e

Critical Thinking Exercises

1. age; rate of metabolism and possible associated conditions

2. therapeutic serum or plasma level

3. below: seizures not controlled; within: seizures controlled; above: toxicity may occur

4. shorter half-life, thus decreased chance of cumulative drug effects

5. highly protein-bound

6. 15-50 mcg/ml

7. nothing related to level if the seizures are controlled with no side effects

8. variable: need to assess current knowledge base regarding anticonvulsants and seizures; understanding of need for regular follow-up and potential consequences of lack of follow-up; proceed accordingly

CHAPTER 22—
Drugs for Neurologic Disorders: Parkinsonism and Alzheimer's Disease

Questions 1-5: refer to text.

6. dopamine and acetylcholine

7. dopamine

8. levodopa

9. carbidopa

10. Aricept (donepezil)

11. enhance

12. selegiline

13. liver

14. ethopropazine (Parsidol) and orphenadrine (Norflex)

15. variable: monitor vital signs, assess for weakness, instruct to eat high-fiber foods,

avoid alcohol, etc.

16. c

17. c

18. b

19. b

20. b

21. d

22. a, b, c

23. b, c, e

24. b, c, e

Critical Thinking Exercises

1. bradykinesia, rigidity, tremors

2. parkinsonism—lack of dopamine and too much acetylcholine at basal ganglia; myasthenia gravis—lack of acetylcholine

3. Levodopa is converted to dopamine in the brain; replaces the lack of dopamine.

4. nausea, vomiting, orthostatic hypotension, cardiac dysrhythmias, psychosis

5. Carbidopa inhibits the enzyme dopa decarboxylase, allowing more dopamine to reach the brain.

6. Used mostly for early cases of parkinsonism and pseudoparkinsonism (drug-induced parkinsonism). D.G. would not be a candidate for anticholinergic antiparkinsonism drug since he had the health problem for 6 years (not newly diagnosed).

7. Amantadine is an antiviral drug for influenza A.
   This drug may be used for early diagnosed parkinsonism and drug-induced parkinsonism. It has fewer side effects than anticholinergics.

8. All are dopamine agonists. They are for early treatment of parkinsonism. Pergolide is more potent than bromocriptine.

9. a. Do not abruptly discontinue the drug as rebound parkinsonism symptoms may occur.
   b. Take drug with food.
   c. Report side effects such as dyskinesia.
   d. Urine may be discolored and darkens when exposed to air. Others: report dizziness.

CHAPTER 23—
Drugs for Neuromuscular Disorders: Myasthenia Gravis, Multiple Sclerosis, and Muscle Spasms

Questions 1-6: refer to text.

7. edrophonium (Tensilon)

8. myelin sheath

9. traumatic, chronic

10. Dantrium

11. pregnancy and lactation

12. neostigmine (Prostigmin)

13. variable: assess for difficulty breathing or swal-
lowing, monitor muscle
strength, observe for
signs and symptoms of
cholinergic crisis, etc.

14. variable: advise not
to drive or operate
hazardous machinery,
avoid alcohol or central
nervous system depres-
sants, take medication
with food, etc.

15. prednisone and/or
immunosuppressive
drugs

16. muscle weakness,
dyspnea, and dysphagia

17. d

18. a

19. b

20. a

21. d

22. c

23. d

24. a

25. b

26. a, b, c

27. a, b, e

28. a, b, d, e

Critical Thinking Exercises

1. centrally acting muscle
relaxants—used to treat
skeletal muscle spastic-
ity; act on the spinal
cord to treat spasticity;
muscle relaxants—used
to treat muscle spasms;
act to decrease pain,
increase range of
motion, and provide a
sedative effect

2. impaired physical
mobility, activity
intolerance

3. CNS depressants to
avoid a potentiated
sedative effect

4. muscle relaxants should
not be abruptly stopped;
advise the client to
avoid alcohol and CNS
depressants; advise the
client to avoid driving
or operating dangerous
machinery when taking
muscle relaxants; these
drugs are contraindicat-
ed for pregnant women
and nursing mothers.

CHAPTER 24— *Antiinflammatory Drugs*

Questions 1-5: refer to text.

6. injury and infection

7. should not

8. redness, heat, swelling,
pain, loss of function

9. aspirin

10. delayed

11. does

12. higher or increased

13. 24

14. NSAIDs act to relieve
inflammation by
inhibiting the COX
enzyme, which is
needed for biosynthesis
of prostaglandins.
Immunomodulators
act to disrupt the
inflammatory process
and delay disease
progression.

15. 250 mg tablets:
2 tablets/dose;
4 tablets/24-hr 500 mg
tablets: 1 tablet/dose;
2 tablets/24 hr

16. 500 mg tablet; only one
tablet twice a day

17. take with food or a full
glass of water

18. b

19. a

20. d

21. c

22. b

23. c

24. b

25. d

26. c

27. c

28. b

29. a

30. b

31. c

32. b

33. d

34. c

35. a

36. b

37. a

38. d

39. c

40. a, c, d, e

41. a, b, c, e

42. b, c, d, e

Critical Thinking Exercises

1. 325-650 mg q4h PRN;

maximum = 4 g/day; >maximum dose

2. 15-30 ng/dl; >30 ng/dl

3. potassium, T_3, T_4, PT, uric acid, AST, ALT

4. inhibition of prostaglandin synthesis

5. Anorexia and stomach pain are side effects of aspirin.

6. tinnitus, agranulocytosis, bronchospasm, leukopenia, anaphylaxis

7. variable: take medicine with meals, notify all providers of high aspirin dosing, keep out of children's reach, avoid alcohol

CHAPTER 25—
Nonnarcotic and Narcotic Analgesics

Questions 1-4: refer to text.

5. c

6. a

7. d

8. e

9. b

10. analgesics

11. propionic acid

12. viral

13. prostaglandins

14. food, mealtime, glass of fluid

15. hepatonecrosis

16. is not

17. variable: keep out of reach of children, avoid

alcohol and highly protein-bound drugs, take ibuprofen and aspirin with food, no aspirin for viral infections

18. central nervous system; peripheral nervous system

19. respiration and coughing

20. antitussive and antidiarrheal

21. head injury and respiratory depression

22. variable: avoid alcohol, increase fluid intake, report dizziness and difficulty breathing

23. MAOIs

24. side effect; health care provider

25. variable: anorexia, nausea, vomiting, constipation, drowsiness, dizziness, sedation, urinary retention, rash, blurred vision, bradycardia, flushing, euphoria, pruritus

26. IV

27. b

28. d

29. d

30. a

31. d

32. d

33. c

34. c

35. b

36. b

37. d

38. d

39. c

40. d

41. a

42. a, b, e, f

43. a, d, e

Critical Thinking Exercises

1. 0.67 ml; intravenously

2. yes

3. inject over 5 minutes

4. side effect of morphine sulfate

5. no; orthostatic hypotension is side effect

6. increases AST and ALT

7. not to take any CNS depressants and alcohol; use nonpharmacologic measures to relieve pain and reduce stress

CHAPTER 26—
Antipsychotics and Anxiolytics

Questions 1-7: refer to text.

8. thought process, behavior; dopamine

9. dihydroindolones, thioxanthenes, butyrophenones, dibenzoxazepines

10. extrapyramidal

11. drowsiness

12. pruritus, photosensitivity

13. decrease

14. are not

15. tolerance

16. sedative-hypnotics

17. dyspnea, heart palpitations, dizziness, trembling

18. relaxation techniques, psychotherapy, support groups

19. buspirone (BuSpar)

20. antihistamines

21. variable: dry mouth (offer throat lozenges); orthostatic hypotension (monitor vital signs); constipation (offer additional fluids); dizziness (teach need to rise slowly); urinary incontinence (offer emotional support)

22. c

23. a

24. a

25. b

26. b

27. c

28. b

29. d

30. b

31. c

32. b

33. c

34. a

35. b

36. b

37. a

38. c

39. a

40. c

41. b

42. b

43. d

44. d

45. c

46. c

47. d

48. b

49. b

50. c

51. a, b

52. a, b, c

Critical Thinking Exercises

1. B.B. is displaying negative symptoms of schizophrenia. Mesoridazine is more effective for treating positive symptoms of schizophrenia, whereas clozapine is effective for both positive and negative symptoms.

2. Agranulocytosis is a life-threatening side effect of clozapine. B.B.'s white blood cell count should be monitored at specified times.

3. The target daily dose is 300-450 mg per day. His prescribed daily dose is within low-normal range. His daily dose may need to be increased; maximum: 900 mg/day.

4. The clozapine should be taken at the prescribed times. Any problem with dosage schedule should be discussed with the health care provider. Use of pill container may be of help to avoid missed doses.

5. Alcohol and CNS depressants with clozapine cause a depressant effect; antihypertensive drugs with clozapine may enhance a hypotensive state; and others.

6. Assess the effects of clozapine and lab results (WBCs). Instruct client to take clozapine as ordered; avoid drugs that may cause drug interaction; avoid orthostatic hypotension; and others.

CHAPTER 27—
Antidepressants and Mood Stabilizers

P	M	T	R	O	V	S	K	L	N	Q	M	B	C	E	I	B
J	A	N	T	I	D	E	P	R	E	S	S	A	N	T	S	W
P	O	X	R	J	T	W	Z	N	A	C	U	Y	K	H	F	L
K	I	W	R	Q	P	U	A	R	I	H	O	E	Y	I	R	W
Q	S	E	C	J	U	T	A	I	E	M	V	O	D	N	Z	S
R	X	C	Y	I	P	L	N	E	N	I	U	B	M	Z	A	I
T	W	R	C	I	O	J	P	X	T	Z	B	V	R	O	P	M
P	H	D	L	P	Y	M	N	C	R	S	B	I	E	W	F	H
R	O	U	I	N	N	M	A	N	I	C	A	P	C	Q	J	W
V	T	B	C	I	S	E	M	N	X	Z	P	O	T	A	W	E
F	R	P	S	S	R	I	S	I	W	T	J	O	B	M	I	A

1. bipolar (affective disorders)
2. SSRIs
3. MAOIs
4. manic
5. antidepressants
6. reactive (depression)
7. tricyclics
8. tricyclic, monoamine oxidase (MAO) inhibitors, and second-generation SSRIs
9. 2 to 4 weeks
10. at night
11. atypical antidepressants
12. major depressive disorders; anxiety disorders (obsessive-compulsive, panic, phobias)
13. MAOIs
14. should not
15. tranylcypromine (Parnate), isocarboxazid (Marplan), phenelzine (Nardil)

16. a
17. a
18. b
19. d
20. c
21. b
22. d
23. b
24. c
25. a
26. d
27. c
28. a
29. b
30. c
31. a
32. d
33. b
34. c
35. b
36. c
37. a

38. a, c, e
39. a, b, c, d

Critical Thinking Exercises

1. history of depression and coping behaviors, vital signs, liver and renal function tests, drug history

2. high end of recommended dosage; should be divided dose with most administered in the morning; avoid nighttime administration

3. three

4. primary

5. variable: grief support group, peer counseling programs, etc.

6. variable: take medicine as prescribed, avoid alcohol, take medicine with food, do not abruptly stop taking medicine, do not operate machinery until dosage is stabilized, etc.

CHAPTER 28—
Penicillins and Cephalosporins

Questions 1-9: refer to text.

10. inhibit

11. kill

12. inhibition of bacterial cell wall synthesis, alteration in cell wall permeability, inhibition of protein synthesis, and interference with metabolism within the cell

13. greater

14. are not

15. 4th-5th

16. 7th

17. acquired

18. nosocomial

19. hypersensitivity reaction, superinfection, organ toxicity

20. resistant

21. absorption, distribution, metabolism, and excretion of the drug

22. drug toxicity

23. constant; time

24. age, white blood cell count, organ function, circulation, immunoglobulins

25. variable: ask client about allergies, culture and sensitivity (C&S) before initiating treatment, monitor for superinfection, monitor for allergic reaction, monitor body temperature, dilute for IV use

26. variable: identification bracelet if allergic, side effects, increase fluids, take all of medicine as prescribed, take medicine with food

27. *Haemophilus influenzae, Neisseria gonorrhoeae, Enterobacter* spp., and anaerobes

28. *Pseudomonas* spp., *Serratia* spp., *Acinetobacter* spp.

29. IM and IV

30. a

31. b

32. d

33. b

34. a

35. a

36. d

37. c

38. a

39. 5 ml; 20 ml

40. d

41. c

42. a

43. b

44. a

45. a, b, d, e

46. a, c, d

Critical Thinking Exercises

1. penicillinase-resistant penicillin

2. 250-500 mg q6h IM; 500 mg-1 g q4-6h IV for severe infection

3. intramuscular, intravenous

4. 2 cc or ml

5. epinephrine

6. broad-spectrum penicillins: to treat both gram-positive and gram-negative bacterias; more costly than penicillinase-resistant penicillin: for treating penicillinase-producing *Staphylococcus aureus*; not effective against gram-negative organisms; less effective than penicillin G against gram-positive organisms

7. variable: monitor for allergic reaction, monitor site of infection, monitor body temperature, dilute antibiotic for IV infusion

CHAPTER 29—
Macrolides, Tetracyclines, Aminoglycosides, and Fluoroquinolones

Questions 1-4: refer to text.

5. bactericidal

6. azithromycin

7. ketolides

8. protein

9. variable: monitor liver enzymes, obtain C&S before initiating treatment, monitor vital signs and intake and output; take with food if gastrointestinal upset

10. vancomycin

11. nephrotoxicity; ototoxicity

12. toxic

13. netilmicin; D

14. ototoxicity and nephrotoxicity

15. variable: C&S before initiating treatment; monitor intake and output; monitor for superinfection; monitor serum peak and trough levels

16. bactericidal

17. chloramphenicol (Chloromycetin)

18. gonorrhea

19. *N. gonorrhoeae* or *H. influenzae*

20. b

21. a

22. a

23. b

24. d

25. first dose = 500 mg + 12.5 ml; daily dose of 250 mg = 6.125 ml

26. decreases; take medication on an empty stomach

27. a, b, d, e

28. a, b, c, d

29. b, c, d, e

Critical Thinking Exercises

1. Yes; one indication is for treatment of lower respiratory tract infections.
    Vital signs; intake and output, renal function tests, drug history, etc.

2. mild to moderate infections:

    A: PO: 250-500 mg q12h
    IV: 200 mg q12h (over 1 hr)

    Severe infections:
    A: PO: 500-750 mg q12h

    IV: 200-400 mg q12h (over 1 hr)

3. seizure disorders, elderly, <1 year, and clients taking theophylline

4. AST, ALT, BUN, serum creatinine

5. variable: monitor intake and output, vital signs; assess for superinfection; monitor BUN and creatinine

6. variable: avoid caffeine; do not operate machinery; use sunblock and sunglasses

CHAPTER 30—
Sulfonamides

Questions 1-3: refer to text.

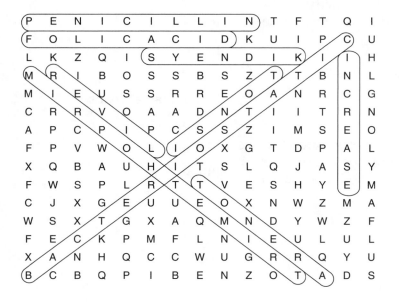

4. folic acid

5. penicillin

6. trimethoprim

7. are not

8. is not

9. liver; kidneys

10. bacteriostatic

11. increase

12. d

13. a

14. b

15. 2; 4

16. d

17. a

18. a, c, d, e

19. b, c, e

Critical Thinking Exercises

1. LD: 75 mg/kg; then 150 mg/kg/day in divided doses; loading dose = 3.75 g

2. more stable in urine

3. variable: administer medicine with full glass of water; monitor intake and output and vital signs; observe for early signs of hematologic reactions including sore throat, purpura, and decreasing WBC and platelet counts; observe for signs and symptoms of superinfection, including stomatitis, furry black tongue, anal or genital discharge or itching

4. variable: instruct Y.M. to drink several quarts of fluid per day; avoid antacids because they decrease absorption rate; alert client and significant others to cross-sensitivity of sulfonamide preparations; take medicine 1 hour before or 2 hours after food; report bruising or bleeding; avoid direct sunlight and wear protective clothing to decrease photosensitivity

5. to prevent crystalluria and formation of kidney stones

CHAPTER 31—
Antituberculars, Antifungals, Peptides, and Metronidazole

Questions 1-5: refer to text.

6. streptomycin

7. is not

8. more

9. B_6 pyridoxine

10. 6-12 months

11. disseminated

12. rifabutin (Mycobutin)

13. polyenes, imidazoles, antimetabolites, topicals

14. lung or central nervous system

15. mouth, skin, intestine, vagina

16. amphotericin B; IV

17. is not

18. increases

19. fluconazole and itraconazole

20. neurotoxicity and nephrotoxicity; BUN and serum creatinine

21. bactericidal

22. gram-negative

23. IV

24. is

25. variable: administer drug 1 hour before or 2 hours after food; administer with pyridoxine; monitor serum levels; collect sputum specimen in morning; schedule eye examinations; stress importance of adherence to drug regimen

26. amebiasis, anaerobic infections, bacterial vaginosis, perioperative prophylaxis, and rosacea

27. d

28. a

29. a

30. b

31. c

32. d

33. b

34. a

35. c

36. d

37. d

38. d

39. a

40. b

41. d

42. c

43. a

44. d

45. 1½ tablets/dose

46. a, b, c

47. a, c, d, e

48. a, b, d, e

Critical Thinking Exercises

1. yes

2. superinfection

3. *Candida*

4. "swish and swallow": put prescribed amount of drug in mouth, swish solution around mouth so that it contacts the mucous membrane, and in a few minutes, swallow the solution (or expectorate the solution after "swishing;" ask health care provider for recommendation)

5. variable: stress adherence to drug regimen to avoid relapse; follow-up with laboratory testing as scheduled; instruct on swish and swallow; report side effects; avoid operating hazardous machinery and ingesting alcohol while taking amphotericin B, ketoconazole, or flucytosine because these may cause visual changes or sleepiness

6. both drugs belong to polyene group; amphotericin B: administered IV in low doses; not absorbed from the GI tract; highly protein-bound; long half-life; highly toxic so urinary output, BUN, and creatinine levels require close monitoring; nystatin: administered orally or topically; poorly absorbed from GI tract; protein-binding and half-life unknown

CHAPTER 32—
Antivirals, Antimalarials, and Anthelmintics

Questions 1-3: refer to text.

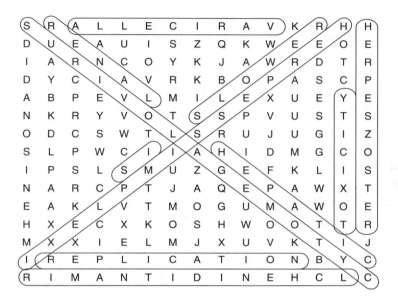

4. replication

5. is

6. slower, toxicity

7. rimantadine hydrochloride, renal, hepatic

8. herpes simplex type 1, herpes zoster, varicella (zoster), cytomegalovirus

9. a

10. erythrocytic

11. trichinosis; muscle biopsy

12. c

13. c

14. yes; one-half tablet

15. b

16. c

17. d

18. c

19. d

20. a

21. c

22. d

23. a

24. d

25. d

26. c

27. b

28. d

29. a, b, c

30. a, c, e

31. a, b, c, d

Critical Thinking Exercises

1. antimetabolite

2. 30-60 minutes before meals with water

3. CBC, BUN, creatinine, liver enzymes

4. decreased urine output, dizziness, anxiety, confusion

5. soft toothbrush, several times each day; prevents gum bleeding and irritation

CHAPTER 33—
Drugs for Urinary Tract Disorders

Questions 1-6: refer to text.

7. tubule and bladder

8. before

9. nitrofurantoin

10. decreases

11. brown, teeth

12. Pyridium

13. decreased

14. micturition

15. contraindicated

16. 5.5

17. Urecholine

18. sulfamethoxazole-trimethoprim (Bactrim, Septra)

19. Monurol (fosfomycin tromethamine)

20. variable: monitor intake and output; obtain urine culture before initiating antiseptic therapy; observe for side effects

of drugs; recognize drug-drug, drug-lab, and drug-food interactions; nitrofurantoin can stain teeth so the client needs to rinse the mouth thoroughly; etc.

21. b

22. c

23. b

24. a

25. d

26. b

27. b

28. d

29. a

30. d

31. c

32. a

33. a, c, d, e

34. a, b, d

35. a, c, d, e

Critical Thinking Exercises

1. urinary antispasmodic

2. 2.5 mg, b.i.d., PO; inform health care provider

3. drowsiness, blurred vision, dry mouth

4. urinary or gastrointestinal obstruction, glaucoma; yes, based on limited data provided

5. none significant

6. Pro-Banthine with frequent dosing may cause urinary hesitancy or retention, so advise the client to void before each dose.

CHAPTER 34—
HIV- and AIDS-Related Drugs

Questions 1-5: refer to text.

6. c

7. a, b

8. c

9. c

10. variable: need for HIV testing, refer as appropriate; chemical signs of depressed immune system; use of prescription, OTC, herbal products; medical care; psychologic support

11. variable: risk for infection; knowledge deficit; disturbed body image; fear; imbalanced nutrition, less than body requirements; social isolation; ineffective coping

12. variable: apply standard precautions; promote adherence; monitor laboratory results; refer for preventive services, nutrition, and spiritual support

13. variable: health teaching how virus damages immune system; need for monitoring health practices; protective precautions (avoid people with URIs); drug therapy plan in writing, establish client/family partnership in plan; how to minimize and manage side effects of drugs; BRAT diet

14. b

15. c

16. d

17. a

18. d

19. a

20. a

21. b

22. a

23. d

24. c

25. b

26. d

27. d

28. c

29. c

30. c

31. b

32. b

33. d

34. a

35. a

36. c

37. a

38. d

39. a

40. a, c, d

41. a, b, c

CHAPTER 35—
Vaccines

Questions 1-5: refer to text.

6. a

7. c

8. d

9. d

10. a

11. c

12. c

13. d

14. b

15. a

16. b

17. d

18. a

19. a

20. c

21. d

22. c

23. d

24. a

25. d

26. a

27. c

28. d

29. b

30. c

31. c

32. a, c, d

Critical Thinking Exercises

1. tetanus

2. headache, irritability, muscle spasms (jaw, neck, arms, legs, back, and abdomen)

3. Td (TDaP is only approved for persons < 64 years old)

4. IM

5. influenza, pneumococcal (PPV), and zoster

6. previous anaphylactic reaction to any of its components, or to eggs; moderate to severe acute illness

CHAPTER 36—
Anticancer Drugs

Questions 1-10: refer to text.

11. h

12. j

13. a

14. d

15. i

16. c

17. g

18. b

19. f

20. e

21. a

22. d

23. b

24. c

25. c

26. a

27. d

28. d

29. a

30. d

31. a

32. a

33. c

34. c

35. d

36. a

37. d

38. c

39. c

40. d

41. c

42. a

43. b

44. d

45. b

46. a

47. c

48. a

49. d

50. c

51. a

52. c

53. c

54. b

55. a, b, d, e, f

56. a, c, e, f, g, i

CHAPTER 37—
Targeted Therapies to Treat Cancer

Questions 1-8: refer to text.

9. d

10. b

11. d

12. d

13. a

14. d

15. d

16. c

17. c

18. a, b, c, d

19. a, b, d

CHAPTER 38—
Biologic Response Modifiers

Questions 1-20: refer to text.

21. b

22. c

23. a

24. d

25. b

26. no; G-CSF does not affect megakaryocyte line

27. report to health care provider; discontinue EPO; assess for signs and symptoms of clotting—prepare client for therapeutic phlebotomy

28. GM-CSF stimulates macrophage production; G-CSF does not.
    GM-CSF can cause more bone pain.
    G-CSF indicated for postchemotherapy administration neutropenia.

29. c

30. a

31. b

32. d

33. d

34. b

35. b

36. a

37. a, b, c

38. b, c, d

39. a, b, d

40. a, b, d

Critical Thinking Exercises

1. Convert 150 pounds to kilograms and multiply these values by 0.037.

2. Accurate fluid balance status will need to be monitored, and pulmonary, renal, and cardiac status assessed. Health care provider may opt not to use IL-2 because of potential side effects.

3. These are side effects of IL-2, but they do need to be assessed by a health care provider and treated with sterroids, antihistamines, and possibly urinary catheterization.

4. Symptoms are related to IL-2. The client should be hospitalized for IV fluids and further evaluation.

CHAPTER 39—
Drugs for Upper Respiratory Disorders

Questions 1-5: refer to text.

```
L Q A D P R U O F O T O W T A
A N Q C L Z I Z D B O P P R S
R Q K S U X Z N O S L Z E T E
Y S R G K T H A P P D N A M D
N I R A L S E P H E O W O G A
G T H Y D T A R T T F N D J T
I I A I P T B C H Q O C P G I
T S U P E W I F Y I J E P A O
I U P K F R V S C R N E J K N
S N I K T L U B B J A I Z H
R I U S D M G W P B U N T Q L
I S N P K V G N U G H G I I N
L O E L F L E F M R U X V R S
C C O M M O N C O L D G B K U
N C E Q S I T I L L I S N O T
```

6. common cold, acute rhinitis, sinusitis, (acute) tonsillitis, (acute) laryngitis

7. common cold

8. two to four

9. constricted

10. sedation

11. urinary

12. rebound

13. six

14. antitussives

15. water or fluids

16. are not

17. minimal

18. variable: observe color of secretions—yellow or green indicates infection; adequate fluid intake; rest; avoid cold remedies at bedtime; read OTC label carefully, especially if you have health problems; etc.

19. b

20. c

21. d

22. a

23. c

24. a

25. c

26. d

27. b

28. a

29. d

30. a, b, c, e

31. a, b, d, e

32. b, d

Critical Thinking Exercises

1. 2-3 gtt in each nostril b.i.d.

2. 3-5 days only

3. rebound congestion; decrease

4. short-term use because frequent use can result in tolerance that results in vasodilation rather than vasoconstriction; take only as prescribed, limit use

5. caffeine, which can increase restlessness and palpitations

6. check with health care provider before using; read labels

CHAPTER 40—
Drugs for Lower Respiratory Disorders

Questions 1-4: refer to text.

5. cyclic adenosine monophosphate (cAMP)

6. epinephrine

7. beta$_2$-adrenergic agonists

8. nonselective

9. cAMP

10. increases

11. synergistic

12. shorter

13. methylxanthine/xanthine; asthma

14. glucocorticoids

15. prophylactic; histamine

16. rebound bronchospasm

17. beta$_2$

18. montelukast (Singulair)
19. evening
20. 10 mg adult; 5 mg child without food
21. mucolytic
22. antibiotic
23. b
24. b
25. c
26. c
27. b
28. a
29. d
30. c
31. a
32. d

33. b
34. a
35. c
36. d
37. b
38. a, b, d, e
39. b, c, d, e
40. a, b, d, e

Critical Thinking Exercises

1. No; it takes 1-4 hours for full effect.
2. Take with food to avoid ulceration.
3. hoarseness, dry mouth, coughing, throat irritation; use of spacer

4. fluid retention, thinning of the skin, purpura, increased blood sugar, impaired immune response
5. variable: obtain medical and drug history, assess breath sounds, theophylline levels, hydration
6. variable: discuss ways to reduce anxiety, report allergic reaction (rash, urticaria) to health care provider, wear ID tag, correct use of inhaler; advise that high-protein, low-carbohydrate diet increases theophylline elimination; low-protein, high-carbohydrate diet prolongs the half-life

CHAPTER 41—
Cardiac Glycosides, Antianginals, and Antidysrhythmics

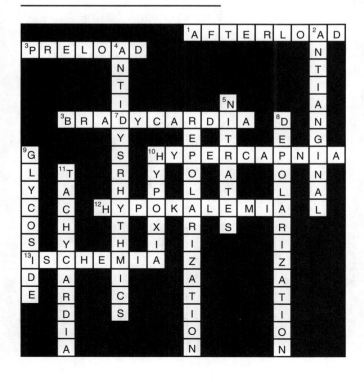

14. weakens; enlarges
15. increase
16. pump
17. digitalis glycosides
18. increase; decrease
19. positive inotropic action (increases heart contraction); negative chronotropic action (decreases heart rate); negative dromotropic action (decreases conduction of the heart cells); and increased stroke volume
20. decrease
21. It undergoes first-pass metabolism by the liver.
22. 2-5 minutes; repeated every 5 minutes three times
23. headache

24. beta blockers
25. verapamil (Calan)
26. reflex tachycardia and pain
27. stressed or exerted
28. at frequent times daily with increasing severity
29. is at rest
30. spasm
31. reduction of venous tone or coronary vasodilator
32. variable: avoid heavy meals, smoking, extremes in weather changes, strenuous exercise, and emotional upset
33. hypoxia; hypercapnia
34. fast sodium channel blockers; beta blockers; calcium channel blockers; also drugs that prolong repolarization
35. alcohol, caffeine-containing fluids, and cigarettes
36. b
37. a
38. b
39. a
40. c
41. d
42. b
43. a
44. d
45. b
46. d
47. b

48. a
49. d
50. b
51. b
52. b
53. d
54. c
55. d
56. c
57. d
58. a
59. b
60. b
61. c
62. c
63. d
64. d
65. a
66. c
67. a
68. c
69. d
70. c
71. b
72. a
73. b
74. b
75. c
76. d
77. d
78. a, d, e
79. b, c, e
80. a, c, d
81. 2 capsules, 0.4 g = 400 mg (move the decimal point 3 spaces to the right)

Critical Thinking Exercises

1. nitroglycerin 0.4 mg, sublingual tablets
2. Take at the onset of angina pain. If pain is not relieved in 5 minutes, repeat dose every 5 minutes for a total of 3 doses. If pain is still present after 15 minutes, notify the health care provider immediately. Do not swallow the SL tablet. Place tablet under the tongue.
3. Beta blockers decrease pulse (heart) rate and blood pressure. At present, J.B. does not have low pulse rate and blood pressure; however, vital signs should be monitored.
4. Both drugs are beta blockers. Propranolol is a nonselective cardiac drug affecting beta$_1$ and beta$_2$, while metoprolol is a cardioselective drug, blocking only beta$_1$. A client with asthma should take metoprolol because it does not block beta$_2$, respiratory.
5. for blood pressure (antihypertensive effect) and for cardiac dysrhythmias
6. relaxation techniques, adequate rest, no smoking, proper nutrition, decrease use of salt, exercise as prescribed
7. Causes similar pharmacologic effects but

is not as potent as nifedipine and verapamil. Blood pressure does not decrease as markedly as with other calcium blockers.

8.   is within normal range; maximum dose 360 mg per day

CHAPTER 42— *Diuretics*

a.   distal tubule: thiazides

b.   proximal tubule: osmotics and carbonic anhydrase inhibitors

c.   descending (loop)

d.   loop of Henle: high-ceiling or loop diuretics

e.   collecting tubule: potassium-sparing

1.   increase in urine output

2.   high blood sugar (glucose) level

3.   serum potassium excess

4.   sodium loss in the urine

5.   decreased urine output

6.   concentration of body fluids

7.   diuretics that promote potassium excretion

8.   to decrease blood pressure in those with hypertension; to decrease edema in those with congestive heart failure

9.   reabsorption; tubules

10. thiazide and thiazide-like, loop or high-ceiling, carbonic anhydrase inhibitors, osmotic, and potassium-sparing

11. potassium

12. digoxin; digitalis toxicity

13. little

14. sparing

15. weaker

16. aldosterone

17. hyperkalemia

18. Dyazide, Moduretic, Aldactazide, and Maxzide

19. less

20. osmotic

21. decrease

22. hypokalemia

23. hypomagnesemia

24. hypercalcemia

25. hypochloremia

26. minimal loss

27. hyperuricemia

28. hyperglycemia

29. cholesterol, LDL, and triglycerides are elevated

30. b

31. b

32. b

33. c

34. b

35. b

36. c

37. b

38. a

39. a

40. a

41. d

42. b

43. d

44. a

45. d

46. d

47. b

48. d

49. b

50. c

51. c

52. c

53. a, c, d

54. a, b, c, e

55. 3 tablets

Critical Thinking Exercises

1.   Hydrochlorothiazide can elevate the blood glucose level. A.D.'s oral antidiabetic drug dose may need to be adjusted.

2.   thiazide

3.   Both act on the kidney by increasing fluid and sodium loss. Thiazides act on the distal tubules of the kidney, while loop diuretics act on the loop of Henle.

4.   Both drugs have similar effects on blood chemistry; however, loop diuretics lower serum calcium level, while thiazides increase the serum calcium level.

5. A.D. should not take hydrochlorothiazide, because it increases serum calcium level.

6. a. Check blood sugar levels frequently.

    b. Eat foods rich in potassium because diuretics cause excretion of potassium.

    c. Emphasize the importance of compliance.

    d. Keep medical appointments; others: rise slowly because of possible blood pressure drop, use sunscreen.

7. A.D.'s serum potassium level is low-average. Diuretics could decrease the level further. A.D. is taking digoxin, and a decrease in serum potassium level (hypokalemia) can cause digitalis toxicity.

8. bradycardia (pulse rate less than 60 beats/min) or a marked decrease in pulse rate; anorexia, nausea, vomiting, blurred vision

9. All potassium-wasting diuretics, such as thiazides, loop diuretics, and osmotic diuretics, decrease serum potassium level; potassium-sparing diuretics can increase serum potassium level.

10. When a client has a low-average serum potassium level, such as with A.D., a combination of drugs prevents excess loss of potassium. If the client's fluid retention is severe, a potassium-wasting diuretic is usually more effective than a potassium-sparing diuretic.

CHAPTER 43— *Antihypertensives*

1. block the alpha-adrenergic receptors, thus causing vasodilation and decrease in blood pressure

2. block $beta_1$ receptors, causing a decrease in heart rate and blood pressure

3. decrease calcium level and promote vasodilation

4. inhibit angiotensin-converting enzyme, which blocks the release of aldosterone

5. block the angiotensin II receptor, causing a decrease in peripheral resistance and vasodilation

6. atrium; overload

7. obesity, aging, family history, hyperlipidemia, and others

8. relaxation techniques, salt restriction, weight reduction, exercise, decrease alcohol use

9. sympatholytics: centrally-acting, peripherally-acting, $alpha_1$ blocker, alpha-beta blocker

10. beta blocker, calcium blocker, angiotensin antagonist (ACE inhibitors), diuretics

11. prehypertension, stage I and stage II

12. diuretic

13. beta blockers and ACE inhibitors, also A-II inhibitors

14. diuretics

15. calcium blockers

16. stage II

17. diminished; lowered

18. African-American

19. cardioselective

20. -olol

21. decreases very-low-density lipoprotein (VLDL) and LDL; increases high-density lipoprotein (HDL)

22. prazosin, doxazosin, terazosin

23. diazoxide and nitroprusside

24. angiotensin II receptor antagonists (A-II blockers)

25. coughing

26. c

27. d

28. b

29. e

30. f

31. g

32. Baseline vital signs for future comparison should first be taken. Blood pressure should

be closely monitored to determine the effectiveness of the drug.

33. BUN, serum creatinine, protein, and potassium levels may be increased when taking an ACE inhibitor. If a client with diabetes mellitus is taking an oral antidiabetic agent, hypoglycemia might result. WBC count should be monitored because neutropenia might occur.

34. ACE inhibitors are usually potent antihypertensive agents and may cause hypotension when the drug is first started. If dizziness persists, health care provider should be notified.

35. Rebound hypertension could result.

36. Severe adverse reaction of ACE inhibitors is petechiae or bleeding.

37. Food could decrease one third of the drug absorption.

38. b

39. b

40. b

41. a

42. d

43. b

44. c

45. a

46. a

47. d

48. b

49. d

50. b

51. d

52. a

53. b

54. c

55. b

56. c

57. b

58. a

59. d

60. d

61. b

62. a

63. c

64. b

65. c

66. b

67. b, c, d

68. a, b, c

69. b, d

Critical Thinking Exercises

1. beta blocker. It is within normal-low range.

2. Atenolol blocks the $beta_1$-adrenergic receptors in the cardiac tissue.

3. It is a diuretic. It complements the atenolol and helps lower S.H.'s blood pressure by decreasing fluid volume.

4. Potassium, sodium, and magnesium imbalance can result. Hydrochlorothiazide is a potassium-wasting diuretic.

5. S.H.'s blood pressure should be closely monitored. His medications should not be discontinued because his blood pressure is not extremely low, nor was there a large blood pressure drop. The health care provider will adjust drug dose as needed.

6. client teaching: the importance of drug compliance and taking drugs at specified times; eating foods rich in potassium and proper nutrition; checking S.H.'s blood pressure; proper rest; exercise if appropriate

7. Atenolol is a beta blocker and amlodipine is a calcium channel blocker. Both drugs lower blood pressure. Amlodipine can also cause sodium and fluid retention.

8. side effects: dizziness, headache, slow heart rate, diaphoresis, cold extremities, fatigue, constipation/diarrhea

9. Serum electrolytes should be checked periodically, and also the liver enzymes.

CHAPTER 44—
Anticoagulants, Antiplatelets, and Thrombolytics

```
P O Q W U D J R S A A B C P S
F A J V I E D R H B E P N M O
I G N S D T Q P T W J K P R V
B G C T H R O M B O L Y T I C
R R J W I S C H E M I A Y Z E
I E A T M C E G E U T F L V A
N G O A W C O P Q C B N J I R
O A J S K A R A W U Z Y A B C
L T W T M N G P G J C D Q I M
Y I K R L H N Y V U E O T U Z
S O Y O J A D H M N L M W H J
I N R K Y B M R T Q W A Z D P
S K N E J Q R T S W Z I N V N
J A C D E P Q R S V C E K T M
```

a. aggregation
b. anticoagulant
c. fibrinolysis
d. ischemia
e. thrombolytic
f. stroke
g. INR
h. LMWH
i. DVT
j. PT
1. artery and vein
2. clot formation
3. do not have
4. venous thrombus that may lead to pulmonary embolism
5. subcutaneously, intravenously
6. standard heparin; lower the risk of bleeding
7. warfarin
8. decrease
9. 4 to 6
10. plasminogen to plasmin
11. hemorrhage
12. fondaparinux (Arixtra)
13. c
14. d
15. a
16. a
17. e
18. d
19. f
20. b
21. f
22. variable: monitor vital signs; check lab test results; check for bleeding gums, injection sites, etc.; keep antagonist vitamin K or protamine available

23. c
24. b
25. c
26. d
27. a
28. d
29. b
30. b
31. d
32. a
33. c
34. b
35. d
36. c
37. a
38. a
39. c
40. a, c, d
41. b, c, e
42. b, d, e, f
43. 0.4 ml

Critical Thinking Exercises

1.   a. either vial

   b. 1 ml of 5000 units/ml or 0.5 ml of 10,000 units/ml

2.   Heparin cannot be given orally because it is poorly absorbed through the gastrointestinal mucosa.

3.   For heparin, the PTT (partial thromboplastin time) and the aPTT (activated partial thromboplastin time) monitor heparin dosage and effect. PTT: 60-70 seconds with 1.5-2 × control in seconds;

aPTT: 40 seconds, with anticoagulant effect in 60-80 seconds.

4. two tablets

5. INR—international normalized ratio, used to monitor the oral anticoagulant warfarin. PT (prothrombin time) values can differ from laboratory to laboratory. INR is the result of reagents used in the PT test and compared to international standard reference.

6. Side effects of warfarin (Coumadin) include bleeding (skin, gums, nose, gastric, rectal), anorexia, nausea, vomiting, diarrhea, abdominal cramps, and fever.

7. warfarin: protein-binding, 99%; half-life, 0.5-3 days; highly protein-bound and long half-life

8. variable: use a soft toothbrush; report adverse effects, such as bruising, marks (ecchymosis); have INR checked; keep medical appointments; etc.

CHAPTER 45—
Antilipidemics and Peripheral Vasodilators

1. HDL

2. chylomicrons, LDL, and VLDL

3. 12-14 hours

4. 30%; 300 mg

5. gastrointestinal discomfort

6. weeks

7. less than 200 mg/dl

8. clofibrate

9. vessel occlusion

10. microcirculation

11. c

12. c

13. a

14. a

15. b

16. d

17. Serum lipid levels (cholesterol, LDL, HDL, and triglycerides) need to be closely monitored, every 3 to 6 months, to determine if drug dose is adequate or needs to be increased or decreased.

18. The ALT, ALP, and GGT values should be checked every 6 months. If liver disorder is present, drug dose should be decreased.
    Antilipidemics are metabolized by the liver.

19. Antilipidemics can cause GI discomfort. Taking antilipidemics with sufficient water and at mealtime decreases the possibility of GI distress.

20. Cataracts have been reported when taking some of the antilipidemics. Annual eye test is advised.

21. Antilipidemics are not a substitute for diet and decreasing the blood lipid levels. Low-fat diet is suggested.

22. When first taking antilipidemics, it takes several weeks before the blood lipid levels decline.

23. c

24. a

25. a

26. b

27. less than 200 mg/dl

28. less than 130 mg/dl (prefer: less than 100 mg/dl)

29. greater than 45 mg/dl (prefer: greater than 60 mg/dl)

30. b

31. c

32. d

33. a

34. variable: take medications with meals; avoid alcohol, smoking, and aspirin; explain possible side effects of drug, such as flushing, headache, and dizziness

35. a, c, d

36. a, c, f

37. a, c

38. a. 10 mg bottle
    b. ½ tablet

Critical Thinking Exercises

1. Desired cholesterol level is less than 200 mg/dl.

Because R.T.'s level is greater than 200 mg/dl, she has been prescribed atorvastatin (Lipitor).

2. Atorvastatin is an antilipidemic drug that inhibits the synthesis of cholesterol. This drug will lower R.T.'s LDL and increase her HDL. R.T.'s drug dose is within therapeutic range.

3. R.T. should know that the pregnancy category for atorvastatin is "X." Therefore she should not take the drug if she is contemplating pregnancy or is already pregnant.

4. Atorvastatin is a highly protein-bound drug at 98%. Two highly protein-bound drugs, such as warfarin and atorvastatin, will compete for protein-binding sites. With insufficient protein sites, one of the highly protein-bound drugs will be a free circulating drug and could cause side effects.

5. Atorvastatin is taken once per day. Many individuals take it in the evening.

6. The serum liver enzymes should be checked periodically. If liver impairment is present, it can cause an increase in liver enzymes and could cause an increase in liver dysfunction.

7. Client teaching for R.T.: lose weight; eat foods low in cholesterol and fat (check food labels); have liver enzymes checked periodically; keep medical appointments; etc.

CHAPTER 46—
Drugs for Gastrointestinal Tract Disorders

Questions 1-7: refer to text.

8. a. oral cavity; b. trachea; c. diaphragm; d. liver; e. gallbladder; f. duodenum; g. ileocecal valve; h. salivary glands; i. superior esophageal sphincter; j. esophagus; k. esophagus; l. stomach; m. pancreas; n. large intestine (colon); o. small intestine; p. rectum; q. anus

9. chemoreceptor trigger zone (CTZ) and vomiting center

10. antihistamines, anticholinergics, phenothiazines, cannabinoids, and miscellaneous

11. antagonists

12. antiemetics

13. gelatin, Gatorade, weak tea, carbonated beverages (flattened), and Pedialyte for children

14. 30

15. are not

16. antihistamines

17. marijuana

18. Ménière's

19. increases

20. to promote adsorption of poison/toxic substance(s)

21. opiates, opiate-related, adsorbents, and combination

22. constipation

23. abuse and misuse

24. soft; soft watery

25. osmotics, contact, bulk-forming, and emollients

26. irritation; diagnostic tests and surgery

27. water accumulation

28. heart failure

29. do not

30. fat soluble; A, D, E, K

31. variable: increase water intake and foods rich in fiber; avoid cathartic-type drugs that may cause electrolyte imbalances and laxative dependence; suggest exercise to increase peristalsis; inform clients that laxatives may cause urine discoloration; and so on

32. b

33. c

34. d

35. b

36. c

37. b

38. c

39. c

40. a

41. d

42. b

43. b

44. a, b, c

45. a, d, e

46. b, c, d, e

Critical Thinking Exercises

1. insufficient water, poor dietary habits, fecal impaction, bowel obstruction, chronic laxative use, neurologic disorders, ignoring urge for defecation, lack of exercise, and certain drugs

2. yes; 10-15 mg PO; max = 30 mg; probably morning to decrease sleep interruption

3. increase peristalsis by direct effect on smooth muscle of intestine

4. draws water into the intestine

5. hypersensitivity, intestinal/biliary obstruction, appendicitis, abdominal pain, nausea, vomiting, rectal fissure

6. decreased effect with antacids, histamine$_2$ blockers, and milk

7. swallow tablets whole; take only with water to promote absorption; not to take within 1 hour of any other drug; take to avoid interfering with sleep or other activities

8. increase fluid intake (if not contraindicated); not for long-term use; increase fiber-rich foods; exercise; keep records of intake; report rectal bleeding, nausea, vomiting, or cramping to health care provider immediately

CHAPTER 47—
Antiulcer Drugs

Questions 1-3: refer to text.

4. 2-5

5. corrosive

6. mechanical disturbances, genetic influence, environmental influence, and drugs

7. gnawing, aching

8. antacids, tranquilizers, anticholinergic, histamine$_2$ blocker, pepsin inhibitor, proton pump inhibitors, and gastric acid secretion suppressants

9. do not

10. are not

11. constipation, diarrhea

12. protective

13. can

14. h

15. i

16. f

17. c

18. g

19. d

20. j

21. b

22. a

23. e

24-32. Refer to nursing process in text.

33. c

34. a

35. a

36. d

37. b

38. b

39. c

40. b

41. a

42. d

43. a

44. d

45. a, b, c, d

46. a, d, e

47. b, c, d

Critical Thinking Exercises

1. no; 600 mg 1 hr p.c. and at bedtime; chewed with water or milk

2. neutralization of gastric acidity; ranitidine: inhibiting histamine at histamine receptors in parietal cells; sucralfate: with gastric acid, forms a protective covering on the ulcer surface

3. increase effect of benzodiazepines; decrease effects with

tetracycline, isoniazid, phenothiazine, phenytoin, digitalis, quinidine, and amphetamines. Lab: increase urine pH, calcium and phosphate levels, and electrolytes may be affected.

4. constipation

5. hypophosphatemia; caution in the elderly

6. variable: avoid foods and liquids that cause gastric irritation such as caffeine-containing beverages, alcohol, and spices

7. variable: encourage drinking 1 ounce of water after antacid to ensure that drug reaches the stomach; do not take antacids at mealtime because they slow the gastric emptying time; report pain, coughing, vomiting blood, diar- rhea, constipation to the health care provider; unlimited amount is contraindicated; read labels if on sodium-restricted diet; contact health care provider after taking self-prescribed antacids for more than 2 weeks; instruct on use of relaxation techniques; advise that stools may become white or speckled

---

CHAPTER 48—
Drugs Disorders of the Eye and Ear

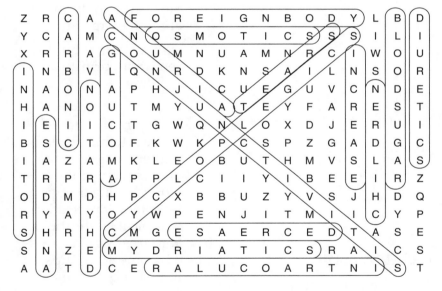

1. foreign body
2. tears
3. intraocular
4. diuretics; (open-angle) glaucoma
5. decrease
6. anuria, dehydration
7. blood sugar
8. cycloplegics
9. children
10. increase
11. conjunctivitis
12. carbonic anhydrase inhibitors
13. increase
14. carbonic anhydrase inhibitors
15. osmotics
16. a
17. c
18. c
19. b
20. b
21. d
22. b
23. c
24. c
25. a, b, d
26. a, b, d
27. a, c, d

Critical Thinking Exercises

1. stimulation of pupillary and ciliary sphincter muscles; to decrease intraocular pressure

2. no; therapeutic range is 1-2 gtt t.i.d./q.i.d.; report immediately to health

care provider; consider dosage adjustment

3. side effect of pilocarpine

4. coronary artery disease, obstruction of GI/GU tract, epilepsy, asthma

5. blurred vision, eye pain, headache, eye irritation, brow ache, stinging and burning, nausea, vomiting, diarrhea, increased salivation and sweating, muscle tremors, contact allergy

6. avoid driving or operating machinery while vision is impaired; check all labels on OTC preparations; need for regular medical follow-up; not to suddenly stop the medication; use of relaxation techniques

7. Ocusert system is an important consideration for D.Z. Advantages: accurate dose, sustained over time, disk changed every week; disadvantages: potential for corneal abrasion

CHAPTER 49—
Drugs for Dermatologic Disorders

1. c
2. d
3. b
4. a
5. epidermis
6. dermis
7. subcutaneous tissue
8. sebaceous gland
9. blood vessel
10. hair shaft
11. sweat gland
12. fatty tissue
13. a
14. a
15. c
16. b
17. c
18. a
19. a
20. a
21. b
22. c
23. c
24. d
25. d
26. a, b, d
27. c, d
28. a, b, c

Critical Thinking Exercises

1. second degree: epidermis, lower dermis; mottled, blistering, intense pain. Third degree: epidermis, dermis, nerve ending involvement, subcutaneous tissue; pearly white, charred, no pain

2. yes

3. inhibits bacterial cell wall synthesis; silver sulfadiazine

4. assess for infection; culture wounds; assess vital signs, fluid status, and pain status

5. administer prescribed analgesia before applying medication as needed; use aseptic technique; monitor fluid and renal function; assess for side effects, vital signs, and acid-base balance. Store drug in dry place at room temperature.

6. rash, urticaria, burning sensation, pruritus, swelling

7. be alert to changes in respiratory status; instruct family, including return demonstration, on care of the wound using aseptic technique; application of topical medications and dressings, as needed; home safety tips; importance of hand exercises

CHAPTER 50—
Endocrine Drugs: Pituitary, Thyroid, Parathyroid, and Adrenal Disorders

a.   acromegaly

b.   adenohypophysis

c.   ACTH

d.   ADH

e.   cretinism

f.   endocrine

g.   gigantism

h.   glucocorticoid

i.   hypophysis

j.   mineralocorticoid

k.   myxedema

l.   neurohypophysis

m.   thyrotoxicosis

n.   thyroxine

o.   triiodothyronine

1.   anterior and posterior

2.   bones and skeletal muscles

3.   dwarfism; gigantism

4.   diabetes mellitus

5.   adrenocorticotropic hormone (ACTH)

6.   primary and secondary

7.   vasopressin

8.   variable: check for edema; monitor weight; monitor vital signs, urine output; adhere to medical regimen; check laboratory results, especially electrolytes and glucose

9.   thyroxine (T_4) and triiodothyronine (T_3)

10.   hypotension and vascular collapse

11.   agranulocytosis

12.   calcium

13.   hypoparathyroidism; hyperparathyroidism

14.   twitching of the mouth, tingling and numbness of fingers, carpopedal spasm, spasmodic contractions, and laryngeal spasm

15.   subcutaneous

16.   glucocorticoids

17.   dexamethasone (Decadron)

18.   tapered over several days. Rationale: to

allow adrenal cortex to produce steroids (cortisol and others)

19. sodium and water retention

20. protein

21. b

22. b

23. a

24. b

25. a

26. b

27. b

28. a

29. b

30. b

31. Cortisone drugs cause increase in sodium and water, and thus an increase in blood pressure.

32. Weight increase can occur as a result of water retention. A weight increase of 2½ to 5 pounds may occur in several days.

33. Glucocorticoid drugs promote sodium retention and potassium loss. These agents also increase blood sugar level.

34. Glucocorticoid drugs can irritate the gastric mucosa and may cause a peptic ulcer.

35. This group of drugs promotes potassium loss. Foods rich in potassium (i.e., fruits, fruit juices, vegetables, meats, nuts) should be eaten.

36. An adrenal crisis could result if the cortisone drug is abruptly stopped. Tapering drug dose permits the adrenal glands to adjust their function of secreting adrenal cortex hormones.

37. High doses of glucocorticoids promote loss of muscle tone and loss of calcium from the bone.

38. High doses of glucocorticoids may cause moon face, puffy eyelids, edema in the feet, increased bruising, dizziness, and menstrual irregularity. Any of these symptoms should be reported.

39. b

40. c

41. b

42. d

43. a

44. c

45. b

46. b

47. b

48. c

49. d

50. c

51. c

52. b

53. a

54. a, b, c, d

55. a, c, e

56. a, c, d, e

Critical Thinking Exercises

1. Yes, safe dosing is between 5 and 60 mg daily in divided doses.

2. Digoxin is a cardiac glycoside, and hydrochlorothiazide is a potassium-wasting diuretic.

3. Prednisone, a glucocorticoid, and hydrochlorothiazide, a potassium-wasting diuretic, promote the loss of potassium via urine excretion.

4. M.N. is taking two drugs that promote potassium loss; therefore, she should be eating foods rich in potassium, such as fruits and vegetables, and should be taking potassium supplements.

5. M.N.'s serum potassium level is low, most likely caused by taking prednisone and hydrochlorothiazide. Hypokalemia enhances the action of digoxin and can cause digitalis toxicity. Potassium replacement is necessary to correct deficit and to prevent recurrence of hypokalemia.

6. Muscle weakness and wasting; thinning of the skin; fat accumulation in the face and trunk (moon face and buffalo hump); elevated cholesterol and glucose levels; hypokalemia

7. Prednisone, prednisolone, and dexa-

methasone are all glucocorticoids. Prednisone is the mildest of the three drugs. Prednisolone and dexamethasone are potent glucocorticoids. Prednisolone may be taken to alleviate severe asthma and may be injected into the joints to alleviate acute inflammation. Dexamethasone can be taken orally or given parenterally for severe allergy or to reduce edema from a head injury.

8. When discontinuing glucocorticoids, the drug dose should be tapered to allow for the adrenal cortex to resume function in secreting cortisol (adrenal cortical hormone). Glucocorticoids such as prednisone suppress adrenal gland function.

9. Teaching points for M.N.: take prednisone with food; eat foods rich in potassium; avoid persons with respiratory tract infections; report side effects such as edema, bleeding.

CHAPTER 51— *Antidiabetics*

1. chronic disease resulting from deficiency in glucose metabolism

2. a protein secreted by the beta cells in the pancreas that is needed for carbohydrate metabolism

3. insulin reaction because of excessive circulating insulin. Client becomes nervous, trembling, uncoordinated, cold and clammy skin, decreased blood pressure, increased pulse rate.

4. insulin-dependent diabetes mellitus, requires insulin

5. non–insulin-dependent diabetes mellitus, usually requires oral antidiabetic drug

6. presence of ketone bodies (fatty acids) in the body as a result of fat catabolism caused by inadequate amount of insulin

7. tissue atrophy or hypertrophy

8. increased thirst

9. increased hunger

10. increased urine output

11. polyuria, polydipsia, and polyphagia

12. a, b, d

13. 0.2 to 0.5 unit/kg/day; clients with type 1 need 0.2 to 1 unit/kg/day to prevent recurrence of hypokalemia

14. insulin and oral hypoglycemic or oral antidiabetic drugs

15. lipodystrophy

16. regular

17. less; more

18. would

19. pork insulin

20. headache, nervousness, tremor, excessive perspiration, tachycardia, slurred speech, memory lapse, and blood sugar <60 mg/dl

21. thirst, polyuria, fruity breath odor, Kussmaul's sign, tachycardia, dry mucous membranes, and blood sugar >250 mg/dl

22. sulfonylureas; are not

23. variable: recognize signs of hypoglycemic reaction; maintain prescribed diet; take insulin at prescribed dose and time; monitor blood sugar level; keep appointments with health care provider; be aware of effect of exercise, infection, and fever

24. variable: monitor blood sugar level; take oral hypoglycemic drug(s) at prescribed dose and time; maintain prescribed diet; monitor weight; participate in regular exercise

25. c

26. e

27. a

28. b

29. f

30. The reference values for blood glucose level are 60-100 mg/dl; for serum glucose level, 70-110 mg/dl. With a blood sugar level <60 mg/dl, hypoglycemia results, and at >110 mg/dl, hyperglycemia is present. It should be monitored periodically.

31. Signs and symptoms of a hypoglycemic reaction include nervousness, tremors, cold and clammy skin, excessive perspiration, slurred speech, tachycardia, and others.

32. Orange juice or a sweetened beverage adds sugar to the body for insulin utilization. Both are a quick source of sugar.

33. Blood sugar test should be checked daily to determine if the blood sugar is within normal range. More or less insulin may be needed.

34. Prescribed diet is calculated according to the amount of insulin given per day. Exchange list of foods should be available to the client.

35. During a severe hypoglycemic reaction, the client may be unable to swallow orange juice. Glucagon would be needed to reverse the hypoglycemic state.

36. Client should have either a medical alert card or tag in case of a severe hypoglycemic reaction in which the client is semiconscious or unconscious.

37. b

38. a

39. b

40. c

41. b

42. d

43. c

44. b

45. c

46. a

47. c

48. a

49. c

50. b

51. a

52. d

53. b

54. d

55. a

56. d

57. a. diminishes serum glucose level following a meal

  b. decreases absorption of glucose from the small intestine

  c. does not produce hypoglycemic or hyperglycemic reactions

  d. answer is correct

58. b

59. c

60. b

61. d

62. b

63. b, c, d

64. a, c, d, e

65. a, b, c, e

Critical Thinking Exercises

1. Humulin insulins have the same amino acids as the client. These insulins have a very low incidence of allergic effects and insulin resistance. Pork insulin has one different amino acid than human insulin, and beef insulin has four different amino acids.

2.

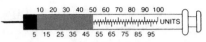

3. Clients taking sulfonylureas usually would need 40 units or less of insulin daily. N.V. has type 1 diabetes or insulin-dependent diabetes mellitus. He is taking a total of 50 units of insulin daily.

4. Instruct N.V. to follow insulin injection site rotation recommended by the American Diabetes Association. This group suggests that insulin should be injected daily at a chosen site for 1 week. The injections should be 1½ inches apart at a site area each day.

5. The average insulin dosage according to weight is: 0.2 unit × 72 kg = 14 units/day; 1.0 unit × 72 kg = 72 units/day. N.V.'s daily insulin is 50 units/day (average: 14-72 units/day).

6. Regular insulin peaks in 2-4 hr, whereas NPH insulin peaks in 6-12 hr. If N.V. receives insulin at 0700, hypoglycemic reaction might occur between 1300 and 1900 (1600 to 1700 is the likely time that hypoglycemia could occur).

7. Most common symptoms include nervousness, tremors, cold or clammy skin, slurred speech, confusion, and, later, seizures.

8. client teaching for N.V.: injection sites, rotation of injections, angle for injections, hypoglycemic reactions, not to withhold insulin during stress and infection, diet, use of a medical alert bracelet or tag, card stating that the client has diabetes

9. When mixing insulins, there may be a loss of regular insulin. NPH does not cause as great a loss of regular insulin as does Lente.

10. a. Client should recognize (if possible) the onset of a hypoglycemic reaction.

    b. Have available orange juice, soda with sugar, or candy.

    Take immediately at the onset of a hypoglycemic reaction. Have glucagon available in case N.V. cannot drink sugar-containing fluid.

CHAPTER 52—
Female Reproductive Cycle I: Pregnancy and Preterm Labor Drugs

1. new-onset grand mal seizure occurring in approximately 5% of women with preeclampsia

2. elevated blood pressure without proteinuria after 20 gestational weeks in clients normotensive before pregnancy

3. hemolysis, elevated liver enzymes, and low platelet count; occurs in about 2%-12% of clients with gestational hypertension

4. Surfactant is made of two major phospholipids: sphingomyelin and lecithin. L/S ratio of 2:1 is a predictor of fetal lung maturity and risk for neonatal RDS.

5. presence of hypertension (systolic blood pressure > 140 mm Hg or diastolic blood pressure > 90 mm Hg) and proteinuria (≥ 300 mg in 24-hour urine collection)

6. labor that occurs between 20 and 37 weeks of pregnancy involving a fetus with an estimated weight between 500 and 2499 g. Regular contractions occur at less than 10-minute intervals over 30 to 60 minutes and are strong enough to result in 2 cm cervical dilation and 80% effacement.

7. hormone of pregnancy, relaxes smooth muscles, resulting in heartburn, constipation during pregnancy.

8. lipoprotein in the alveoli that reduces surface tension of pulmonary fluids and keeps alveoli open during expiration

9. substances that cause developmental abnormalities

10. drug therapy to decrease uterine muscle contractions

11. are not

12. effect of circulating steroid hormones on the liver's metabolism of drugs, increased glomeular filtration rate and increased renal perfusion resulting in more rapid renal excretion of drugs, alteration in the clearance of drugs in later pregnancy resulting in a decrease in serum and tissue concentrations of drugs

13. do not

14. does

15. slower

16. breast

17. timing, dose, duration of exposure

18. sphingomyelin, lecithin

19. lung maturity, prevention of neonatal RDS

20. a. betamethasone (Celestone), 24, 7, 24-34

    b. to accelerate lung maturation with resultant surfactant development in the fetus, decreasing the incidence and severity of RDS with increased survival of preterm infants

21. seizures (eclampsia), HELLP syndrome

22. nutritional supplementation with iron, vitamins, and minerals; treatment of nausea and vomiting, gastric acidity, and mild discomforts

23. 18, 27, 120, 6, 1-3, reticulocytosis values

24. will not

25. Mexico

26. eating crackers, dry toast, bread, dry cereal, or other complex carbohydrates before rising; avoiding fatty or highly seasoned foods; eating small, frequent meals; eating a high-protein bedtime snack

27. limiting the size of meals; avoiding highly seasoned, fried, or greasy foods; avoiding gas-forming foods; drinking adequate fluids but during meals

28. instruct client to lie on left side; signs and symptoms of progressive preeclampsia and when to seek medical assistance; pharmacologic and nonpharmacologic treatment measures for preeclampsia; diet with additional protein (90 g), normal sodium diet and adequate fluid intake

29. a

30. d, e

31. c

32. c

33. g

34. b

35. d

36. h

37. f

38. d

39. d

40. a

41. b

42. b

43. d

44. d

45. c

46. a

47. d

48. b

49. a

50. c

51. a, c, d

52. c

53. a, c, d

Critical Thinking Exercises

1. PTL occurs between 20 and 37 weeks' gestation with regular contractions occurring at less than 10 minute intervals over 30-60 minutes; she is 28 weeks' gestation, having contractions every 8 minutes

2. vaginal exam—2 cm dilation and 80% effacement

3. low socioeconomic status and previous history of preterm delivery

4. (Note: Consider the biopsychosocial implications for the children and employer while constructing your plan of action.) Initially, suggest she drink water (1-2 glasses/hour), lie down on her left side, empty her bladder every 2 hours, and rest. In addition, does she have any vaginal bleeding, is the fetus moving, or is there a change in the fetal movement? Instruct her not to insert anything in her vagina. Does she have anyone (friend, neighbor, church) who can meet her children? Does she have transportation to the local hospital?

5. pregnancy of less than 20 weeks' gestation (confirmed by ultrasound), bulging or premature rupture membranes (PROM), confirmed fetal death or anomalies incompatible with life, maternal hemorrhage and evidence of severe fetal compromise, chorioamnionitis

6. decrease; uterine contractions, stop preterm labor, lung maturation, uterine

7. changes in heart rate >100 beats/min, ausculated cardiac dysrhythmias, respirations >30 breaths/min or change in quality (wheezes, rales, coughing), FHR >180 beats/min and significant increased in uterine contractions, leaking of amniotic fluid, any vaginal bleeding or discharge or complaints of rectal pressure

8. contractions decrease to 6 or fewer per hour. Cervical dilation and/or effacement or no further change in dilation and/or effacement

9. stop/prevent preterm labor

10. a. Because terbutaline is to be taken every 3-4 hours, she may take it with her meals.

  b. She may take the dose, because it has a peak plasma/serum concentration of 1-2 hours and a duration of action of 4-8 hours. In addition, we would discuss the importance of taking the medication as scheduled.

CHAPTER 53—
Female Reproductive Cycle II: Labor, Delivery, and Preterm Neonatal Drugs

1. Analgesics alter the client's perception and sensation of pain without producing unconsciousness/sedation—these drugs minimize maternal anxiety and fear and promote rest and relaxation, but they do not provide pain relief.

2. loss of painful sensations with or without the loss of consciousness

3. scoring system to assist in predicting whether labor induction may be successful

4. softening of the cervix

5. Additional drug doses do not increase the degree of respiratory depression, maternal or neonatal.

6. one of a large group of alkaloids derived from a fungus, act by direct smooth muscle cell receptor stimulation. These drugs are not used in labor but are used postpartally in the prevention or control of postpartum hemorrhage and the promotion of uterine involution.

7. analgesia, decreased GI motility, miosis, and sedation

8. stimulation of effective uterine contractions once labor has begun

9. stimulation of uterine contractions before the spontaneous onset of labor, with or without ruptured fetal membranes

10. result in analgesia, decreased GI motility, euphoria, respiratory depression, sedation, and physiologic dependence

11. drugs given to enhance uterine contractility; Pitocin, Syntocinon

12. synthetic form of the hormone Pitocin. Used in labor induction and labor augmentation.

13. chemical hormone, myriad of actions in the body. Prostaglandins E_2 and F_2 are primarily associated with the reproductive system.

14. caused by pressure of the presenting part and stretching of the perineum and vagina. Pain of the transition phase and the second stage of labor is transmitted to the S1, S3, and S4 areas by the pudendal nerve

15. breaking the membranes with an amniotic hook with subsequent release of prostaglandin F_2 from the decidua or prostaglandin E_2 from the cervix

16. lipoprotein in the alveoli that reduces surface tension of pulmonary fluids and keeps alveoli open during expiration

17. uterine inactivity or hypotonic contractions

18. Pain from the cervix and uterus is carried by sympathetic fibers and enters the neuraxis at T10, T11, T12, and L1 spinal levels. Early labor pain is transmitted to T11 to T12 with later progression to T10 and L1.

19. Survanta, Infasurf

20. endotracheal tube, intrathecally

21. 1-3; 3-4; to prevent fetal or neonatal depression

22. to minimize transfer to the fetus via the placenta

23. dose ceiling. This means additional doses do not increase the degree of respiratory depression, maternal or neonatal.

24. kappa, mu

25. hydroxyzine (Vistaril)

26. 25

27. local, episiotomy; regional blocks; epidural

28. spinal headaches

29. a. analgesics

    b. increased fluids

    c. bed rest
    Other treatment methods include 500 mg of caffeine in 500 ml of normal saline given over 2 hours and blood patching.

30. achieve pain relief

31. Bishop

    a. dilation

    b. effacement

    c. station

    d. cervical consistency

    e. cervical position

32. a. insertion of a Foley catheter through an undilated cervix and internal os with subsequent inflation of the bulb. The Foley catheter bulb provides a mechanical stimulation similar to "stripping of the membranes." When the Foley "falls out," the client is started on IV oxytocin.

    b. Extra-amniotic saline infusion with a balloon catheter may be used to induce labor.

    c. membrane stripping—with release of prostaglandin F_2

from the decidua or prostaglandin E_2 from the cervix

33. uterine hyperstimulation, uterine rupture

34. Can cause sustained uterine contractions (tetanic contractions), which would result in fetal hypoxia and possibly uterine rupture.

35. a

36. c

37. d

38. b

39. a

40. c

41. c

42. c

43. d

44. d

45. b

46. d

47. c

48. c

49. c

50. c

51. c

52. b

53. b

54. a

55. d

56. d

57. b, c, d

58. a, b, d, e

59. d, e

60. a, c, e

Critical Thinking Exercises

1. uterine contractions every 2-3 minutes with an intensity of 55-65 mm Hg

2. rating of pain as 8 on scale of 1-10, described as "intense cramping," in "my lower belly," or "Can't you do something?"

3. morbid obesity, severe preeclampsia, coagulation disorders, and/or generalized sepsis

4. "Yes, women do have a longer labor, approximately 15-30 minutes longer. They can feel movement and pressure but not pain."

5. Nubain will be given at the beginning of the uterine contraction to minimize the narcotic transfer to the fetus via the placenta.

6. It depends.

7. 500-1000; dextrose-free IV fluids; prevent hypotension

8. Turn her on her left side, and place a wedge under her left hip.

9. Administer ephedrine 5-15 mg IV. Monitor BP every 1-2 min for the first 10 min, then every 10-30 min until the block wears off.

10. 10-20 units of oxytocin added to 1000 ml of normal saline, lactated Ringer's, or dextrose (D_5) solution

CHAPTER 54—
Postpartum and Newborn Drugs

1. incision made to enlarge the vaginal opening to facilitate newborn delivery

2. ointment administered to prevent gonococcal conjunctivitis and chlamydial conjunctivitis (ophthalmia neonatorum), which can cause blindness

3. Estimated 30%-40% of chronic infections are believed to have resulted from perinatal or early childhood transmission; AAP recommends universal HBV immunization for all newborns.

4. Hepatitis B immunoglobulin (HBIG) should be given within 12 hours of birth, concurrently with hepatitis B vaccine at a different site; it provides temporary protection in postexposure situations.

5. breast-feeding or milk production

6. Parenteral injection is administered to the newborn in the vastus lateralis muscle; newborn is unable to synthesize vitamin K during the first 7-10 days of life because the gut is sterile at birth and requires bacteria to synthesize vitamin K.

7. released from anterior pituitary, responsible for increase in and maturation of ducts and alveoli in the breasts and for initiation of lactation after birth

8. the period from delivery until 6 weeks' postpartum

9. newborn vaccine recommended by AAP to be given within 12 hours of birth, provides long-term protection; to be given at birth, then 12 months later, and the third dose by 6-18 months

10. drug to prevent sensitization based upon the infant's direct Coombs' test

11. development of protective antibodies against Rh-positive blood.

12. congenital syndrome; cataracts, glaucoma, deafness, heart defects, and mental retardation

13. rubella titer during pregnancy, <1:8 or <1:10 (lab dependent) or susceptible or negative titer is an indication that the woman needs the rubella vaccine postpartum

14. benzocaine (Americaine Dermoplast), Tucks

15. witch hazel compresses, Nupercainal ointment, benzocaine spray

16. prolactin

17. to minimize perineal discomfort and facilitate stool passage secondary to decreased peristalsis following delivery

18. Question; milk or antacid should not be used with administration as enteric coating of Dulcolax may dissolve, resulting in abdominal cramping and vomiting.

19. No; the use of the heat lamp with benzocaine topical spray may cause tissue burns.

20. Apply ointment externally; apply small quantity of ointment onto 2 × 2 inch square, place inside peripad against swollen anorectal tissue 5 times/day; wear gloves to administer; may cause burning sensation if anal tissue not intact. It may be inserted in the rectum of nonobstetrical clients, as they do not have perianal wounds that extend into the anus.

21. mineral oil

22. conjunctivitis; ophthalmia neonatorum; blindness

23. redness, ecchymosis, edema, discharge, approximation

24. apply witch hazel pads with peripads and reapply witch hazel pads; change both frequently

25. tympany; bowel; over four quadrants of the abdomen; simethicone (Mylicon); chew thoroughly before swallowing; 6-8; laxative

26. b, c

27. a, b

28. c

29. b

30. a

31. d

32. b

33. a

34. a

35. c

36.

13. blood component and safety factors

14. With either documentation, this indicates the need for rubella vaccine administration.

15. Administration of both drugs may result in suppression of rubella antibodies with need to recheck rubella titer in approximately 3 months.

16. Discuss importance of using effective contraception for 4 weeks after vaccine injection as rubella vaccine is teratogenic. Identify contraceptive method of choice and document instruction. Rubella titer may be assessed approximately 3 months after administration.

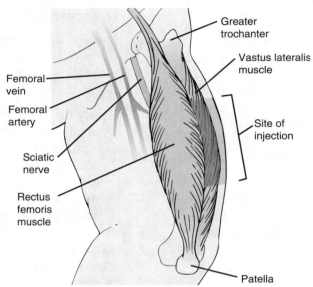

From Nichols F, Zwelling E: *Maternal-newborn nursing: theory and practice*, Philadelphia, 1997, Saunders.

CHAPTER 55—
Drugs for Women's Health and Reproductive Disorders

Questions 1-4: refer to text.

5. estrogen progestin; progestin-only

6. A = abdominal pain (severe)

   C = chest pain or shortness of breath

   H = headache, dizziness, weakness, numbness, speech difficulties

   E = eye disorders including blurring or loss of vision

Critical Thinking Exercises

1. obstetrical history—previous pregnancies and their outcome, father's Rh status, mother's Rh status, whether she has had RhoGAM in the past, religious beliefs

2. Rh incompatibility and sensitization; understanding of the relationship of Rh status to Rh disease, relationship of the Coombs tests (direct and indirect), understanding of the doses specific to pregnancy and postpartum

3. antibodies; antigen; antibody nonsensitized; prevent; sensitized; antibody; antigen

4. b

5. a

6. b

7. a

8. b

9. a

10. a

11. b

12. positive; antibodies; antigen; negative; negative; 72

S = severe leg pain or swelling of calf or thigh

7. triphasics

8. altering the cervical mucus

9. suppressing ovulation; changing pH of vaginal mucosa; sperm

10. Disagree; nurse did not calculate re-injection dates correctly because she did not use a wheel that takes variable numbers of days in month into account; thus client will progressively be late in getting re-injected and level of protection could be compromised; also, nurse did not document site of injection (important with re-injections that need rotation).

11. weight gain, increased appetite, migraine, breast soreness, sleep disorder, backache, joint pain, constipation, emotional lability, depression, difficulty concentrating on tasks

12. exercise—aerobic; increase water in diet—limit salty foods, alcohol, caffeine, chocolate; eat 4-6 small high-carbohydrate meals (low fat); pack portable snacks (rice cakes, vegetables, bagels, fresh fruit, pasta, soups, cereals); increase dietary magnesium; use of NSAIDs from symptoms to beginning of menses in conjunction with vitamins (Mg, Ca, pyridoxine, vitamin E, and zinc) acknowledge reality base of symptoms; convey research to client, family, community; start and keep a feeling log; discuss issues of drug dependency/withdrawal if alprazolam is used

13. irregular menses, vasodilation, vaginal alterations, decreased bone mass

14. hormone replacement therapy

15. advantages: decreased ovarian cysts, decreased menstrual migraine headache, easy to use, low failure rate, minimal risks, not linked to sex act, decreased dysmenorrhea, decreased chance of endometrial cancer

disadvantages: risky for fetus if pregnancy occurs; may perceive side effects as bothersome; if nonmonogamous, there is increased risk of STDs

16. variable: teach ACHES, moderate caffeine intake, advise use of barrier method for first month of use and for 3 months after discontinuing use, instruct about missed pills, take pill with food, report breakthrough bleeding, perform monthly breast self-exam

17. variable: monthly breast self-exam, notify health care provider immediately of headache, visual disturbances, chest pain, or signs of thrombophlebitis; take medication with meals to avoid nausea and vomiting

18. a

19. b, d, e

20. a, c

21. e

22. c

23. a

24. c

25. d

26. c

27. c

28. d

29. c

30. d

31. a

32. a

33. c

34. d

35. b

36. b

37. c

38. b

39. a

40. a

41. d

42. a

43. a, b, c

44. a, c, d

45. b, c, d

Critical Thinking Exercises

1. reduced estrogen support for the vaginal tissue; has estrogen therapy in the vagina, such as a cream or ring, may alleviate some of her vaginal symptoms without the systemic effects and risks of oral medications.

2. vascular changes she may be experiencing: hot flashes, tachycardia, sleep disturbances, changes in height, backache

3. fractures resulting from decreased bone mass associated with osteoporosis. C.W. has been menopausal for over a year and it is known that the most rapid decrease in bone mass occurs in the first 3-5 years postmenopause (thus time is of the essence).

4. fear of breast cancer and resumption of withdrawal bleeding; include decreased risk of osteoporosis and colorectal cancer as well as relief of menopausal vasomotor symptoms, may not be achieved if women opt not to use estrogen replacement therapy

5. reduction in incidence of coronary artery disease; retardation of osteoporosis; reduction in vasodilation symptoms; thicker vagina with increased moisture and lubrication with decreased discomfort; placed in this order because (A) coronary artery disease is the major health problem for older women, as it is for men, and research studies show significant decreases in heart attacks and possibly strokes; total cholesterol is lowered and HDL is increased; (B) acceleration in loss of bone density caused by estrogen loss results in pain, suffering, lost productivity, and diminished life quality for hundreds of thousands of women each year with high personal and health care costs for women ages 75-85, often with diminished resources. Therefore need to start early to have an impact on the problem. (C) sleep deprivation and somatic discomforts from vasodilation manageable and not life-threatening or as costly; same with vaginal discomforts.

6. added to minimize the risk of endometrial hyperplasia, endometrial cancer, and breast cancer from use of unopposed estrogen alone; goal is to use the lowest effective dose of the least metabolically active progestin to oppose the stimulation of the endometrium

7. plan for at least 10 years postmenopause and probably longer for cardiovascular benefits; explain that it is true that the goal for initiating HRT has a bearing on the dosage form. Explain that the best bone protection will be through prolonged systemic therapy, which will also aid vaginally; tell her that she could use just local estrogen cream for the vaginal problem but that this will not help with the other aspects; you could also use systemic HRT and a product such as K-Y jelly.

8. breast cancer (known or suspected), thrombophlebitis, liver disease (acute), undiagnosed genital bleeding; pregnancy

9. the progestin component; communicate with the health care provider regarding individualizing the dose; also may consider use of cyclic versus combined continuous approach with health care provider

10. normal finding to bleed days 25-30, last 2-3 days, be lighter and have less premenstrual symptoms; normal to have an occasional hot flash while going through withdrawal bleeding (she should report any headache, visual changes, thrombophlebitis signs, or chest pain)

CHAPTER 56—
Drugs for Men's Health and Reproductive Disorders

Questions 1-5: refer to text.

6. testosterone

7. plateau, orgasm, resolution

8. negative feedback loop

9. longer

10. one-third to one-fifth

11. monitoring of endocrine status

12. decreased muscle tone, polyuria, and increased urine and serum calcium

13. antiandrogens

14. menotropins, immediately

15. GnR, LH, FSH

16. adulthood; surgical excision, radiation therapy, and chemotherapy

17. L-dopa

18. b

19. d

20. b

21. b

22. a

23. d

24. b, c, d

25. a, b, d

26. a, b, c

Critical Thinking Exercises

1. The motivation for treatment and M.T.'s self-esteem should be assessed.

2. There is no evidence that treatment results in greater growth.

3. A drug is selected on the basis of the desired balance of growth and sexual maturation.

4. At minimum, endocrine, renal, and gastrointestinal effects should be monitored.

5. Treatment can be expected to last 3-6 months.

CHAPTER 57—
Drugs for Infertility and Sexually Transmitted Diseases

Questions 1-6: refer to text.

7. infertility, life-threatening illness, and neonatal illness and death

8. vertical

9. syphilis

10. predominantly sexual, sexual and nonsexual

11. gonococcal conjunctivitis neonatorum

12. hepatitis A and B, HIV

13. syphilis, penicillin

14. abstinence, one faithful partner

15. diabetes, HIV/AIDS

16. acyclovir, famciclovir, or valacyclovir

17. 1 year

18. hormone replacement therapy

19. 15

20. danazol, suppress gonadotropin output

21. progesterone

22. emotionally, financially

23. thins cervical mucus

24. c

25. a

26. b

27. b

28. a

29. a

30. a

31. a, b, d

32. a, b, c

33. a

34. c

35. a, b, d

Critical Thinking Exercises

1. Tess might have incurred fallopian tube scarring if the infection ascended her reproductive tract.

2. HIV more readily enters the body through lesions such as those associated with other STDs; the fact that a partner transferred gonorrhea indicates that he could have transferred another STD, including HIV.

3. Side effects include breast discomfort, fatigue, dizziness, depression, nausea, vomiting, increased appetite, weight gain, urticaria, dermatitis, anxiety, restlessness, weakness, heavier menses, vasomotor flushing, abdominal bloating, pain, and gas.

    Adverse effects that may require interruption of therapy include visual impairment, ovarian hyperstimulation resulting in ovarian enlargement, midcycle ovarian pain, and cysts.

4. Ovulation is predicted by a 0.5° F drop in basal body temperature, followed by a 1° F rise. The couple should engage in coitus every other day from 4 days before ovulation to 3 days after. Sex on schedule might become a chore and feel dehumanizing to one or both partners.

5. One or both partners may feel inadequate as a man or woman and self-esteem may be damaged; they and their families may engage in blaming of the other partner.

    Alternatives might include adoption, becoming a foster parent, becoming involved with family members' children, and volunteering in youth organizations or services.

CHAPTER 58—
Adult and Pediatric Emergency Drugs

Questions 1-6: refer to text.

7. PSVT (paroxysmal supraventricular tachycardia)

8. confusion, drowsiness, hearing impairment, muscle twitching, and/or seizures

9. opiate; morphine, meperidine, codeine, Darvon, heroin

10. milk or milk products

11. false

12. true

13. bronchodilator; asthma and anaphylaxis/allergic reactions

14. b

15. c

16. b

17. a

18. a

19. c

20. c

21. b

22. d

23. d

24. c

25. b

26. c

27. b

28. d

29. c

30. a

31. d

32. c

33. a

34. b

35. c

36. c

37. a

38. a, b, d

39. a, b, d

40. a, b, c

*Critical Thinking Exercises—
Case Study #1*

1. The initial CVP reading was low, indicating the client was "dry" or volume-depleted; a component of his shock state was hypovolemic in origin. The fluids corrected the hypovolemia as evidenced by the CVP increasing to 9 cm of H_2O. Administering dopamine when hypovolemia is present worsens the low perfusion state by causing further vasoconstriction that is detrimental.

2. enhanced cardiac output by increased myocardial contractility (beta$_1$ effect) and elevation of blood pressure through vasoconstriction (alpha-adrenergic effect)

3. by IV infusion through an electronic infusion pump for accuracy

4. Continuous heart and blood pressure monitoring are

essential. Carefully document vital signs and intake/output as ordered (usually at least q1-2 hours in the acute period). Assess for significant adverse effects: tachycardia, dysrhythmias, myocardial ischemia, nausea, and vomiting. Assess IV site for signs/symptoms of drug infiltration. Do not abruptly discontinue dopamine; severe hypotension can result.

5. Notify primary health care provider immediately; restart infusion in another site as soon as possible to prevent hypotension from abrupt discontinuation of the drug (central access sites are preferred). The site must be infiltrated with phentolamine (Regitine), 5-10 mg diluted in 10-15 ml of normal saline, to prevent or

reduce tissue damage. Surgical debridement and skin grafting may be required if tissue necrosis occurs.

6. No. The high rate was most likely related to fever and hypovolemia; it was best treated with methods to reduce fever and correct the client's fluid status. Verapamil and adenosine are indicated for paroxysmal supraventricular tachycardia (PSVT). As an aside, the rate of PSVT is usually >150 beats/min.

Critical Thinking Exercises—Case Study #2

1. Yes. C.S.'s chest pain should be considered to be cardiac in origin.

2. Heart rate and blood pressure. A full description of the chest pain and any associated signs/symptoms (i.e., nausea, vomiting,

dyspnea, diaphoresis) will also be useful.

3. naloxone (Narcan)

4. continuous cardiac and blood pressure monitoring; use of a volumetric infusion pump for accuracy of drug delivery

5. Decrease the NTG infusion until BP is >100 mm Hg.

6. Turn off the NTG infusion. Place the client's head down and elevate his legs until his BP increases. (The half-life of NTG is short; if the BP drop is due to the NTG alone, it should be of short duration once these actions are taken.)

7. atropine: minimum adult dose = 0.5 mg IV; maximum adult dose = 3 mg IV

8. It blocks the effects of the vagus nerve (vagolytic action).

Appendix A
Basic Math Review

OBJECTIVES

- Convert Roman numerals to Arabic numbers
- Convert Arabic numbers to Roman numerals
- Solve problems with fractions
- Solve ratio and proportion problems
- Convert percentages to decimals, fractions, and ratios and proportions
- Complete the math review test with a grade of 80% or higher

TERMS

Roman numerals	divisor
Arabic numbers	dividend
ratio	least common denominator
proportion	

INTRODUCTION

Principles of basic mathematics surround us each day; they are part of life. Knowledge of arithmetic and how to do basic mathematical calculations is needed in everyday living and throughout one's nursing career.

Keep in mind that your goal is to prepare and administer medications in a safe and correct manner. The following recommendations are offered:

- **Think.** Focus on each step of the problem. This applies to simple as well as difficult problems.
- **Read accurately.** Pay particular attention to the location of the decimal point and the operation to be done (i.e., addition, subtraction, multiplication, division).
- **Picture the problem.**
- **Identify an expected range for the answer.**
- **Seek to understand the problem**, not merely the mechanics of how to do it.

The basic math review describes arithmetical operations that form the foundation that nurses use to calculate ordered dosages of medications. Specific information includes converting Roman and Arabic numerals; addition, subtraction, multiplication, and division of fractions and decimals; and solving percentage and ratio and proportion problems.

The basic math review is followed by a test on the material (in the Instructor's Electronic Resource). You may want to review this section first or go directly to take the test. It is strongly recommended that you attain a test score of at least 80% before going ahead. In reality, aim to score 100% on the test because it is essential material for understanding future chapters and calculating medication dosages.

NUMBER SYSTEMS

Arabic and Roman are the two systems of numbers associated with drug administration.

The *Arabic System* is expressed in numbers 0, 1, 2, 3, 4, 5, 6, 7, 8, and 9. Each has a place value reading from right to left. For example, the number 123 has 3 in the one's place, 2 in the ten's place, and 1 in the hundred's place. Each successive numeral indicates a value ten times more than the preceding one.

The *Roman System* is expressed by selected capital or lowercase letters (e. g., I, V, X, i, v, x). The Roman letters may be changed to equivalent Arabic numbers:

The equivalents are:

Roman Numerals		Arabic Number
I	i	1
V	v	5
X	x	10
L	l	50
C	c	100
D	d	500
M	m	1000

Roman numerals are commonly used when writing drug dosages in the Apothecary System. The Roman numerals are written in lowercase letters (e.g., i, v, ix). The lowercase letters may be written with a line above the letters (e.g., ī, v̄, īx̄) and a dot above each (e.g., i̇, i̇i̇, i̇i̇i̇).

Roman numerals may appear in combination, such as xi and ix. Addition and subtraction are used to read multiple Roman numerals.

Expressing Roman numerals:

#1. When the first Roman numeral is greater than (>) the following numeral(s), then ADD them together.

Examples: xiii = 10 + 3 = 13
vi = 5 + 1 = 6

#2. When the first Roman numeral is less than (<) the following numeral(s), then SUBTRACT the first number from the second.

Examples: ix = 10 − 1 = 9
XL = 50 − 10 = 40

#3. Numerals are never repeated more than three times in a sequence.

Examples: iii = 3
xxx = 30

#4. When a smaller numeral is between two numerals of greater value, the smaller numeral is subtracted from the numeral following it.

Examples: xix = 10 + (10 − 1) = 19
mcmxci = 1000 + (1000 − 100) + (100 − 10) + 1 = 1000 + (900) + (90) + 1 = 1991

Practice Problems I

Express the following as Arabic numbers:

1. XVI _____
2. XC _____
3. XIV _____

4. XXII _____
5. L _____
6. MXL _____

Express the following as Roman numbers:

7. 100 _____
8. 36 _____
9. 30 _____

10. 259 _____
11. 85 _____
12. 60 _____

FRACTIONS

A fraction is one or more of the equal parts of a unit. In the fraction ½, the 2 is the denominator and indicates into how many parts the whole is divided. The 1 is the numerator and indicates how many of the equal parts are taken.

The value of a fraction depends mainly on the denominator, and when it increases, the value of the fraction decreases because it takes more parts to make a whole. For example: with the fractions ⅓ and ½, the larger value is ⅓ because three parts make the whole, whereas for ½ it takes 12 parts to make a whole.

Proper, Improper, and Mixed Fractions

A **proper faction** has a numerator less than the denominator.

Examples: ¾, ⅞, ½

An **improper fraction** has a numerator equal to or greater than the denominator.

Examples: %, ¹¹⁄₁₁, ⅝

An improper fraction may be changed to a whole or mixed number by dividing the numerator by the denominator.

Examples: % = 1% or 1⅓
               ¹¹⁄₁₁ = 1
               % = 2

A **mixed number** is a whole number and a fraction (e.g., 2 ⅛, 3 ⅓, 6 ½). Mixed numbers can be changed to improper fractions by multiplying the denominator by the whole number, then adding the numerator.

Examples: 2 ½ = 1 ¹⁷⁄₈; 3 ⅓ = ¹⁰⁄₃; 6 ½ = ¹³⁄₂.

Addition/Subtraction of Fractions

To ADD fractions with the same denominator, add the numerators, keep the same denominator, and reduce to lowest terms.

Examples: $\frac{1}{2} + \frac{1}{2} = \frac{2}{2} = 1$
$\frac{3}{8} + \frac{7}{8} = \frac{10}{8} = 1\frac{2}{8} = 1\frac{1}{4}$
$\frac{5}{6} + \frac{4}{6} = \frac{9}{6} = 1\frac{3}{6} = 1\frac{1}{2}$

To ADD fractions with different denominators, change to fractions having the least common denominator (LCD), which is the smallest whole number that contains the denominator of each of the fractions. Divide the LCD by the denominator of each fraction and multiply both terms of the fraction by the quotient.

Example: $\frac{1}{6} + \frac{3}{8} + \frac{3}{4} + \frac{5}{12}$

Twenty-four is the smallest number that yields a whole number when divided by denominators in the example: 6, 8, 4, and 12. Then multiply both numerator and denominator by the same number. Then add as you would with fractions of the same denominator and reduce to lowest terms.

$\frac{1}{6} = \frac{4}{24}$
$\frac{3}{8} = \frac{9}{24}$
$\frac{3}{4} = \frac{18}{24}$
$\frac{1}{2} = \frac{10}{24}$
$\frac{44}{24} = 1\frac{17}{24}$

To SUBTRACT fractions with the same denominator, subtract the smaller numerator from the larger, keep the denominator, and reduce to lowest terms.

Example: $\frac{9}{10} - \frac{1}{10} = \frac{8}{10} = \frac{4}{5}$

To SUBTRACT fractions with different denominators, change fractions to LCD, subtract the numerator, and keep the denominator.

Examples: $\frac{5}{6} - \frac{1}{3} = \frac{5}{6} - \frac{2}{6} = \frac{3}{6} = \frac{1}{2}$ (LCD = 6)
$\frac{5}{8} - \frac{1}{4} = \frac{5}{8} - \frac{2}{8} = \frac{3}{8}$ (LCD = 8)

Multiplying Fractions

To MULTIPLY fractions:
- a) multiply the numerator
- b) multiply the denominator
- c) reduce fraction to lowest terms

Example 1: $\frac{1}{3} \times \frac{3}{8} = \frac{3}{24} = \frac{1}{8}$

Answer is $\frac{3}{24}$, which is reduced to $\frac{1}{8}$. To reduce to lowest terms, 3 goes into both numbers evenly (i.e., $3 \div 3 = 1$ and $24 \div 3 = 8$).

Example 2: $\frac{1}{8} \times 4 = \frac{1}{8} \times \frac{4}{1} = \frac{4}{8} = \frac{1}{2}$

A whole number is considered the numerator over one ($\frac{4}{1}$). Four divided by eight $(4 \div 8) = \frac{1}{2}$. $(0.5 = \frac{5}{10} = \frac{1}{2})$.

Dividing Fractions

To DIVIDE fractions, invert the second fraction (or divisor) and then multiply.

Copyright © 2009, 2006, 2003, 2000, 1997, 1993 by Saunders, an imprint of Elsevier Inc. All rights reserved.

Example 1: $\frac{1}{2} \div \frac{1}{4} = \frac{1}{2} \times \frac{4}{1} = \frac{4}{2} = 2$

Example 2: $\frac{9}{10} \div \frac{1}{3} = \frac{9}{10} \times \frac{3}{1} = \frac{27}{10} = 2\frac{7}{10}$

Decimal fractions: To change fractions to decimals, divide the numerator by the denominator (e.g., $\frac{1}{2} = 1:2 = 0.5$; $\frac{1}{8} = 0.125$).

Practice Problems II

1. Which has the greatest value, $\frac{1}{6}$ or $\frac{1}{8}$?

2. Reduce improper fractions to whole or mixed numbers:

     a. $\frac{16}{4} =$ c. $\frac{7}{3} =$

     b. $\frac{36}{6} =$ d. $\frac{21}{8} =$

3. Add fractions:

     a. $\frac{1}{10} + \frac{3}{10} =$ c. $\frac{1}{16} + \frac{5}{8} =$

     b. $\frac{1}{8} + \frac{3}{24} =$

4. Subtract fractions:

     a. $\frac{7}{8} - \frac{1}{8} =$ c. $2\frac{1}{4} - 1\frac{3}{8} =$

     b. $\frac{3}{8} - \frac{1}{16} =$

5. Multiply fractions:

     a. $\frac{3}{8} \times \frac{1}{6} =$

     b. $6\frac{1}{4} \times 2\frac{1}{3} =$

6. Divide fractions:

     a. $\frac{1}{3} \div 2 =$ c. $4\frac{1}{2} \div 4 =$

     b. $\frac{7}{8} \div \frac{1}{3} =$ d. $6\frac{3}{5} \div 3 =$

7. Change each fraction to a decimal:

     a. $\frac{1}{3} =$ c. $\frac{3}{10} =$

     b. $\frac{3}{5} =$

DECIMALS

Decimals are referred to as (1) whole numbers and (2) decimal fractions. The following number, 1234.8765, is an example of the division of units for a whole number with a decimal fraction.

     Decimal fractions are written in tenths, hundredths, thousandths, and ten thousandths. Decimal fractions are rounded off to tenths after solving problems using decimals. To round off in tenths, when the hundredth column is five or greater, the number in the tenth column is increased by one (e.g., $0.47 = 0.5$, $0.12 = 0.1$).

Decimal fractions are an integral part of the metric system. Tenths refers to the first decimal place 0.1 or ¹⁄₁₀; hundredths, the second decimal place 0.01 or ¹⁄₁₀₀; and thousandths, the third decimal place 0.001 or ¹⁄₁₀₀₀; When a decimal fraction is changed to a fraction, the denominator is based on the number of digits to the right of the decimal point (first = 10; second = 100; third = 1000).

Examples:
1. 0.9 = ⁹⁄₁₀ or 9 tenths
2. 0.33 = ³³⁄₁₀₀ or 33 hundredths
3. 0.444 = ⁴⁴⁴⁄₁₀₀₀ or 444 thousandths

Multiplying Decimals

To multiply decimal numbers, multiply the multiplicand by the multiplier as you would two numbers. Identify how many numerals are to the right of the decimals in both numbers. Counting from right to left, mark off the same number of spaces in the answer. Round off to tenths.

Example: 1.65   multiplicand
              4.4   multiplier
              660
              660
              7.260

Answer: 7.3. Since 6 is greater than 5, the "tenth" number is increased by 1.

Dividing Decimals

The decimal point in the divisor is moved to the right to make a whole number. The decimal point in the dividend is then moved to the right an equal number of decimal spaces. Carry number to two places beyond the decimal point.

Example: 3.69 ÷ 1.2 or 3.69 dividend
                              1.2 divisor

                      3.075   = 3.1
    divisor   1.2)3.6900   dividend
                      36
                       90
                       84
                       60

Practice Problems III

1. Multiply   a.   4.7 × 0.284

              b.   6.1 × 1.052

2. Divide   a.   74 ÷ 3.6

              b.   18.7 ÷ 0.41

3. Change the decimals to fractions:
   a.   0.21 =
   b.   0.02 =
   c.   0.068 =

RATIO AND PROPORTION

A **ratio** is the relationship between two numbers and is expressed with a colon separating the numbers (e.g., 3 : 4 [3 is to 4]). A ratio is another way of expressing a fraction (e.g., 3 : 4 = 3/4). Proportion is the relationship between two ratios and is expressed with a double colon or equal sign separating the ratios (e.g., 3 : 4 [:: or =] 6 : 8). The middle numbers of the proportion example are called *means* and the end numbers are called *extremes*. The product of the means equals the product of the extremes.

Example 1:

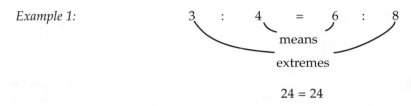

$$24 = 24$$

When the value of one number of the proportion is not known, it is represented by an "X". To solve for "X", the means are multiplied and the extremes are multiplied. The number with the X is always the divisor. Check: substitute the answer for "X"

Examples:

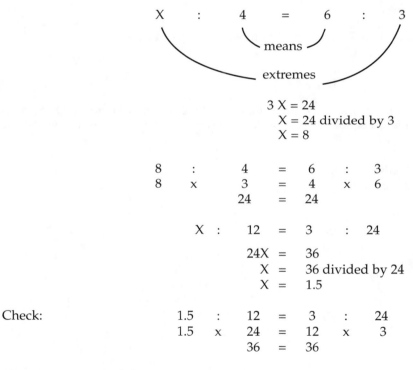

$$3 X = 24$$
$$X = 24 \text{ divided by } 3$$
$$X = 8$$

8	:	4	=	6	:	3
8	x	3	=	4	x	6
		24	=	24		

X	:	12	=	3	:	24
		24X	=	36		
		X	=	36 divided by 24		
		X	=	1.5		

Check:

1.5	:	12	=	3	:	24
1.5	x	24	=	12	x	3
		36	=	36		

The ratio and proportion problem may be set up as a fraction. Cross multiply to solve for X or to prove the computation.

Example: Ratio and proportion

X	:	4	=	3	:	1
		X	=	12		

Fraction

$$\frac{X}{4} = \frac{3}{1}$$
$$X = 12$$

Check:

$$\frac{12}{4} = \frac{3}{1}$$
$$12 = 12$$

Practice Problems IV

Solve for "X":

1.   2   :   20   ::   5   :   X

2.   0.8   :   100   ::   X   :   1000

3.   Change the ratio and proportion to a fraction:

                         1   :   3   ::   X   :   18

4.   It is 1500 miles from New York City to Miami, Florida. Your car uses one gallon of gasoline per 32 miles on average. How many gallons of gasoline are required for the trip?

PERCENTAGE

Percent means parts of 100; thus 4% means four parts of 100 and 0.4% means 0.4 parts (less than 1) of 100. A percent may be expressed as a fraction, a decimal, or a ratio.

    Example:

Percent	Fraction	Decimal	Ratio
20	$^{20}/_{100}$	0.20	20 : 100
0.5	$^{0.5}/_{100}$	0.005	0.5 : 100

    To change percent to decimal, move the decimal point two places to the LEFT. Unless noted otherwise, the decimal point is assumed to be after the number (e.g., 20% = 20.%).

Practice Problems V

Change each percent to a fraction, a decimal, and a ratio

Percent	Fraction	Decimal	Ratio
1			
¾			
300			

ANSWERS

Practice Problems I

1. $10 + 5 + 1 = 16$

2. $100 - 10 = 90$

3. $10 + 4 = 14$

4. $10 + 10 + 2 = 22$

5. 50

6. $1000 + (50 - 10) = 1040$

7. C

8. XXXVI

9. XXX

10. CCLIX

11. LXXXV

12. LX

Practice Problems II

1. ⅙ has the greater value; there are six parts in a whole and not eight.

2. a. 4   b. 6   c. $2\frac{1}{3}$ d. $2\frac{5}{8}$

3. a. $\frac{1}{10} + \frac{3}{10} = \frac{4}{10} = \frac{2}{5}$

   b. $\frac{1}{8} + \frac{3}{24} = \frac{3}{24} + \frac{3}{24} = \frac{6}{24} = \frac{1}{4}$

   c. $\frac{1}{16} + \frac{5}{8} = \frac{1}{16} + \frac{10}{16} = \frac{11}{16}$

4. a. $\frac{7}{9} - \frac{1}{9} = \frac{6}{9} = \frac{2}{3}$

   b. $\frac{3}{8} - \frac{1}{16} = \frac{6}{16} - \frac{1}{16} = \frac{5}{16}$

   c. $2\frac{1}{4} - 1\frac{3}{8} = \frac{9}{4} - \frac{11}{8} = \frac{18}{8} - \frac{11}{8} = \frac{7}{8}$

5. a. $\frac{3}{48} = \frac{1}{16}$

   b. $\frac{25}{4} \times \frac{7}{3} = \frac{175}{12} = 14\frac{7}{12}$

6. a. $\frac{1}{3} \times \frac{1}{2} = \frac{1}{6}$

   b. $\frac{7}{8} \times \frac{3}{1} = \frac{21}{8} = 2\frac{5}{8}$

   c. $\frac{9}{2} \times \frac{1}{4} = \frac{9}{8} = 1\frac{1}{8}$

   d. $\frac{33}{5} \times \frac{1}{3} = \frac{33}{15} = 2\frac{3}{15} = 2\frac{1}{5}$

7. a. 0.33   b. 0.60   c. 0.30

Practice Problems III

1. a. $1.3348 = 1.33$

   b. $6.4172 = 6.42$

2. a. 20.5

   b. 45.6

3. a. $\frac{21}{100}$

   b. $\frac{2}{100}$

   c. $\frac{68}{1000}$

Practice Problems IV

1. $2X = 100$
   $X = 50$

2. $100\,X = 800$
   $X = 8$

3. $\frac{1}{3} = \frac{X}{18}$
   $3X = 18$
   $X = 6$

4. 1 gal : 32 mi :: X gal : 1500 mi
   $32\,X = 1500$
   $X = 46.875$ gal
   $X = 47$ gallons

Practice Problems V

	Percent	Fraction	Decimal	Ratio
1.	1	$\frac{1}{100}$	0.01	1 : 100
2.	¾	$\frac{0.75}{100}$	0.0075	0.75 : 100
3.	300	$\frac{300}{100}$	3.00	300 : 100

Appendix B
Prototype Drug Chart

Prototype Drug Chart **Generic name:** _____

Drug Class:	**Dosage:**
Trade Name:	
Pregnancy Category:	
Contraindications:	**Drug-Lab-Food Interactions:**
Caution:	

Pharmacokinetics:	**Pharmacodynamics:**
Absorption:	*Onset:*
Distribution:	*Peak:*
Metabolism:	*Duration:*
Excretion:	

Therapeutic Effects/Uses:

Mode of Action:

Side Effects:	**Adverse Reactions:**
	Life-Threatening: